BECOMING A HEALTHCARE LEADER

SECOND EDITION

by Steven B. Reed, FACHE
Indiana University – Purdue University Indianapolis

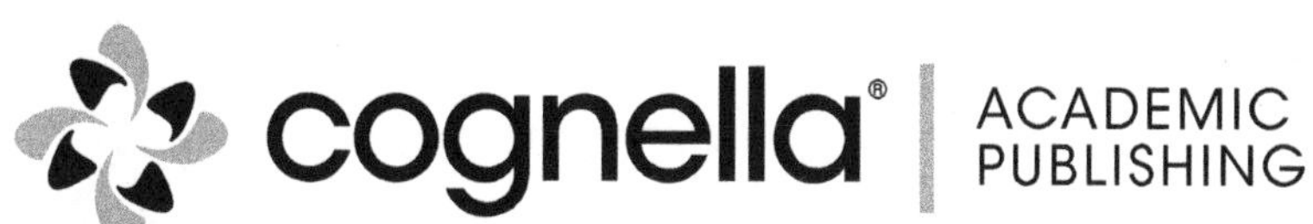

Bassim Hamadeh, CEO and Publisher
Carrie Montoya, Manager, Author Care and Revisions
Kaela Martin, Project Editor
Alia Bales, Production Editor
Miguel Macias, Senior Graphic Designer
Alexa Lucido, Senior Licensing Specialist
Claire Yee, Interior Designer
Natalie Piccotti, Director of Marketing
Kassie Graves, Vice President of Editorial
Jamie Giganti, Director of Academic Publishing

Printed in the United States of America.

ISBN: 978-1-5165-2900-1 (pbk) / 978-1-5165-2901-8 (br) / 978-1-5165-4515-5 (al)

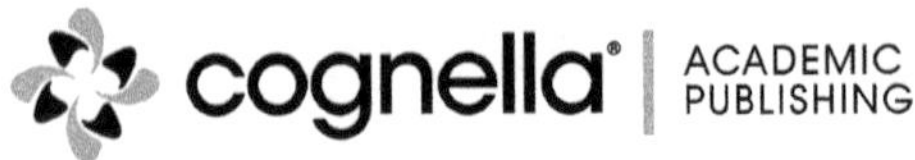

Contents

Foreword

Healthcare, as we know it, is changing. This is not a cerebral statement as healthcare has undergone constant change. But today, it's different. A fairly high level of uncertainty exists and our industry will continue to change—maybe even more dramatically than we've seen in recent years—and become a more demanding and challenging proposition for any aspiring healthcare leader for the foreseeable future. That being said, how does a healthcare leader prepare to navigate these waters—much of which are uncharted?

This book presents a creative approach for all of those who aspire to a level of leadership in healthcare. As the Director of a Master of Healthcare Administration (MHA) Program, I regularly interview prospective students who have exhibited a strong academic record. At some time during the interviews, I ask them where they want to be 15 years after graduating from our MHA Program. Invariably, the answer is a CEO of a hospital. As I probe more deeply into their answer, we arrive at the inevitable outcome: They want to be leaders in the healthcare system and make a difference. After some discussion and reflection by prospective students, many indicate they may or may not become a leader of a hospital, but they still want to be a healthcare leader at some level and make a difference for others. I believe our job, as educators and teachers, is to prepare them for a soft landing into the healthcare marketplace and provide them with a foundation of knowledge and skills they can apply in the field and further develop and refine through experience. Becoming a healthcare leader is more than just having knowledge or holding a position. Becoming a healthcare leader is a journey, and I believe a leader matures into being the leader he or she is capable of being through experience and mistakes.

Experience is the greatest teacher for all of us, and mistakes are an excellent guide, as long as we learn from them. We have all made them, and some of us have turned our errors into teachable moments through which we learned to improve our own performance. Some of the teachable moments in this book come from some experienced, highly-respected and successful hospital and healthcare leaders who offer their insight, wisdom, and lessons learned from their own experiences and careers.

This book presents a viable outline of the issues confronting a healthcare leader, and the skills, abilities, and techniques that can help a leader be as effective as possible in his or her leadership. It captures the depth and breadth of the concerns challenging the delivery of healthcare services and its leadership and provides a detailed approach, which someone aspiring to that role can follow.

Paul Lang, MPA, Past Program Director
IU MHA Program, Richard M. Fairbanks School of Public Health

Foreword: Effective Leadership

With all the changes occurring in the healthcare industry, including the increasing expectations of patients, consumers, and other stakeholders and the growing sentiment that hospitals and other health service organizations must improve their patient quality, service, cost structure, and overall performance, there is a greater need for effective healthcare leadership today than in any other time in our country's history. What exactly is effective leadership? We all know what it is when we experience it. But what exactly constitutes effective leadership, and how do you describe it? You can't see it, touch it, or have a conversation with it. But you know it when it is present. Steve has spent most of a lifetime studying, practicing, and teaching leadership in a variety of different settings, environments, and scenarios. One of his beliefs is, in order to be an effective leader—or to realize your potential as a leader—you must be a student of leadership throughout your career. His personal journey of leadership has been one with both setbacks and successes, always learning, growing, and developing as a leader along the way. As a student of leadership, Steve has spent a lifetime trying to prepare himself and others for the challenge of being the best leader they can be.

Healthcare leadership gets even more complicated. Government intervention with some of the most intellectual people on the planet presents situations that are unfathomable in most other industries. To be an effective leader in healthcare, you must accept and truly embrace the myriad of different challenges that confront you and your organization on a daily basis. Most effective leaders in healthcare view challenges as opportunities. With the growing challenges and demands of healthcare, the next generation of healthcare leaders must be better prepared than ever to embrace this new world of healthcare and thrive in this environment of challenge and opportunity. And it takes other leaders and teachers, like Steve, to help prepare and push future leaders to work hard and be as prepared as possible to effectively lead in this new world of healthcare.

In his book, Steve has tried to establish the difference between those who have been effective and those who wish they would have been effective. It takes courage to lead from the front. It also takes a whole lot of honesty, a little bit of luck, and a lot of preparation and hard work. It takes a commitment to a career of learning, growth, and development, as much of leadership is learned through its actual practice. This book will explore some of the key traits and elements of leadership practice and how these can be effectively applied by a healthcare leader in the real world of healthcare leadership.

This book can play a significant role in the classroom and academic setting, helping students in their learning, understanding, and preparation for healthcare leadership. The lessons provided in this book are designed to help students establish a foundation based on some theory and a lot of practical application. But, this book also has use and application for practitioners in the field who want to continue to develop and augment their leadership philosophy and refine their leadership style and skills. If you read what is presented in this book—and adopt and follow the principals and techniques that you believe will work best for you—it will make an impact on your career. This book provides an abundance of leadership insight and lessons learned through experienced healthcare professionals sharing their wisdom. Practicing healthcare leaders can use this book as a guide or reference on a variety of pertinent leadership topics.

Whether you are a healthcare administrative student studying a profession you aspire to join someday; a young, aspiring healthcare leader working in an entry level administrative position; or even a seasoned veteran; reading this book can help you advance your career as a healthcare leader. As a CPA, Healthcare Consultant, and Director with Blue and Co., LLC, and with over 30 years of experience in the healthcare field, I can also tell you that any of my hospital or health service clients could benefit, as well, from reading this book.

Ed Abel, CPA
Director, Healthcare Division
Blue and Co., LLC

A Few Things I Have Learned in My Healthcare Career

Becoming a healthcare leader—and becoming as effective of a leader as you can—is a journey. Above all, this journey is an ongoing process of active learning and discovery. The journey of becoming the most effective healthcare leader you can be is filled with a lot of self-discovery and reflection; learning through experience; and learning from others. It takes an attitude or mental construct and desire to learn as much as you can each and every time a learning opportunity presents itself. And, learning opportunities present themselves all the time, every day, in most every encounter or experience you have. The door of learning is always knocking; we just don't always hear it.

Below is a list of some of the lessons I've learned along my own journey of healthcare leadership. I am still adding to this list and actively look for opportunities to learn and grow each and every day. I hope there are some points of learning on this list that resonate with you and that you take to heart. Some of these points you may already recognize, as several come in the form of quotes from other people whose point of learning has touched or inspired me in some way: maybe some of these have already done the same for you, as well.

Sometimes learning is fun and easy, and sometime learning is a bit painful or difficult. Hey, learning is part of life, and life isn't always fun or easy either. I've always believed the hard times make us appreciate our work and efforts that much more.

Here's my list:

- Healthcare leadership is not for everyone. If it was easy, anybody could do it.
- Good really is the enemy of great—it breeds complacency.
- Mastering your profession through total dedication has become unfashionable—be a trend setter.
- You can personally make all the difference in the world—but only if you believe you can.
- Seeing isn't believing—believing is seeing.
- A person doesn't build character when everything is going well. It is when the chips are down, when your back is against the wall, and your world is crashing down that true character is revealed.
- Things are never as good as you think or as bad as they seem at the time.
- The answer to any problem or decision is usually right in front of you, but sometimes, you have to look closely and carefully to find it.
- Every single person you meet has something to teach you if you are willing to observe, listen, and learn.
- There is one person more interested and willing to teach you about leadership and life than anyone else. This person can be your personal tutor and the best teacher you'll find in the world—and that person is you.
- "***Quitters don't win, and winners don't quit at quitting time.***" (Peyton Manning speech, 2004)
- "***There is no way to happiness: happiness is the way.***" (Wayne Dyer audio tape—*The Power of Intention*)
- "***People thrive by focusing on who they really are, and connecting that to work they truly love.***" (Po Bronson, freelance writer)
- How does a big-league hitter batting .350 go into a hitting slump? Practice building your confidence—everyday.
- Always have a contingency plan for your work and your career—you just never know when you'll need it.
- When you are confronted with the choice to take the high road or the easy way, remember one thing—your legacy might just be at stake.
- Your life's work as a healthcare leader culminates into what will become the most important aspect of your career: your leadership legacy.
- You are never too smart, too wise, or too experienced to have a mentor.
- "***What good is success if you don't share it with others?***" (Karl Malone, NBA player, during Hall of Fame speech).
- Be first in line to acknowledge and praise the work of others
- Every organization is perfectly designed to generate the performance that it is generating.
- Never be afraid to walk in someone else's shoes—it will provide you with more perspective than you ever imagined.
- Never criticize someone in writing or in front of others.

- You won't receive what you don't give: be very respectful of others.
- Trust always matters. Be good to your word—even if it kills you.
- Stay connected to your passion and you'll never work a day in your life.
- Don't be in too big a hurry to get to the "top"—it will be waiting when you get there.
- ***"The door of opportunity doesn't just knock once or twice, it knocks all the time. It's just that, most of the time, we aren't listening". (***Patricia Fripp)
- "***The only thing more important than the will to succeed is the will to prepare to succeed."*** Vince Lombardi)
- Communication fosters understanding. Understanding fosters acceptance. Acceptance fosters support. Communicate until it hurts.
- People accept or reject change for their own reasons. Understand this, and you can change the world.
- You'll make the biggest improvements in leadership development and effectiveness by tapping into what you don't know you don't know, and to do this, you need to get out of your comfort zone and get outside insight.
- Great leaders help develop those around them. Remember, management is about getting work done through others.
- As a leader, you must hold yourself accountable for holding others accountable. This is one area where employees are constantly keeping score.
- If you can't fire someone when you need to, then management may not be for you.
- Always give people a second chance to succeed when you can. We all make mistakes and deserve a second chance.
- Let your dreams, not your failures, set your course.
- "***Failure is the opportunity to start again more intelligently***." ("Henry Ford")
- Embrace failure—it is the only way you'll ever succeed.
- **"It's not your expertise that blesses others, it's your humanness.**" ("Rachel Naomi Remen, MD, *Care For The Journey* CD")
- *In life, and in healthcare leadership, you get what you give.*

1

US Healthcare: An Industry Under Transformation

The U.S. healthcare industry—the largest industry in the world—is experiencing unprecedented change. The fundamental, sweeping change the healthcare industry is experiencing has implications for every single aspect of healthcare and the healthcare consumer, including how care is delivered, the types of delivery settings in which care is delivered, coordination of care, how care is billed and reimbursed, whether healthcare is a right or a privilege, financial incentives and regulations, and management and leadership. There continues to be growing emphasis/pressure on improving the quality of care, as well as the patient's safety and experience. These changes and more are impacting an industry that has historically been described as a "cottage" industry consisting of private, public, voluntary, and governmental organizations involved in the development, manufacturing, and distribution of healthcare supplies, equipment, and technologies; the delivery of health services; the education, training and development of healthcare manpower; the insuring, financing, and paying for health service delivery; the rule makers and regulators; and the vendors and consultants. In short, the healthcare industry has been, and remains, fragmented. Should healthcare truly become an interconnected system of organizations and services? Will it do so under healthcare reform?

OBJECTIVES

1. Appreciate how the U.S. healthcare industry is structured and organized and how its evolution has created the industry as it exists today.
2. Learn about some of the fundamental changes brought about by the Affordable Care Act and the healthcare reform movement.
3. Understand the roles and functions of various health service organizations.

U.S. HEALTHCARE'S EARLY PERIODS

U.S. healthcare's early periods—in the late 1800s and early 1900s—are that of a very humble, inauspicious beginning. Healthcare during this early time period involved sometimes crude and unsanitary environments and conditions, with clinical practitioners having minimal to no real medical or clinical education or training. It wasn't until around World War I when medical discoveries, such as the x-ray machine, penicillin, and ether (for anesthesia), came about and more advanced clinical diagnostic and therapeutic interventions came into being. Granted, the "tools" of medicine during the 1920s and 1930s were still somewhat primitive by today's standards. However, as our clinical knowledge and understanding of the human body grew, so did our medical research and new discoveries and advancements in medicine, surgery, and infection control, which spawned the growth of the healthcare system as we know it today. The development of public health also accelerated along with its initial primary emphasis on clean drinking water and modern sewage treatment facilities. New hospital construction, spurred by the Hill–Burton Act of 1946, also helped make improvements in healthcare delivery. Hill–Burton provided federal funding primarily for the construction of new hospitals in rural areas.

In 1965, Social Security Amendments—referred to as Title 18 and Title 19 and otherwise known as Medicare and Medicaid—were signed into law by President Lyndon B. Johnson. This legislation focused on what were considered to be two vulnerable populations: the elderly and the poor. As with today's healthcare reform, much of the provider community at that time was skeptical of these programs. However, Medicare and Medicaid began in 1966 as cost-based reimbursement programs. This meant that, when participating providers rendered covered healthcare services to Medicare or Medicaid beneficiaries, they billed the respective governmental healthcare program full charges, which were then paid in full. Cost-based reimbursement lasted from 1966 through 1982. Starting in 1983, Medicare began reimbursing hospitals for inpatient care using a new reimbursement system called prospective payment, or PPS, which used a new payment methodology featuring diagnostic-related groups, or DRGs. Under PPS, reimbursement rates were set in advance using a somewhat complicated formula that accounted for a hospital's area wage index and patient acuity level among other factors. For the first time, there was a hospital reimbursement system that provided an incentive for hospitals to manage their costs—a sign of things to come.

PRIMARY GOVERNMENT HEALTHCARE PROGRAMS

MEDICARE

A federal healthcare program for the elderly, people entitled to Social Security payments under the Social Security Disability Insurance (SSDI) for two or more years, people with end-stage renal disease requiring kidney dialysis or a kidney transplant, or people eligible or receiving Railroad Retirement Board benefits. Reimbursement under Medicare is in four distinct parts, as outlined below. Eligibility under Medicare is not means tested; therefore, eligibility is not based on income.

Part A—reimburses for hospital and outpatient care under a cost-sharing program.

Part B—voluntary part of Medicare where participating beneficiaries pay a monthly premium payment. Part B reimburses for physician and related professional services.

Part C—Medicare managed care program available in selected markets.

Part D—voluntary part of Medicare where participating beneficiaries pay a monthly premium payment. Part D reimburses for prescription drugs.

Medicare is administered through the Department of Health and Human Services (DHHS) and the Centers for Medicare and Medicaid Services (CMS). Medicare is primarily financed through both employer and employee taxes, along with premiums, co-payments, and coinsurance payments from beneficiaries.

MEDICAID

A federal healthcare program for low income families, women, and children, Medicaid is financed jointly through federal dollars and state dollars under a formula that is based on the states per capita income level (poorer states get more federal dollars for Medicaid under the formula). Medicaid is administered by each state, and each state is required to provide a basic set of benefits. States have the option of enriching their Medicaid benefits but are then required to pay a greater share of the cost for those benefits.

HEALTHCARE'S UNSOLVED PROBLEMS

It is true the US healthcare system has many challenges, problems, and areas where improvements need to be made. In this author's opinion, it is also true the US healthcare system is the greatest healthcare system in the world. The US healthcare system has the most advanced specialty care available: the best-quality outcomes; the best-trained physicians, nurses, and other ancillary and medical personnel; the best quality improvement and quality control with our licensing and accreditation bodies and standards; and so on. However, with all its virtues, the US healthcare system has many challenges and problems that have never been solved—and probably never will be. In many ways, this is just the nature of healthcare.

Supply doesn't always equal demand, whether it's manpower, drug supplies, bed availability or usage, patient volumes, medical equipment, medical supplies, excess or unused capacity in an area such as the emergency department, distribution of physicians (particularly primary care physicians), the number or location of acute care hospitals, or even the availability of health plans. There is an inherent, ongoing tension between the supply (accessibility) and demand (need or desire) for healthcare services. There are a myriad of factors that affect both the supply and the demand for healthcare services. As one thinks critically about this paradigm around a never-ending search for a balance between supply and demand, one observation can be made: supply and demand will never be exactly even, and there has been, and always will be, an ongoing tension in this regard. Some tension is probably a healthy thing, as it drives society toward a more optimum balance which—at least in theory—should produce the best access, quality, and service at the lowest cost.

LEVELS OF CARE

There are four recognized levels of care: primary care, secondary care, tertiary care, and quaternary care.

PRIMARY CARE

Primary care can be provided by a primary care physician; a mid-level provider, such as a nurse practitioner or physician assistant; an advanced practice nurse; dentist; mental health therapist, or counselor; physical, speech, or occupational therapist; chiropractor; home health nurse; or other appropriate clinical or ancillary health service provider. Primary care services include diagnosis and referral to a specialist. Primary care can be provided in a hospital, outpatient department or clinic; nursing home or assisted living facility; physician or doctor's office; therapy center; or even in a private home or residence.

SECONDARY CARE

Secondary care can be provided by a physician or surgeon, invasive radiologist, specialized ancillary health service provider, or other medical specialist, such as an emergency medical technologist or oral surgeon. Secondary care includes surgical procedures, such as a colonoscopy; removal of tonsils and adenoids or gallbladder; or oral and maxillofacial surgical procedure performed in a hospital or surgery center.

TERTIARY CARE

In most instances, tertiary care is provided in a hospital. Tertiary care is typically provided by a physician specialist, typically by a surgeon and other specialized nursing and ancillary health service personnel who are part of the tertiary care treatment team. Tertiary care is usually more costly, resource intensive, and uses advanced technologies. Patients receiving tertiary level care typically have higher levels of acuity and longer lengths of stay and recovery times.

QUATERNARY CARE

Quaternary care is the most advanced and costly care and treatment available and includes highly specialized physicians and sub-specialty surgeons, nursing and ancillary health service providers. Quaternary care is provided in Academic Health Centers (AHCs), Veteran's Administration Hospitals, and large community hospitals and includes burn units, transplantation services, and maternal–fetal surgery.

DELIVERY SETTINGS

Delivery settings where health services are rendered are quite varied and range from the private home to an academic health center. Delivery settings include short-term residential facilities, like a skilled nursing facility, psychiatric hospital, mental health center, or acute care hospital and diagnostic centers, ambulatory surgery centers, outpatient departments, physician offices, air or ground ambulances, or homes. Delivery settings also include long-term residential facilities, such as an intermediate care nursing home or adolescent home. As medical technologies advance, higher levels of patient acuity and care are being performed and rendered in less institutional, less restrictive environments to reduce overall costs and provide greater patient convenience. Ambulatory care is not a level of care but rather care delivered on an outpatient basis. Ambulatory care can be provided in virtually any delivery setting.

LONG-TERM CARE

Long-term care can be provided in virtually any delivery setting. Long term care is predominantly but not exclusively provided to the elderly. Other populations that can receive long term care include the physically or mentally disabled, as well as those recovering from a major injury or disease, such as a brain or spinal cord injury or severe stroke. Much of the long-term care being provided to the elderly is supporting or assisting patients with activities of daily living, or ADLs. These activities include bathing, using the restroom, brushing teeth, eating, getting dressed, or even ambulating. When assessing patients and determining their level of need in a long-term care setting, it is principally based on assessment of ADLs and their level of independence or dependence on others for their ADLs.

COST SHIFTING

Cost shifting is a phrase commonly used to describe the net effect of private payers' subsidizing the cost of care provided to Medicare and Medicaid beneficiaries as well as indigent patients, all of whom typically reimburse hospitals and other providers less than the actual cost of providing that care. Cost shifting lies at the heart of provider pricing strategies and negotiation tactics with health insurance carriers, managed care companies, and preferred provider organizations (PPOs).

MEDICARE/MEDICAID EXAMPLE OF COST SHIFTING

Providers who participate in the Medicare and Medicaid programs agree to accept the reimbursement payment from these entitlement programs as payment in full—excluding any portion the patient or guarantor may owe in the form of deductions, copayments, and coinsurance. For example, a hospital's prevailing charge for a minor surgical procedure is $10,000. Assume the hospital's overall net revenue (what it expects to be paid from all payer's sources) is 45 percent of full charges (gross revenue); then the average reimbursement for the surgical procedure in this example would be $4,500. Let's assume that Medicare, under the prospective payment system (PPS), reimburses $2,500 for this surgical procedure, and Medicaid reimburses $2,000 for this same surgical procedure. Let's further assume the hospital's operating margin (defined as net operating income divided by total net operating revenue) is 5 percent. This means, in general, that the hospital generates a 5 percent net operating margin on every dollar of net revenue collected. This type of operating margin would be considered good, and necessary to sustain long-term financial viability. However, let's assume the actual cost of producing this same surgical procedure costs, on average, $4,275. Under these assumptions—which are realistic for many hospitals today—all the hospital's private payers are subsidizing these same surgical procedures by $2,000 (Medicare) and $2,500 (Medicaid), respectively. Since the actual average cost of rendering these surgical procedures to all patients is $4,275 per case, the net loss per surgical case rendered to every Medicare patient is $2,000, while the net loss per surgical case rendered to every Medicaid patient is $2,500. If the average reimbursement through insurance and managed care contracts if 75% of full charge, the average reimbursement per surgical case would be $7,500 from commercial payers. Therefore, one can see how commercial payers are subsidizing the actual cost of care for these government programs. Moreover, the cost shift to private payers from indigent patients who can't pay any or much of the actual charge is even much greater than that from Medicare and Medicaid.

IMPLICATIONS AND NET EFFECTS OF COST SHIFTING

Healthcare reimbursement is complex, ever changing, and difficult to understand—a specialty unto its own. Nevertheless, this example above shows the net effect of cost shifting. Here are a few of cost shifting's implications.

1. Hospital operating costs—salaries, wages, benefits, medical/surgical supplies, medications, new equipment and technology, and facility improvements—continue to increase every year. Assuming no change in patient volume, the hospital will need to realize more reimbursement from the same number of patients previously served in order to maintain its net income (total net operating revenue minus total operating expenses) and overall financial operating performance (all other things remaining the same).
2. As Medicare and Medicaid shortfalls grow (mainly due to stagnant or even declining reimbursement rates), there is a corresponding increase in pressure placed on hospitals and other providers in rate negotiations with private payers. Why? Because the only place additional net revenue can be generated is through rate increases to private payers.
3. Private payers—particularly American businesses, which have traditionally provided the overwhelming preponderance of private health insurance through employer-sponsored group health plans to their eligible employees and their dependents—are pushing back against the ever-increasing high cost of healthcare. Moreover, the more healthcare consumes a greater portion of American businesses' operating expenses (and, subsequently, profits), the less businesses can afford to subsidize the cost of healthcare. In some cases, employers have chosen to shift more of the actual cost of their group health plans to their employees or even discontinue offering their group health plans altogether.

4. The continued growth in high-deductible health plans has shifted more of the financial risk and overall cost of a group health plan to participating employees. This is called cost sharing. The trend for employers offering high-deductible health plans in lieu of more traditional indemnity health insurance plans continues and is a major force driving healthcare consumerism, resulting in a more knowledgeable and informed healthcare consumer who is increasingly shopping for value.
5. With high-deductible health plans, providers are forced to bill and collect a greater portion of the healthcare bill from the patient or guarantor, resulting in a bit of a different dynamic and relationship between the provider and consumer. Moreover, this can be a significant amount, given that high-deductible health plans can have annual deductibles of up to $10,000 or more. One impact this has is on bad debt as well as on different types of direct discounting to the consumer to try and drive prompt payments.
6. High-deductible health plans have also played a role in softening consumer demand somewhat, as consumers may think twice or do additional research before going to a provider for an elective medical or surgical need. When consumers pay a larger portion of the healthcare bill, they are less quick to pursue non-urgent healthcare.
7. In particular, hospitals have historically set rate increases by focusing more on departments and services having a higher percentage or mix of private-pay patients. In effect, hospital rate increases in departments and services predominantly serving a higher percentage or mix of Medicare or Medicaid patients results in little or no impact on net revenue.
8. The difference between full charges and what Medicare and Medicaid reimburse is called contractual allowance. Every year, as hospitals and other providers raise their rates and Medicare and Medicaid reimbursement rates stay flat or even decline, contractual allowance grows. Contractual allowance is a line item on the income statement and represents the aggregate shortfall in Medicare and Medicaid reimbursement from full charges.

THE ROLE OF COST SHIFTING IN THE HEALTHCARE INDUSTRY

In summary, hospital and provider operating expenses increase every year. At the same time, Medicare and Medicaid reimbursement, which can represent 50–85 percent of a community hospital's payer mix, are staying flat or even declining. When hospitals raise their rates, contractual allowance goes up. The only place to increase reimbursement is with private-payer contracts, and it is American business that is footing the majority of the bill for private-pay patients. And as employers push more group health plan costs to participating employees through high-deductible health plans, it is becoming increasingly difficult for hospitals to generate a net income from operations—income needed for any organization to have adequate working capital and money to purchase new equipment, make facility improvements, or provide any type of annual increase in employees' salaries or wages. Overall, cost shifting is created by significant and growing shortfalls in Medicare and Medicaid reimbursement, increasing contractual allowance and putting more and more pressure on providers to go back to the well of private payers to solicit the increases in reimbursement needed to remain financially sustainable. Unfortunately, it appears that cost shifting in its current form is simply not sustainable long-term. At the same time, recent projections have Medicare running out of money in approximately fifteen years. On the other hand, Medicaid is jointly funded through federal and state dollars, and neither the federal government nor most states will be able to afford or fund the dollars needed to continue most state Medicaid programs, especially given their recent expansion under the Accountable Care Act.

HEALTHCARE MANPOWER

PHYSICIANS

A physician is someone who has, at a minimum, graduated from an allopathic or osteopathic medical school, either in the U.S. or a recognized international medical school. (International Medical Graduate). Upon graduation from medical school, the physician can then use the acronym "MD" (medical doctor) or "DO" (doctor of osteopathy) after his name. However, a physician cannot provide or render direct clinical care to patients unless they have completed at least one year in residency and received a license to practice as a physician in a respective U.S. state. However, a general pediatric, family practice, or internal medicine residency program is three years. Completing one of these three residency programs provides the physician with the clinical training to be a primary care physician in one of these three specialties. There are four primary care physician specialties: general practice (a physician who completed one, but less than three, years in residency training), family practice, pediatrician, and internist. There are a few general differences between family practice and internal medicine residency training. Family practice residency training includes pediatric and adolescent medicine. Family practice residency training programs in rural areas can include obstetrics, minor procedures in dermatology, and even surgical procedures in gastroenterology. Internal medicine residency training doesn't include pediatrics and usually doesn't include adolescent medicine, while there is typically more extensive training in critical care medicine, including cardiology and pulmonology.

Board certification is a voluntary process whereby the physician completes the highest academic and clinical standards as designed and promulgated by his medical or surgical specialty association. For some specialties, this means passing a written and oral exam. For other specialties, it means documenting and presenting clinical case studies from their practice to a board of peers, including diagnoses and treatment provided. This type of process is completed several years post clinical training. Board certification is increasingly being used as the standard that must be met by physicians when applying for hospital privileges or participation in health insurance networks.

PHYSICIAN SPECIALTIES AND SPECIALISTS

Physician specialists receive additional training after completing either a three-year internal medicine or pediatric residency training program. Training in a medical or surgical specialty can include three additional years of training in the specialty area. Sub-specialty training can include one to four additional years of post-residency training in a highly specialized area, such as spinal surgery for an orthopedic surgeon or cancer surgery training for a general surgeon. Primary care physicians include the following four specialties: family practice, internal medicine, pediatrics, and general practice. All other physicians are considered physician specialists. Almost one-third of all physicians are primary care physicians, while over two-thirds of all physicians are specialists. The ratio of primary care to physician specialists in the U.S. is completely opposite of most every other country in the world.

Anesthesiologist—specialist who administers local and general anesthesia. Puts patients to sleep using general anesthesia or conscious sedation or local anesthesia for surgical procedures.

Breast Surgeon—specialist in general surgery who has either completed additional fellowship training in breast surgery or has limited his practice to the care and treatment of breast cancer and related diseases of the breast.

Cardiologist—specialist who provides care and treatment of the heart and cardiovascular system and typically provides cardiac catheterization procedures in the cardiac catheterization laboratory.

Cardiovascular Surgeon—specialist who performs open heart (coronary artery bypass graft (CABG)) and related vascular surgery procedures.

Dermatologist—specialist who provides care and treatment of the skin.

Ear, Nose, and Throat (ENT)—specialist who provides medical and surgical care and treatment of the ears, nose, and throat. Some ENT physicians also provide head and neck cancer surgical procedures, and treatment of allergies.

Emergency Medicine—specialist who provides care and treatment to patients in a hospital emergency department, including coordinating pre-hospital emergency care via communication with emergency medical technicians providing emergency medical services in the field.

Endocrinologist—specialist who provides care to patients with diabetes and other associated metabolic diseases.

Family Practitioner—primary care physician trained to care for patients and families of all ages. Family Practitioners typically receive residency training that includes pediatrics, adolescent, adult, and geriatric medicine. In addition, some family practice residencies teach obstetrics, minor dermatology procedures, sigmoidoscopies, or other minor surgical procedures—especially those training physicians for a rural medicine practice.

Fertility Specialist—specialist in obstetrics and gynecology who has additional training in infertility and related medicine and surgical procedures.

Gastroenterologist—specialist in the medical and surgical care and treatment of the digestive system, including stomach and colon.

General Practitioner—primary care physician who has completed at least one year of family practice or internal medicine training, but has not completed a three-year residency program.

General Surgeon—specialist who provides a variety of surgical procedures in a hospital or ambulatory surgery center. Most general surgery procedures are performed between the waist and the neck of a patient, including colon, stomach, and breast.

Hand Surgeon—Orthopedic Surgeon or Plastic Surgeon who specializes in the medical and surgical care and treatment of the hand and elbow.

Hospitalist—physician who provides care to patients in an inpatient hospital setting. Hospitalists are typically internists, cardiologists, or pulmonologists.

Internist—primary care physician trained to care for patients and families of adult ages through geriatrics. Some internal medicine residencies include adolescent medicine training (ages 12 and above). An internal medicine residency is taken prior to any specialty adult residency training program in surgery or other specialty.

Intensivist—physician who specializes in hospital intensive care medicine and who predominantly or exclusively limits his practice to caring for patients in a hospital intensive care unit. Intensivists are typically internists, cardiologists, or pulmonologists.

Interventional Radiologist—Radiologist who has additional training in performing invasive and surgical procedures in the invasive radiology suite of a hospital or diagnostic imaging center.

Joint Replacement Specialist—Orthopedic Surgeon who specializes in performing total joint replacement of the hip and/or knee.

Medical Oncologist—specialist who provides care and treatment for cancer and other blood-related diseases. Prescribes and manages the care and treatment of chemotherapy infusions.

Nephrologist—specialist who provides care and treatment for patients with end-stage kidney disease and related disorders.

Neonatologist—specialist who provides inpatient hospital critical care medicine and treatment to newborn infants, including multiple births and babies born prematurely.

Neurologist—non-invasive specialist in the brain, nervous system, and some muscle disorders, such as multiple sclerosis.

Neurosurgeon—specialist who provides surgical care and treatment for the brain, neck, and spine.

Obstetrician and Gynecologist (OB/Gyn)—specialist who provides obstetrics and gynecological services and is considered a specialist in women's health.

Ophthalmologist—specialist who provides medical and surgical care and treatment for diseases of the eye.

Orthopedic Surgeon—specialist who provides medical and surgical care for the musculoskeletal system (bone, joints, and muscles).

Pathologist—specialist in the hospital or freestanding clinical laboratory who provides clinical diagnoses on patients to attending and consulting physicians based upon blood and tissue samples. May also performs autopsies.

Pediatrician—primary care physician trained to care for newborns and infants, toddlers, and adolescents through 16 or 18 years of age. A pediatric residency training program is required prior to taking any specialty pediatric residency training program in surgery or other specialty.

Physiatrist (PM&R)—specialist in physical medicine and rehabilitation. Many times, a Physiatrist provides outpatient pain management care and treatment, as well as inpatient medical rehabilitation.

Plastic Surgeon—specialist who provides surgical care in the area of plastic and cosmetic surgery that can include skin grafts and reconstructive surgery.

Psychiatrist—specialist in the diagnosis, care, and treatment of psychiatric, mental health, and alcohol and substance abuse diseases. Typically works in close collaboration with psychologists, and non-physician mental health providers and counselors in regards to the treatment of mental health patients.

Pulmonologist—specialist who provides medical and surgical care and treatment for breathing and lung conditions, such as severe asthma and chronic pulmonary obstructive disease (COPD).

Radiation Oncologist—Radiologist who has completed additional training in the field of oncology and directs and manages the care and treatment of cancer patients receiving treatment via a linear accelerator.

Radiologist—specialist who reads and interprets x-rays, including plain film, computerized tomography, magnetic resonance imaging, and sometimes, nuclear medicine scans and provides diagnoses to attending and consulting physicians and their patients.

Rheumatologist—specialist in the care and treatment of rheumatoid arthritis and related conditions of joints and the musculoskeletal system.

Surgical Oncologist—specialist in general surgery typically with fellowship training in surgical oncology who provides surgical care for patients with cancer and related diseases.

Uro-Gynecologist—Urologist or Gynecologist who has limited his practice to the medical and surgical care and treatment of the female bladder and urinary tract system.

Urologist—specialist who provides medical and surgical care and treatment for diseases of the bladder, urinary, and reproductive systems.

Vascular Surgeon—typically a General or Cardiovascular Surgeon who has limited his practice to the care and treatment of vascular disease, including surgical procedures for life-threatening conditions or cosmetic cases, such as for varicose veins.

NURSES

The largest segment of health care workers in the U.S. is nurses. Approximately two-thirds of all healthcare workers are nurses, and approximately two-thirds of all nurses work in hospitals. Nurses can receive on-the-job training and be certified but unlicensed; such is the case with a certified nurse assistant. Nurses that must be licensed are licensed practical nurses and registered nurses. Licensed practical nurses (LPNs) receive education and training in a two-year community college. Registered nurses receive their education and training in one of three ways: a four-year college or university, a three-year hospital diploma program, or a two-year associate's degree program in a community college. Nurses are licensed by each respective state. In order to be licensed, a nurse must complete a nursing program, pass the state's nursing licensure examination, and pay a license fee. Reciprocity is the term for when some states honor the nursing licensure of one or more other states whereby only a fee must be paid to obtain a license that recognizes another state's nursing licensure program.

Advanced practice nurses are those who receive advanced clinical training toward a master's degree in nursing in a recognized program that trains the nurse to perform higher-level clinical functions. A Nurse Practitioner (NP) is a registered nurse with advance training—typically receiving a master's degree with this additional training. Examples of advanced practice nurses include Nurse Anesthetists, Midwifes, Clinical Nurse Specialists, and Nurse Practitioners. Advanced practice nurses function according to the respective state's Nurse Practice Act or body of law that governs the practice of nursing within the state.

- **Nurse Anesthetist**—nurses who render local anesthesia, conscious sedation, and general anesthesia for surgery patients and patients in labor/delivery.
- **Midwifes**—nurses who provide prenatal care and obstetrical services.
- **Clinical Nurse Specialists**—nurses who provide advanced care in a specialized area of a hospital, such as surgery, adult intensive care, psychiatric, or neonatal intensive care.
- **Nurse Practitioners**—nurses who provide advanced care in hospitals and outpatient clinic and office settings, typically as primary care providers.

OTHER DOCTORS PROVIDING HEALTH SERVICES

- **Acupuncturist**—physician or doctor who has completed advanced training in acupuncture using thin needles to eliminate or reduce pain or treat other diseases or conditions.
- **Chiropractor (DC)**—doctor who specializes in the care and treatment of the neck and spine, providing diagnosis, spinal manipulation, and physiotherapy.
- **Dentist (DDM)**—there are general dentists and eight recognized dental specialists: endodontics, oral and maxillofacial surgery, oral pathology, orthodontics, pediatrics, periodontics, prosthodontics, and public health.
- **Optometrist (OD)**—doctor who specializes in the diagnosis of eye disorders and vision problems proscribing eye glass wear.
- **Physician Assistant (PA)**—mid-level provider with 20 to 36 months of didactic and clinical training who typically provides primary clinical care and treatment and functions as a physician extender under the supervision of a physician.
- **Podiatrist (DPM)**—doctor who specializes in the medical and surgical care and treatment of the foot and ankle.

ANCILLARY HEALTH SERVICE PROVIDERS

Ancillary health service providers are licensed (but are neither a physician nor nurse) and work in a specialized area of healthcare delivery. Examples include psychologists; mental health or substance abuse counselors; physical, occupational, or speech therapists; athletic trainers; medical laboratory technologists; social workers; and registered dieticians. Some ancillary health service providers cannot provide services without an order from a physician, while some can. This is determined by each respective state's laws.

THIRD-PARTY PAYERS

Third-party payers are organizations who pay the healthcare bill, or healthcare claims as they are known in the industry, for covered services rendered to a health plan or program beneficiary. Third-party payers are organizations such as Medicare; Medicaid; private health insurance companies, referred to as "carriers;" and third-party administrators, referred to as "TPAs." In the U. S. today, there are hundreds of third-party payers in operation. The abundance of third-party payers has been one of the factors cited as creating inefficiencies in the healthcare system, in addition to contributing to healthcare inflation.

Under an employer-sponsored group health plan, a health insurance contract or policy is executed between the carrier, who underwrites the health insurance policy, and the employer or sponsoring organization of the health plan. The health plan document is what governs the health plan and includes specifics on all the details about the health insurance plan, including what services are covered by the plan, policies and procedures governing the plan, designation of the plan year, provider networks that are used, etc. This is in contrast to an individual health policy where a health insurance policy is executed between the carrier and the individual covered plan beneficiary. In the case of a self-funded, employer-sponsored group health plan, an agreement is entered between the employer and the participating employee.

When a healthcare provider renders services to a patient that has some type of public or private health insurance coverage, the patient is typically asked to sign a form, called the assignment of benefits, authorizing the healthcare provider to bill the patient's third-party payer on behalf of the patient. The assignment of benefits also authorizes the third-party payer to pay the charges for covered services directly to the provider on behalf of the beneficiary or patient from the healthcare claim the provider generates when services are rendered. This is an important distinction to note: the third-party payer is making payment to a provider on behalf of the beneficiary or patient. Although most providers have separate contracts for participation in Medicare, Medicaid, private health insurance plans offered by carriers, and other PPO networks, health insurance policies that beneficiaries or patients have are between the beneficiaries or patients and their respective third-party payer—not with the provider who renders healthcare services. In other words, the provider of healthcare services becomes a "middle man" in this reimbursement transaction. When a provider agrees to bill the beneficiary or patient's third-party payer, and the assignment of benefits authorization is provided, they are doing so as a service to the beneficiary or patient. If a third-party payer does not make payment for a covered healthcare service to a provider, the beneficiary or patient remains ultimately responsible for payment of the bill.

HEALTH INSURANCE COMPANIES/CARRIERS AND THIRD-PARTY ADMINISTRATORS

Health insurance companies—also referred to as "carriers," provide two types of health insurance policies, an individual policy and a group policy. Carriers typically provide two different types of health insurance plans, a fully insured plan and administrative services only, or ASO, plan. A fully insured health plan is the traditional health insurance plan that "insures" the beneficiary by providing reimbursement coverage for a pre-established list of healthcare services. A traditional, fully insured health plan is called a defined benefit plan. Defined benefit plans are those that define the benefits in advance that will be covered. This type of traditional health plan has the carrier assuming all the financial risk for paying all healthcare claims covered by the plan and incurred by the beneficiaries during any given plan year. A plan year is any given 12-month period designated by the health plan in the plan document. Under a fully insured health plan, the financial risk for the plan has been transferred from the employer (under a group health plan) or individual policyholder (under an individual health plan policy) to the carrier in exchange for the payment of a pre-established monthly premium.

When the carrier is providing ASO services, there is a significant difference: the carrier doesn't actually provide insurance, which means the carrier doesn't underwrite the plan or assume any financial risk, as the financial risk is maintained by the self-funded, employer-sponsored group health plan. Again, please note that ASO services refer to a carrier providing administrative services only—with no underwriting or actual insurance provided. Therefore, a carrier providing ASO services to a self-funded, employer-sponsored group health plan, is providing similar services to that of a third-party administrator, or TPA.

PAYER MIX

A term frequently used in healthcare is the term payer mix. Payer mix refers to the respective percentage of reimbursement a provider receives from the general categories of payers: Medicare, Medicaid, commercial insurance companies, preferred provider organizations, self-pay, donations, grants, and charity and indigent care. The way healthcare is funded and reimbursed today, payer mix is an important indicator of a healthcare provider's financial picture. As a general rule, the greater the percentage of commercial or private pay patients, the higher a health service organization's reimbursement on a per-unit basis. The type and mix of services offered, location and number of competitors, demographics of the organization's service area, type of hospital and organizational mission, number of employers in the service area, and types of health insurance plans they offer all help determine the health service organization's payer mix.

HOSPITALS

There are many different types of hospitals and hospital settings in which health care services are rendered. Hospitals can be categorized as governmental, private, or public. What determines a hospital's legal status as a corporate entity—including whether it is a governmental, private, or public hospital or if it is not-for-profit or tax-paying—is how it is created/organized as a legal entity when it was created. Hospitals can also be categorized as academic health centers, tertiary care provider, teaching, community, and critical access. The board of directors is the ultimate decision-making body with the overall responsibility for the hospital and its assets.

- **Academic Health Center (AHC)**—a large, urban, tertiary care hospital that is operated in conjunction with a university medical school; provides numerous medical and surgical residencies, clinical nursing training, and a variety of other ancillary health service training programs; receives patients through referrals from outlying areas; is extensively involved in clinical research; and typically serves a higher level of Medicaid and indigent care patients.
- **Affiliated hospital**—a hospital that has a contractual relationship with another hospital or hospital system to collaborate on one or more areas of strategy or operations.
- **City hospital**—created as a city-sponsored hospital that is controlled/governed through a public Board of Directors, typically with participation or control by city officials, such as the city or town council members.
- **Community hospital**—a hospital that is not an academic health center, U.S. Department of Veteran's Affairs (VA), or specialty hospital and exists to serve the healthcare needs of the community in which it resides.
- **County hospital**—created as a county-sponsored hospital that is controlled/governed through a public Board of Directors, typically with participation or control by county officials, such as the county commissioners.
- **Critical Access hospital**—a small, rural, not-for-profit community hospital with 25-beds (or less) that has been designated as a critical access hospital by the federal government and is reimbursed at 101% of allowable costs by Medicare.
- **For-profit hospital**—a hospital that is tax-paying and is not organized as a charitable organization with a charitable mission, also referred to as a proprietary hospital.
- **Freestanding hospital**—a hospital that is not part of a hospital system and is operated independently on its own.
- **Government hospital**—created as a hospital owned, operated, or sponsored by the government. This could be a VA hospital, a military hospital, or a city or county hospital.
- **Long-term acute care hospital**—a hospital that specializes in the care and treatment of acute care patients who typically have longer lengths of stay, such as a patient on a ventilator for an extended period of time.

- **Not-for-profit hospital**—a hospital that is exempt from paying taxes due to its charitable mission. Also referred to as a tax-exempt hospital or 501 (c)(3) hospital (IRS tax code for tax exemption).
- **Private hospital**—created through a private initiative, either as a not-for-profit or tax-paying hospital, and governed privately by a Board of Directors.
- **Psychiatric hospital**—hospital that specializes in the care and treatment of behavioral health and/or alcohol and substance abuse patients.
- **Public hospital**—a governmental or community not-for-profit hospital that was created through a public initiative with a charitable mission and is owned or controlled/governed through a public Board of Directors.
- **Rehabilitation hospital**—a medical, inpatient rehabilitation hospital that specializes in providing intensive rehabilitation services of patients with stroke, neurological impairment, or surgical rehabilitation needs.
- **Safety net hospital**—typically a large city or county hospital in an urban area that treats a high number of Medicaid and indigent care patients seen as vulnerable populations.
- **Single specialty hospital**—a hospital that only offers care and treatment in one major service line, such as a women's hospital, cardiac hospital, or orthopedic hospital.
- **Sole community provider**—the only hospital serving a defined area, market, or geographic population.
- **Substance abuse hospital**—a hospital that specializes in the care and treatment of alcohol and chemical dependency services.
- **Teaching hospital**—any hospital that offers at least one or more clinic training programs for physicians, nurses, or ancillary health service specialties.
- **Tertiary care hospital**—a hospital that provides tertiary care, such as open heart surgery, joint replacement, neurosurgery, or other tertiary care–level services.

DISPROPORTIONATE SHARE HOSPITALS

Disproportionate Share Hospitals (DSH) is a federal program that provides additional reimbursement, through the Medicare and Medicaid program, for hospitals that have a higher payer mix of Medicare and Medicaid and indigent care patients and meets pre-established levels for Medicaid and indigent patient care utilization under a somewhat complex formula.

HOSPITAL INPATIENT REIMBURSEMENT METHODOLOGIES

The following chart categorizes and describes most of the major hospital inpatient reimbursement methodologies.

HOSPITAL INPATIENT REIMBURSEMENT SYSTEM	HOSPITAL INPATIENT REIMBURSEMENT METHODOLOGY	HOSPITAL AND PAYER RESPECTIVE INCENTIVES
Cost-based	Reimbursement paid at 100% full charges or some percentage of allowable costs	Hospital: ↑ patient volume and costs Payer: ↓ volume and utilization
Prospective payment system	Set reimbursement amount for inpatient care based on respective diagnostic-related group or DRG	Hospital: ↑ patient volume and ↓costs Payer: ↓ volume and utilization
Case rates	Set reimbursement amount for inpatient care based upon respective case rate payment	Hospital: ↑ patient volume and ↓ costs Payer: ↓ volume and utilization
Per diem rates	Set daily payment amount per inpatient unit or service	Hospital: ↑ patient volume and ↓ costs Payer: ↓ volume and utilization
Global payment	Flat fee amount based upon respective diagnosis or procedure, including hospital, physician and all ancillaries services	Hospital: ↑ patient volume and ↓ costs. Negotiate with other providers for payment share. Payer: ↓ volume and utilization
Bundled payment	Flat fee amount based upon respective diagnosis or procedure including hospital, physician, and all ancillaries services. One check cut for entire bundled service payment.	Hospital: ↑ patient volume and ↓ costs. Negotiate with other providers for payment share. Payer: ↓ volume and utilization. May financially incentivize providers based upon quality and service performance/outcomes.
Bundled payment for episodes of care	Flat fee amount based upon respective diagnosis or procedure, including hospital, physician, and some or all ancillary services. Can include all pre- and post-hospital care associated with the episode, including service provided by multiple entities and providers. One check cut for entire bundled service payment.	Hospital: ↑ patient volume and ↓ costs. Negotiate with other providers for payment share. Payer: ↓ volume and utilization. May financially incentivize providers based upon quality and service performance/ outcomes.
Capitation	Flat monthly amount to cover any and all covered healthcare services required by a population of insureds.	Hospital: ↓ patient volume and costs Payer: May financially incentivize providers based upon quality and service performance/outcomes.

PERFORMANCE IMPROVEMENT

The emphasis placed on quality assurance and improving the quality, service, and performance of hospitals has been an evolutionary process in hospitals, as well as with other health service providers. From the initial efforts of Edward Deming examining quality to today's use of Lean, Six Sigma, or similar structured processes to identify opportunities to improve quality, service, and costs, performance improvement, or PI, is a philosophy, and most organizations are trying to make it part of their culture and everyday operations. With the incentives and pressures on providers to improve patient safety and quality outcomes, patient satisfaction outcomes, and organizational operating performance, PI is becoming a top priority in most hospitals and health service organizations. External pressures for improved outcomes by providers are sure to continue the drive for PI.

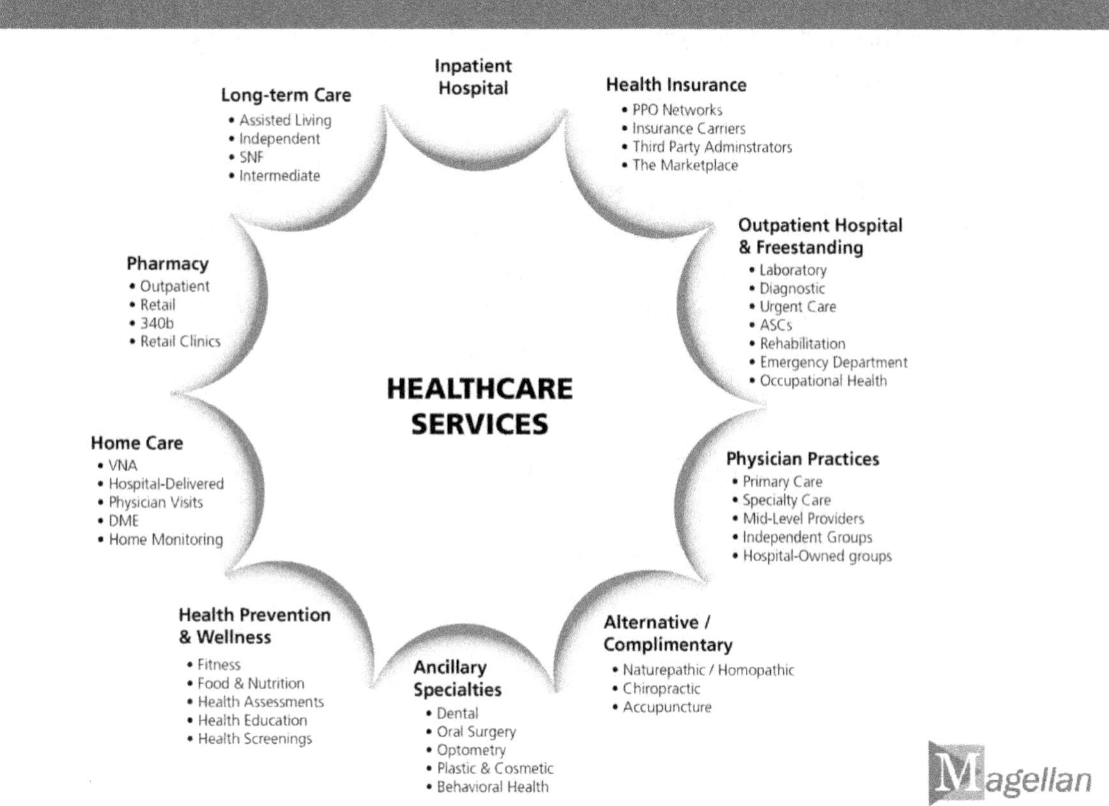

FIGURE 1.1 The Healthcare Continuum

DISCUSSION QUESTIONS

1. What are the two primary government-sponsored healthcare programs, and how do they differ?
2. Explain what tertiary care is.
3. Describe cost-shifting.
4. What are activities of daily living of ADLs?
5. What is the main difference between a primary care physician and a physician specialist?
6. What are third-party payers and third-party administrators?
7. Describe two or three of the major categories of change promulgated by Healthcare Reform. Describe the elements of access to care.
8. Which government healthcare program is funded with federal and state dollars, and is administered on a state-by-by-state basis?
9. What criteria are traditionally used to measure the health status of a defined population, and therefore the quality and effectiveness of a healthcare system?
10. Why does the economic support of a healthcare system determine the level of access, quality, specialization, use of technology, outcomes and effectiveness overall?

2

US Healthcare Reform

HEALTHCARE REFORM

Clearly, healthcare reform has been a mandate for significant change and action. The Patient Protection and Affordable Care Act of 2010 (PPACA), or public law 111–148, along with the Healthcare and Education Reconciliation Act of 2010 (HCER), or public law 111–152, provide for the most sweeping change in the healthcare industry since the passage of Medicare and Medicaid in 1965. The initial legislation of PPACA is approximately 2,700 pages or more in length with predictions that range anywhere from 20,000 to 200,000 pages of implementing regulations that will be involved over the 10-year period of implementation. Signed into law on March 23, 2010, and made retroactive to January 1, 2010, this legislation is commonly referred to as "Obamacare," "Healthcare Reform," or the ACA. This sweeping piece of legislation impacts every aspect of the general and specific environments, and all stakeholders in the U.S. In other words, it impacts everybody and everything. Healthcare reform impacts the three major dimensions of healthcare, cost, quality, and access, in a very significant way. Healthcare reform can be described using the three "C's:" comprehensive, complex, and contentious. Many of the changes are widely viewed as both positive and negative, much of which is determined by your respective perspective as a healthcare stakeholder.

The thinking for reform is found in the three major dimensions of healthcare: reduce the cost, improve the quality, and increase the access. Initial projections were that healthcare reform would cost $938 billion over the 10-year implementation period; provide health insurance coverage to approximately 26 to 32 million of the estimated 45 to 50 million uninsured; and offer a variety of mechanisms and demonstration projects to help incentivize providers to control or reduce healthcare costs and improve quality. The Congressional Budget Office (CBO) initially estimated that healthcare reform would reduce the U.S. deficit by $124 billion. The principle costs for healthcare reform were to be paid for in two ways: higher taxes and significant cuts in Medicare and Medicaid reimbursement payments to providers—namely hospitals and doctors. The original "Business Case" for reform made to providers was that significant cuts in Medicare and Medicaid reimbursement would be offset by the 26 to 32 million additional insureds projected, in essence significantly reducing charity care and bad debt to providers. The estimated 26 to 32 million additional insureds would come about through two mechanisms: the expansion of Medicaid on a state-by-state basis and additional insureds through the health insurance exchanges/marketplace.

It is difficult to do justice to healthcare reform due to its comprehensive nature, as well as the fact that so many elements are not yet defined as of this writing; however, we've broken healthcare reform into seven categories:

- Significant changes in payment and reimbursement
- Incentives for integration, care coordination, and accountability
- Mandate to providers for significant operating cost reductions
- Information technology enhancements, electronic health record implementation, and improved cost and quality outcomes tracking and reporting
- Public and private health insurance reform
- Quality outcomes reporting, benchmarking, and pay-for-performance
- Increase in regulatory and compliance and related monitoring and scrutiny

One of the demonstration projects most discussed and debated in the provider community has been the creation of accountable care organizations, or ACOs. An ACO is a formal legal entity of hospitals and physicians who become accountable for the cost and quality of care delivered to assigned Medicare patients (at least 5,000 or more per ACO) for a geographic area. Requirements for becoming an ACO include being a legal entity, employing adequate numbers of primary care physicians and providers for the assigned Medicare beneficiary population serviced, promote evidenced-based medicine and coordination of care across the entire continuum of care, demonstrate the adoption of patient-centered care, agree to a three-year term of participation, administer beneficiary and plan data to include determination of payment for shared savings, and provide information on quality and cost outcomes.

A feature of ACA that significantly impacted almost every hospital and physician practice has been the requirement to implement an electronic health record (EHR) and meet published standards for "meaningful use" of the EHR system. Meaningful use is defined as a common language to ensure accurate and secure health information exchange across different EHR modules. Meaningful use is using certified electronic health record technology to improve quality, safety, efficiency; reduce health disparities; engage patients and families; improve care coordination, along with population and public health; and maintain privacy and security of patient health information. Meaningful use sets specific objectives that eligible professionals and hospitals must achieve to qualify for CMS incentive programs, and subsequently not be penalized via government reimbursement (www.healthIT.gov). The government financially incentivized providers to meet the meaningful use standards by providing incentive payments to those who did. Alternatively, the government also financially incentivizes providers by reducing reimbursement to those providers who do not meet the meaningful use standards. While these EHR systems can greatly improve access to clinical information for providers, they come with a hefty price tag and involve not just the cost of acquisition of the system, but significant implementation and ongoing operation and maintenance costs as well. Moreover, there are advantages and disadvantages to all the major EHR systems available to providers on the market today.

With major reform to both public and private health insurance, it also includes—for the first time in the history of the U.S.—the requirement for virtually every citizen to have health insurance coverage as of 2014 (a provision which was rescinded in 2017). It also creates health insurance exchanges or marketplace over the internet—administered by the respective state or federally facilitated by the federal government—making individual insurance policies available to those not otherwise eligible for any public or private health insurance plan. Another first features the benchmarking of providers using quality and service outcome data in payment calculations for reimbursing hospitals.

Examples of a few other major provisions of healthcare reform include greater funding for fraud and abuse monitoring; tort reform development; community benefit requirements for 501 (c) (3) hospitals to complete a community health needs assessment every three years; a national healthcare workforce commission; data centers to report hospital and physician outcomes and related performance data, as well as health insurance reimbursement data; a state review process for "unreasonable health insurance premium increases;" and various new fines and penalties.

DISCUSSION QUESTIONS

1. What are the three major dimensions of healthcare?
2. What were the two pieces of healthcare reform legislation totally 2,700 pages signed into law on March 23, 2010 known as "Obamacare"?
3. How many new insureds were projected with Obamacare?
4. What were the two primary ways in which 26 to 32 million people would become insured under Obamacare?
5. What were the two primary ways in which Obamacare was to be paid for?
6. As of January 1, 2018, how many states elected to expand Medicaid?
7. What is an accountable care organization (ACO) and what is its main goal or objectives?
8. What was the time period Obamacare was initially scheduled to be implemented?
9. How many people were estimated to have purchased health insurance through a state-based health insurance exchange or the federally-facilitated health insurance marketplace in 2017?
10. Define what is meant by the term "meaningful use," and the central role it played in the implementation of electronic health records (EHR's) in healthcare.

FIGURE CREDIT

3

Rural Healthcare in the US

RURAL HEALTHCARE

Most healthcare in the US today is rural healthcare. While it is the larger hospitals, such as academic health centers, religious-affiliated hospitals, and other large hospital systems that get most of the national attention and notoriety, the majority of the US is rural, and therefore the majority of hospitals in the US are smaller, not-for-profit, county/community hospitals. Healthcare services available in a given market or geographic area are largely determined by the area's population. As it stands to reason, larger, more densely populated urban areas tend to have more healthcare services, including larger hospitals with more services available. However, many other factors come into play and influence the quantity, level of care or specialization, and availability and accessibility of healthcare services in a given area. For example, one of these factors affecting the supply and type of available healthcare services is the general attractiveness or desirability of the area. Another factor is the local economy, particularly the availability of jobs and a suitable workforce. Even the sociocultural characteristics can have some influence on the amount and type of healthcare services available in a given area.

LIMITED RESOURCES

PATIENT SAFETY & CHANGE MANAGEMENT

A major trend that has influenced the provision of healthcare service delivery in the US has been the continuing advancements made in the area of medical technology, along with the availability of new discoveries and advancements in drugs, medical supplies, and related medical information and knowledge regarding medical and surgical procedures, protocols, and best-demonstrated clinical practices. One area that has received much attention and focus, both inside and outside the healthcare industry, is on patient safety. In recent times, there has been a growing body of knowledge and information on developing a patient safety culture, including use of policies, procedures, and checklists; education and training; and monitoring techniques that hospitals are embracing nationally. Statistically, rural hospitals are just as safe in terms of the frequency of medical errors and adverse events as their larger urban hospital counterparts (for the same services and procedures). It stands to reason that implementing change in a complex organization like a hospital is a multifaceted, complex process; however, change management is typically easier to expedite in a rural hospital with three hundred employees, fewer departments, and less specialization than in an academic health center with five thousand employees, over one hundred departments, one hundred or more physician residents in training, and highly advanced tertiary and quaternary care being provided, along with research and clinical trials being performed.

MAJOR ECONOMIC EMPLOYERS IN THEIR RESPECTIVE LOCATIONS

Rural providers face many different challenges than those in urban areas. Rural providers—especially rural hospitals—are major employers in their respective communities, representing a substantial force driving the local economy. In many cases, rural communities are at risk without their major healthcare providers, as they relate to access to quality healthcare, economic support for the local businesses, and quality of life. At the same time, rural providers often face the "grass is greener" phenomenon (which is really an aspect of human nature): a belief that most services, including healthcare, are superior in a bigger city. The result is typically an ongoing marketing and public relations challenge to curtail outmigration of patients traveling to the bigger city for healthcare services available locally. While, as a rule, larger hospitals, health systems, and other health service providers in bigger communities typically offer a greater breadth and depth of services and specialties, there is no clear evidence that urban providers offer a higher level of quality for the same services provided in a rural area.

EMPLOYEE POOL

Another issue is skilled healthcare manpower. While recruitment and retention of healthcare manpower is an ongoing challenge in any organization, it is of particular concern in most rural areas of the country. There are many factors at play, including the number of jobs and related employment opportunities, perceived quality of life and cultural opportunities, education or entertainment opportunities, etc. Moreover, in many circumstances, a healthcare worker may perceive they have limited career mobility or growth opportunities in a rural setting and relocate to a larger community. Whatever the case, the ability to recruit and retain highly skilled healthcare manpower in rural areas can be quite challenging.

As a result, many rural areas suffer from manpower shortages in a number of areas, including nurses, surgical technicians, X-ray technologists, physical therapists, and more. A particular challenge is the recruitment and retention of physicians in rural areas. A growing shortage of primary care physicians nationally makes this a more acute challenge in rural areas, particularly since the majority of graduating residents from primary care residencies indicate their desire to practice in larger communities. Moreover, with modern medicine being so highly specialized, physicians are trained with a plethora of physician specialists and subspecialists readily available, which is not the case in most rural areas. In addition, rural areas suffer from a shortage of other healthcare providers, such as dentists, optometrists, chiropractors, and podiatrists. One area of particular need that many rural areas experience shortages in is behavioral health and substance abuse treatment.

MENTAL ILLNESS SUPPORT RESOURCES

According to the National Institute of Mental Health (NIMH) in the 2015 *National Survey on Drug Use and Health*, there were an estimated 43.4 million adults aged eighteen or older in the US with some type of mental illness. Mental illness is generally defined as any mental, behavioral, or emotional disorder (excluding substance abuse). Survey results report the prevalence of mental illness as being the highest among females ages eighteen to twenty-five (https://www.nimh.nih.gov/health/statistics/prevalence/any-mental-illness-ami-among-us-adults.shtml).

While the abuse of opioids has received considerable attention recently, substance abuse has undoubtedly been a national problem that has no geographic, economic, or sociocultural boundaries. Alcohol, prescription drugs, illegal drugs such as heroin and cocaine—the list goes on—are all drugs abused daily in the US by literally millions of people. The *National Survey on Drug Use and Health*, conducted in 2015, found that nearly twenty-one million Americans ages twelve and older had a substance use problem, with an estimated 27.1 million Americans having used an illegal drug in the month prior to the survey. The survey also revealed that about one in twelve Americans needed some form of substance abuse treatment, but only 11 percent of them actually received treatment (https://www.livescience.com/56026-drug-use-america-2015-report.html). It can easily be argued that substance abuse is a national epidemic.

BEHAVIORAL AND SUBSTANCE ABUSE SERVICES

Rural areas are particularly problematic in that many suffer from a lack of behavioral and substance abuse providers and services. As a result, a number of patients who need and seek behavioral health or substance abuse care and treatment do so from their primary care provider, local urgent care center, or hospital emergency department. While this occurs in urban communities as well, the ability to refer patients for help to mental health and substance abuse providers is either limited or not available locally at all. As a result, primary care providers, urgent care center providers, and hospital emergency departments diagnose and treat these conditions as best they can on an ongoing basis. In addition, patients find it difficult to access mental health and substance abuse service providers when they are available locally because of long wait times or other restrictions to access, including the provider not accepting all forms of insurance payments. Clearly, this situation impacts the health status of any community.

Other determinants of health status—such as smoking, obesity, physical activity or exercise, accessing preventative health services, and access to fresh fruits, vegetables, and other nutrient-dense fresh foods—all tend to be worse in rural areas. Approximately half or more of premature deaths can be attributed to lifestyle, and these factors—as well as others—contribute to higher morbidity and mortality rates, on average, in rural populations. Moreover, as a general rule, a higher percentage of the population in rural areas have Medicare and Medicaid coverage (versus private insurance), which provide lower reimbursements to healthcare providers on a per-unit-of-service basis.

An example of one of the challenges facing rural hospitals is told by a well-known rural hospital CEO about why the hospital opened a renal dialysis center providing hemodialysis—even though they knew it would always lose money. In this southern Indiana community of approximately 6,700, someone with end-stage renal disease (ESRD) or needing hemodialysis would be forced to travel over an hour (one way), typically three days a week for hemodialysis treatment. Patients would have to travel to one of two large urban areas for the treatment. Given a typical three-hour hemodialysis treatment procedure time, this would be a whole-day affair. Moreover, some dialysis patients would not be able to drive or make the trip alone, requiring at least one other person—likely a family member or good friend—to drive them for the life-sustaining treatment. Time, travel, traffic, anxiety, cost, inconvenience—a number of factors must be confronted and overcome for this to work. And for some dialysis patients in this rural community, it didn't work. The option for some where this didn't work? In essence, to stay home, in their community, and face certain death.

The rural hospital CEO realized it was up to him and the hospital to provide hemodialysis locally—a money-losing venture—or more people in the community who needed hemodialysis would die from a lack of access to the life-sustaining treatment. In the case of this rural hospital, it had the financial strength to invest the capital into a money-losing service like hemodialysis to provide this essential service.

Many rural hospitals in the US would not have been able to do this, given the negative financial return and significant capital required to start this type of service. This type of decision differs from one being considered in a typical urban area in several ways. In many urban areas, there are one or more hospitals or health service providers already offering a service such as hemodialysis. Conversely, in most cases, the rural hospital is the sole community provider. Moreover, most rural hospitals have limited financial resources and would just not be able to subsidize a new money-losing service—even though it might be needed. Most rural hospitals do not have access to required capital to build a new (or remodel an existing) area of the hospital or purchase the needed equipment for such a capital-intensive venture.

DISCUSSION QUESTIONS

1. What is the major defining difference between an area considered urban versus one considered rural?
2. Small rural hospitals and other small rural health services organizations lack economies of scale. What does economies of scale refer to?
3. What has been the trend for recruiting and retaining primary care physicians in rural areas, and what are the factors supporting this trend?
4. Identify one or two elements or characteristics that make operating in today's environment more challenging for rural hospitals or health services organizations.
5. For the same or similar services rendered, how do rural hospital's quality of care and clinic outcomes compare to their urban counter parts?
6. On average, do rural hospitals have a lower or higher percentage of Medicare and Medicaid patients as compared to their urban hospital counter parts?
7. On average overall, how does the health status of rural populations compare to those in urban areas?
8. Provide an example of why the primary care physician shortage may be more acute in rural areas versus urban areas.
9. How do the characteristics of human nature – referred to as the "grass is greener / bigger is better" syndrome impact rural hospitals?
10. In general terms, descrie access to behavioral helath and substance abuse services in many rural areas of the US.

4

Health Insurance and Employer-Sponsored Group Health Plans

HEALTH INSURANCE & EMPLOYER-SPONSORED GROUP HEALTH PLANS

The most important benefit, in terms of the needs of the majority of working Americans, is health insurance. The large majority of private health insurance in the US is provided by businesses and other employers through employer-sponsored group health plans. As the cost of healthcare continues to rise over time, having access to private health insurance through employment has increasingly become more valuable to Americans and more expensive to provide on the part of employers. Until the advent of Obamacare, the employer's decision to offer a group health plan to employees and their dependents was exclusively the employer's—no strings attached. However, Obamacare mandated that all employers with fifty or more employees offer a group health plan, with associated parameters to meet and significant taxes to pay. Those employers large enough to meet this requirement are required to pay a tax if they don't meet the requirement. Prior to Obamacare, approximately two-thirds of the US population had some type of health insurance. After the implementation of Obamacare, the percentage of the US population with some type of health insurance increased, but not by the numbers originally projected.

Health insurance is regulated on a state-by-state basis. Group health insurance plans are also governed by a federal regulation called ERISA (the Employee Retirement Income Security Act of 1974). ERISA is a federal US tax and labor law that establishes minimum standards for pension plans in private industry as well as regulation surrounding employee benefits. Among a number of provisions promulgated by ERISA, a group health plan must meet the criteria that it not be considered nondiscriminatory; this includes both fully insured and self-insured plans. The health plan document is the controlling document that spells out all the policies, procedures, and provisions of the group health plan, including covered services and benefits, the specific plan year, and other important features and aspects governing the health plan.

RISK TRANSFER

At the basis of any type of insurance is the concept of risk transfer: the transferring of financial risk for a future claim covered by the respective insurance policy in exchange for a monthly, quarterly, or annual premium payment from the insured to the insurance company. However, health insurance is different from most other types of insurance. For example, when someone purchases property insurance or care insurance, they do so with the hope they won't have a claim; however, the insurance provides them with a sense of security, knowing if they do have a claim, it shouldn't be financially catastrophic to them personally, as their policy will provide some level of coverage and financial protection. While health insurance can clearly provide financial protection from a catastrophic episode requiring significant healthcare interventions and services, there are other drivers for the purchase of health insurance. Here is a short list of ways that health insurance differs from other types of insurance.

1. Spreads out financial outlays, helping to make payments more affordable and manageable
2. Purchased with the intent to actually use it
3. Mitigates financial outlays from a catastrophic event with significant costs requiring significant outlays
4. Utilization is somewhat self-determined for health issues and concerns that are elective in nature
5. Typically offered through place of employment, making it easily accessible

Today, group health insurance is a significant cost to both employers and employees alike. As healthcare costs have continued to rise at a rate that exceeds general inflation year in and year out, employers have implemented a number of changes in order to contain the spiraling cost of healthcare. The 1980s saw the onset of managed care, an umbrella term under which the financing and delivery of healthcare are somehow integrated in an effort to reduce unnecessary or unwarranted healthcare. Managed care has taken many different forms, including precertification for medical necessity prior to a healthcare service being rendered; drug formularies whereby certain high-priced brand-name drugs are restricted from coverage when suitable brand-name and generic alternatives are available; restrictions on access to providers through contracted networks; required second-opinion provisions to validate medical necessity; utilization-review provisions whereby expensive inpatient treatment plans and care rendered are reviewed daily for medical necessity; gatekeeping provisions requiring the patient's designated primary care provider (PCP) to authorize referrals to specialty care or other services; and more. While managed care has become a permanent aspect of insurance embedded in virtually all health plans, its effectiveness in controlling unnecessary healthcare, and therefore containing costs, can be debated.

Another strategy employer-sponsored group health plans utilize to try and slow their growing cost of providing a group health plan is cost sharing. "Cost sharing" is a term that refers to employer efforts to move a greater amount of the growing cost of sponsoring group health plan coverage to participating employees. While there are a number of mechanisms employers have used in this regard (including those mentioned above as examples of managed care), here are several other primary mechanisms used:

Coinsurance—a percentage of the healthcare service or claim that is paid by beneficiary.

Copayment—a flat/set amount of the healthcare service, prescription drug, or physician office visit that is paid by the beneficiary.

Deductible—an annual amount (per plan year) the beneficiary must pay for covered healthcare services before insurance coverage begins—excluding insurance payments for preventive services, physician office visits, and prescription drugs.

Premium—the monthly amount a health plan enrollee pays for health insurance coverage, typically paid via payroll deduction through the enrollee's employer under the enrolled group health plan.

High-deductible health plans (HDHPs)—defined by the IRS for 2018, a health plan with a minimum annual deductible of $1,300 for an individual and $2,600 for a family. An HDHP's total yearly out-of-pocket expenses (including deductibles, copayments and coinsurance) can't be more than $6,550 for an individual or $13,100 for a family.

Health savings accounts (HSAs)—HSAs can be made available with qualifying HDHPs. HSAs allow participants to make tax-free contributions into their HSA account and then use money from the account to pay for qualifying healthcare expenditures not otherwise covered under an enrollee's health plan. Employers may also make contributions to an employee's HSA. HDHPs must meet the following criteria to qualify for an HSA to be offered:

- Minimum levels for single and family deductibles must be met.
- Maximum limits on total employee stop-loss amounts—including deductibles, copayments and coinsurance—must be met.

- No insurance coverage is provided until the deductible is met, except for health insurance premiums, wellness and preventive care, expenses resulting from accidents, and dental or vision expenses.

The prevalence of high-deductible health plans continue to increase. The Kaiser Family Foundation reports that employee deductibles have increased, on average, by 67 percent from 2010 to 2015 (Becker's Hospital CFO Report, May 19, 2016). High-deductible health plans have impacted the healthcare industry in a variety of ways, as the healthcare consumer is spending more of his own money for healthcare services, driving the healthcare consumer to be a more informed purchaser than he has been historically. Under a high-deductible health plan, the beneficiary is required to satisfy the annual deductible with his own money before the coinsurance is applied. This financial incentive is driving health consumers to become more educated about their healthcare purchasing decisions, shopping more than ever for value. While it can be argued this changing behavior driving healthcare consumerism is good overall, it is not without side effects. Some high-deductible health plans' participants may delay needed care or avoid accessing it altogether, given the initial up-front costs associated with satisfying the deductible. Moreover, the healthcare industry is only in its infancy with regard to the publication and accessibility of meaningful competitive data on quality outcomes, service delivery, and costs. However, as the industry evolves with quality, service, and cost reporting, so will benchmarking of these same key elements, thus equipping healthcare consumers with more of the information they need to be informed purchasers of healthcare services.

Many group health plans also offer a health savings account (HSA) along with the high-deductible health plan. An HSA can only be offered in conjunction with a qualified high-deductible health plan. An HSA acts as a personal savings account: employee contributions are made pretax, and the funds can be used for eligible health services not otherwise covered or reimbursed by the group health plan, including deductibles, copayments, coinsurance, and eligible over-the-counter drugs and medical supplies. Also eligible for reimbursement from an HSA account are dental and vision care, including contacts and eye glasses. Annual contribution limits in 2018 to an HSA account are $3,450 for single medical coverage and $6,900 for family medical coverage. Those fifty-five years of age or older can contribute an additional $1,000, for an annual total of $4,450 to an HSA account for single medical coverage and $7,900 for family medical coverage (Ray Martin, *MoneyWatch*, October 24, 2017).

A unique feature of the HSA is that at age sixty-five, participants can receive penalty-free distributions for any reason. In other words, the HSA acts like an Individual Retirement Account (IRA) once the account holder turns sixty-five years of age. However, like an IRA, funds withdrawn for nonqualified medical expenses are subject to ordinary income tax.

A somewhat similar account that has been around for decades is called the flexible spending account. A flexible spending account, like an HSA, is contributed to on a voluntary basis by an employee covered under a health insurance plan offered under a qualified cafeteria benefits structure. A flexible spending account is offered for two purposes: 1) dependent-care coverage expenses, and 2) uncovered or otherwise unreimbursed medical expenses that are eligible for reimbursement under flexible spending (these reimbursable services are similar to those listed under the HSA). All employee contributions are pretax, up to an annual contribution limit of $2,650 in 2018. However, unlike the HSA, contributions to a flexible spending account that are not used in the plan year they are made are forfeited; therefore, plan participants should carefully plan out their annual contributions with this important caveat in mind. Another feature of the flexible spending account is that it can be offered in conjunction with an HSA; however, when the group health plan enrollee is a participant in both the HSA and the flexible spending account, flexible spending account contributions are restricted to dental and vision services reimbursements only (Stephen Miller, "2018 FSA Contribution Cap Rises to $2,650," *Society for Human Resource Management*, October 23, 2017).

SELF-INSURED AND SELF-FUNDED GROUP HEALTH PLANS

The majority of employer-sponsored group health plans today are self-insured or self-funded and contract with an outside third-party administrator (TPA) to administer the health plan. Under this methodology, the employer does not actually purchase insurance and maintains the financial risk for health plan utilization and expenditures. One of the biggest variables in self-insuring or self-funding an employer-sponsored group health plan is the plan experience: the number of health claims incurred and the total cost for same. The projected expenditure in any group health plan is determined as a function of the age and health status of the insureds or health plan participants; the health plan's benefit design; related incentives that drive the behavior of the insureds regarding how and when they access health services; and the overall plan experience rating based on its historical plan experience for utilization and expenditures.

Most of the large carriers have what is referred to as two different "books of business": fully insured and ASO. Fully insured is what most think of as traditional health insurance whereby the carrier underwrites the plan, accepts all the financial risk for plan utilization and health claim expenditures incurred, and charges a premium structure based on the provisions, benefits, and design of the health plan, including services covered and the experience rating of the group being insured, based on factors used to assess and determine projected health claim outlays and administrative expenses. Monthly premiums charged are typically for individual coverage, individual plus spouse coverage, or family coverage. Under a fully insured group health plan, the carrier sets the monthly premium rates to cover all projected health claim expenditures to be incurred in the upcoming plan year, plus the "administrative load," which includes various marketing and administrative expenses plus profit. Under a fully insured plan, the employer is purchasing the group health plan as designed, including premiums to be charged and the portion of the premium that will be paid by the employer versus what is paid for by the participating employee (although sometimes the portions of the premium paid for by the employer and employee can be modified in some cases). In a fully insured group health plan, the carrier "owns" the health plan, which means the employer typically can't make changes to the design of the health plan. Under a self-insured group health plan, the employer owns the health plan and can make whatever modifications to plan design, premiums charged, etc., as deemed appropriate. Therefore, under a self-insured group health plan, the employer can determine what services will be covered under the plan; the premiums that will be charged to employees under the different coverage options; other benefits that will or will not be offered, such as wellness and health-promotion services; and what, if any, financial incentives will be used to drive or promote healthy behaviors.

Therefore, the two primary reasons why an employer would choose to self-insure its group health plan are: 1) it is less expensive in the long run versus paying a carrier for marketing, administrative expenses, and profit under a fully insured plan; and 2) the employer has the ability to make plan-design changes, employ incentives, and generally control key elements of the health plan. However, one major consideration for self-insuring is the inherent volatility in any group health plan regarding utilization, catastrophic high-dollar claims, or just experiencing a particularly bad plan year in terms of total aggregate claim expenditures. The basis of insurance is spreading risk over a larger base of insureds; therefore, as a general rule, the greater the number of group health plan participants, the less volatility the plan should experience overall. Why? Because a few large, high-dollar, or catastrophic health claims can be more easily absorbed or buffered by the size of a larger group health plan. The opposite of this is also true as well. While there is no set minimum number of group health plan participants that make self-funding preferred over a fully insured plan, at least 150 to 200 group health plan participants is generally thought to be the minimum number needed to make good financial sense to self-insure. However, in most all cases, the use of reinsurance is essential for the self-insured group health plan to mitigate its risk exposure.

In most cases, employers mitigate their financial risk by purchasing reinsurance through a reinsurance company. Reinsurance can be thought of as "insurance on top of insurance." Many reinsurance carriers specialize in this type of insurance and don't offer other types. In many instances, it is the insurance broker, health benefits consultant, or third-party administrator who brings the reinsurer to the group health plan. This reinsurance provides insurance coverage at two levels: 1) specific or individual claim stop-loss coverage for high-dollar claims, and 2) aggregate or total claim expenditures in a plan year.

In the world of health insurance, the term "stop loss" refers to two things. For the employer, stop loss refers to the individual and aggregate thresholds where reinsurance kicks in. For example, the individual or specific stop loss might be set at a threshold of $75,000. This means that any individual claim that exceeds $75,000, the self-funded plan will pay the first $75,000 and the reinsurer will pay any amount over $75,000. All claims less than $75,000 are the responsibility of the group health plan. The lower the individual claim threshold, the more individual claims will be reimbursed by the reinsurer and the higher the cost of the reinsurance premium will be to the employer. The higher the individual claim threshold, the fewer individual claims will be reimbursed by the reinsurer and the lower the cost of the reinsurance premium will be to the employer. This process is called risk transfer; the more risk that is transferred to the reinsurer, the greater the cost for the reinsurance coverage, which is paid in the form of a premium by the employer.

Typically, the aggregate stop loss is set at 125% of total anticipated/projected claims for the plan year. Therefore, all claims that exceed 125% of the anticipated/projected total amount of claims paid in a plan year will be reimbursed to the employer by the reinsurer. While the individual stop-loss amount is typically hit numerous times in a plan year (of course, this depends on the number of health plan participants and other related variables), it is less common for the aggregate stop loss to be realized.

For covered employees/plan beneficiaries, stop loss refers to the total maximum out-of-pocket amount the employee has to pay in any given plan year before insurance will pay 100% of all subsequent covered health claims for the remainder of the plan year. For the employer, stop loss refers to the dollar amount of the threshold for individual or aggregate reinsurance coverage. For example, the individual coverage annual stop loss may be $10,000 for a given plan year and $15,000 for family coverage. After the stop-loss threshold has been met by the employee through copayments, coinsurance, and deductible payments, the insurance plan will pay all remaining covered healthcare services for the remainder of the plan year. This stop-loss provision protects the employee from catastrophic financial outlays and financial loss.

THIRD-PARTY ADMINISTRATORS

Third-party administrators (TPAs) are organizations that contract with self-insured employers to administer most or all aspects of the employer's group health plan. Like most industries, the TPA industry continues to experience changes, including consolidation. Today, there are several hundred TPAs operating in the US, from small individually or family-owned firms to large corporations administering benefits for hundreds of employers and thousands of group health plan participants. TPAs do not take any financial risk of the group health plan they administer—they act more like a bank, using the employer's own money to pay health claims incurred by group health plan participants on behalf of the group health plan.

Employers who choose to self-insure or self-fund their group health plan typically contract with an outside third-party administrator (TPA) to administer all aspects of the employer's group health plan. Fundamentally, there are two different types of TPAs. One is an organization designed to provide TPA services to self-insured groups and is not an insurance company. These TPAs are not licensed as insurance companies and don't underwrite or provide any insurance per se—they administer group health plans. These organizations are simply referred to as TPAs. The other type of organization that administers group health plans for self-insured employers is the large health insurance companies—referred to as health insurance carriers, or just "carriers" for short—that also provide TPA services. However, when a carrier provides TPA services, it is referred to as providing "administrative services only," or ASO services. ASO refers to the fact that the carrier is not underwriting the group health plan and is not providing insurance or accepting any financial risk for utilization or claims incurred by the group health plan; it is providing administrative services only, just like a TPA. Therefore, by definition, only a carrier that provides one or more fully insured health insurance products is referred to as providing ASO when administering a group health plan on behalf of a self-funded group health plan.

TPAs can provide a multitude of different services in the administration of a group health plan, and their charges for doing so are typically rendered on a per-employee-per-month basis (that is, per employee participating in the group health plan each month). Moreover, most TPAs charge a set fee per participating employee for a set package of services provided; however, the more services provided beyond this set package the TPA provides, the greater the per-employee fee will be. This is because many TPAs typically provide a number of additional or value-added services to self-insured group health plans.

TPAs typically provide some or all of the following services:

- Health plan document writing, revisions, and maintenance
- Recommendations regarding health plan benefits design
- Support and assistance during open enrollment of employees
- Issuance of health plan beneficiary cards
- Health claims processing and adjudication
- Health claim accuracy validation
- Health claim code editing
- Contracting with a preferred provider organization (PPO) network
- Repricing and payment of healthcare claims
- Issuance of explanations of benefits (EOBs) to beneficiaries and explanations of payment (EOPs) to providers
- Contracting and administration of annual deductibles, coinsurance, and copayments
- Calculations and administration of flexible spending accounts and health savings accounts (HSAs)
- Medical-necessity determinations and utilization review
- Contracting with a reinsurance company

EMPLOYER COST-CONTAINMENT STRATEGIES

Employers are using a variety of cost-containment and cost-sharing strategies to try and reduce the escalating cost of their group health plans. Some examples of these strategies—several of which have already been mentioned—include:

1. Providing plan participants with price and quality data on available providers. An increasing number of third-party services are available that provide current price and quality-outcomes data on providers in a variety of specialty areas.
2. Through defined-contribution health plans in which the employer funds an HSA or some other vehicle in order to "cap" the employer's annual contribution and costs.
3. Use of pharmacy benefit managers (PBMs) and specialty drug or other prescription drug programs to help reduce costs, especially given the increasing number of drugs available on the market and their associated high costs.
4. The purchase of group health plan coverage through private health insurance exchanges.
5. Narrow provider networks, including for specialty, tertiary, and high-cost quaternary care services where preferred pricing has been prenegotiated.
6. Use of drug formularies.
7. Adoption of employee wellness, health promotion, and fitness programs.
8. Conversion to a self-funded group health plan.

9. Establishment and operation of on-site primary care clinics.
10. Use of education and training to help enrollees become better educated and informed purchasers of healthcare services.

EMPLOYEE HEALTH & WELLNESS

Employers are increasingly searching for ways to slow the continually spiraling costs of providing group health plans. This is true for companies that compete domestically as well as companies that compete internationally. One area receiving more attention is promoting and incentivizing employees and dependents to be as healthy as possible. One of the challenges for employers is measuring the success of their health promotion and wellness efforts in a quantifiable way. What plan-design changes, incentives, and other promotional efforts make the biggest impact? How do you balance necessary mandates or requirements versus options and alternatives? How do we assess short-term versus long-term objectives and performance? While employer efforts to promote employee and dependent health and wellness are really in their infancy nationwide, these efforts are almost sure to intensify as the cost of sponsoring a group health plan continue to rise.

HEALTH BENEFIT CONSULTANTS

Healthcare is complex. Navigating the world of health plans and health services can be a daunting task, to say the least. Analysis and decision-making around fully insured versus self-insured options; plan design and administration; going to the market for bids; setting premiums under a self-insured plan; securing the services of a TPA and reinsurer; and more. Many employers use the services of a professional health benefit consultant to assist and provide the expertise and advice that most employers need to navigate the group health plan waters. For example, understanding the differences, including advantages and disadvantages, between preferred provider organizations, narrow provider networks, and carve-outs for selected tertiary care services takes real knowledge, understanding, insight, and expertise about many different aspects of the complex healthcare system.

REFERENCES CITED

Indiana Hospital Association. "Eleven Ways Indiana Businesses Are Attempting to Cut Health Care Costs." *Harmony*.

Pennza, Amy. "How to Tell If Your High-Deductible Health Plan Is HSA Qualified." PeopleKeep. February 13, 2017. https://www.zanebenefits.com/blog/how-to-tell-if-your-high-deductible-health-plan-is-hsa-qualified.

DISCUSSION QUESTIONS

1. Describe several ways in which health insurance is different from other types of insurance.
2. Describe what is meant by risk transfer, and how it relates to health insurance.
3. Explain what is meant by the term adverse selection.
4. What is the fundamental difference between a fully-insured group health plan and a self-insured group health plan?
5. What is reinsurance and what role does it play in a group health plan that is self-insured?
6. What does the term stop loss mean in terms of reinsurance?
7. What does the term stop loss mean to an employee who has individual coverage through his/her employer's group health plan?
8. Explain what the term stop loss means.
9. Explain the difference between a traditional indemnity health insurance policy and a high deductible health plan.
10. Describe what is meant by out-of-pocket payment.

5

The Role of Healthcare Leadership

The decision to become a healthcare leader, like any career decision, is one that shouldn't be made lightly. Why become a healthcare leader? There are many reasons why someone would want to become a healthcare leader. In general, healthcare leaders are in a position to make a tremendous impact on countless lives inside the organization, as well as in the community. It is hard to imagine another profession that has such an opportunity to make the lives of others better; help employees achieve their hopes, dreams, and career goals; be an integral part of a team that saves lives and improve the functioning and overall physical and mental health of everyday people during their time of need. However, the path to becoming a healthcare leader is not easy or without its own challenges.

Although the role and functions of healthcare leaders can vary greatly, there are some common themes that typically apply across the healthcare leadership spectrum. This chapter will discuss the role, functions, and typical daily activities of a healthcare leader.

OBJECTIVES

1. Learn the four basic functions of management.
2. Explore the activities common to many healthcare leaders and what they spend their time doing on a daily basis.
3. Understand why a team or organization is a reflection of leadership and compare and contrast the leadership role of a football coach with that of a healthcare leader.

Most people who become a healthcare leader won't experience much, if any, fame or glory; probably won't get rich; work long, hard, and mostly thankless hours; are responsible for the actions and behaviors of others, especially when things go wrong; deal with the "politics" of working any people-oriented business; and typically deal with a high level of pressure and stress for delivering results and performance. Nonetheless, a career in healthcare leadership can be tremendously satisfying and rewarding knowing the impact that can be made in service to others.

WHAT DO HEALTHCARE LEADERS DO?

Management is getting work done through others. What healthcare leaders do can be categorized into the four basic functions of management: planning, organizing, leading, and controlling.

Planning—To determine a goal and the means to accomplish it.

Organizing—To coordinate and carry-out tasks. Deciding where decisions will be made, who will do what jobs and tasks, and who will work with or for whom.

Leading—To be in charge of and responsible for people and/or tasks. Motivating and inspiring others to work hard and achieve organizational, departmental, team, or individual goals.

Controlling—To guide or check; the act of fostering accountability. Monitoring progress toward goal achievement and taking corrective action, when needed.

There are many other functions and activities of management that healthcare leaders undertake; however, each of these fits into one of the four basic functions of management.

Healthcare leaders, especially those in senior management roles, get involved in a myriad of functions, decisions, projects, and management activities. Although all healthcare leaders have their own professional areas of strength and weakness, along with areas of special expertise or experience, many would be considered management "generalists"—a manager with a broad scope of knowledge, skill, and ability covering a wide variety of important functions and pertinent tangible and intangible areas of management. As a senior manager of a hospital or health service organization, you may have overall organizational responsibility for the Quality Improvement (QI) process, state licensure, Healthcare Facilities Accreditation Program or Joint Commission on Accreditation of Healthcare Organizations accreditation, and Medicare conditions of participation; overall staffing and productivity in nursing, ancillary, or support service departments; quality of patient care and clinical outcomes, customer service, and patient satisfaction results; employee morale, satisfaction, and engagement; capital and operating budgets and financial performance; organizational change and innovation; marketing and sales outreach; public relations and community service involvement; salary, wage, and benefits administration, including retirement plan(s); human resource policy and procedure administration; recruitment, candidate screening, and hiring; infection control; employee health; plant operations, maintenance, or bio-medical engineering management; clinical protocols in specialty areas, such as cardiology; or information technology system planning, implementation, and management. The variety of subject matter can be both vast and complex; consequently, some senior healthcare leaders become very conversant—even experts—in one or more specialty areas of healthcare. However, many senior healthcare leaders become more of a management generalist—with special knowledge, experience, or interest in one or more areas of healthcare leadership.

Vince Caponi, CEO of Ascension Health in Indiana talks about some of the most important skills and attributes of a leader. Mr. Caponi states that "***Our ability to lead is not as important as people's willingness to follow. It demands great relationship skills. But none is going to take an interest in you until you take an interest in them. To have a friend you have to be a friend. They are never going to hear, listen to you, or take your leadership until you open up and listen to them first.***"

Mr. Caponi has a flip chart in his office that has the following key points for his leadership team written on it:

- Simplicity
- Accountability
- Standardization
  - Business
  - Clinical
- Managing across the continuum
- Reaction time improvement

The ways in which leadership will accomplish these goals is through:

- Talent
- Leverage
- Information
- Execution

Mr. Caponi goes on to explain a bit about what is written on the flip chart. "***Healthcare is very complex. Our jobs many times are to try and simplify the complex. And begin to map out a plan of how we might***

address that, and how that plan sinks-up with our mission, vision, values and strategic plan. Many times, however, you are going down the path, and you think you're on the right path, and then there are a thousand distractions that come upon you. I think the leader has to filter through that. And there may be 2 or 3 things you really do need to pay attention to."

> **Healthcare is very complex. Our jobs many times are to try and simplify the complex.**

Back to the question: what do healthcare leaders do? The typical healthcare leader gets involved in a lot of different management functions, processes, decisions, and activities, as previously stated. Of course, the actual involvement will depend on a myriad of variables, including the organization and its culture, size, scope of services, and problems and resources; the actual job and direct responsibilities of the leader; the needs of the organization, along with its mission, vision, strategy, goals, and priorities; and a host of other variables, including the leader's own initiative, management philosophy, and leadership style. A healthcare manager can receive a request or suggestion to do something or even order from a superior to take some kind of action. Additionally, a healthcare leader may take the initiative to do something through his own volition—typically referred to as being "self-motivated" to take action that is needed. This is also referred to as healthcare leader who is a "self-starter," or a leader who doesn't need or wait for someone to suggest or tell them what needs to be done or accomplished, but rather, who is in-tuned with the needs of the organization and its people and takes the initiative to move action forward, as needed.

Management is about getting work done through others, so much of what a typical healthcare leader does involves working with employees and providing them the training, support, resources, guidance, direction, motivation and coaching they need to perform their work at a high level—individually and collectively as a team. This requires the leader to know and understand the nature of the work to be performed along with policies, procedures, protocols, work processes and general expectations regarding the work and desired performance. Naturally, there will be problems, issues, and various decisions that will need to be addressed from time to time. How the healthcare leader approaches these are a matter of leadership philosophy and style, along with the organizational culture, or the way business is typically handled in the organization.

Healthcare leaders also are typically involved in staffing and scheduling of employees by shift, as well as orienting, training, supervising, coaching, developing, and supporting employees in their respective jobs and work. Healthcare leaders strive to create an atmosphere and working environment that motivates, encourages, and inspires employees to give their best, help solve problems, and make improvements to work processes, so the work performed is as efficient and effective as possible. Leadership is motivating and inspiring others to work hard to achieve organizational, departmental, service, team, and individual goals. Creating a working environment where employees are engaged to give their best effort and performance is, therefore, a critical function and goal of healthcare leadership.

Sam Odle talks about the time a leader spends with his employees. ***"It's not making time for your employees. Spending time with your employees should be how you do your work. If you look at six sigma, or lean, or Studer, Leland Kaiser's work around the uncommon leader; all of those drive behaviors that cause you [(the leader)] to spend more time with the front line staff who are dealing with the customer. It's all about getting out there and spending more time—back in engagement with the people who are doing the work."***

Healthcare leaders get involved in a lot of activities that relate to and involve communication of the organization's mission, vision, strategy, goals, and priorities and what they mean for the work being done in the respective department, function, or service and the employee's job, role, function, responsibilities, objectives, tasks, and related activities. Leaders must be skilled at communication and interpersonal skills, as these are paramount to workers' understanding what is expected and required and getting efficient, high-quality work done through others by motivating and inspiring them to work hard and give their best. There is a whole chapter in this text devoted to leadership communication.

Part of being an effective healthcare leader involves conceptual skills—the ability to see the organization as a whole, understand how the different areas, departments, functions, services, and decisions affect each other, and recognize how the company fits into or is affected by its environment. Conceptual skills are vital to being an effective healthcare leader, and can be learned and developed—primarily through observation and experience, but also through coaching and mentoring, as well as self-study.

Healthcare leaders are typically working on one or more projects, usually involving other employees or leaders, and increasingly, involving physicians as the role of the physician and his or her integration with the hospital and clinical operations evolves. Projects can include a multitude of possible areas and needs of the organization, from clinical process or service improvements to cost reduction efforts, regulation, and compliance-related issues to business or service development and a myriad of other functions or topics. Leaders should always be open to and on the lookout for opportunities to make the situation better, and sometimes, these opportunities cross lines of department or service functions and leadership responsibilities. The functions and services provided by hospitals and health service organizations are highly interconnected and dependent upon each other for a patient's overall service experience to be optimal and the operations to be both efficient and effective. Therefore, healthcare leaders, particularly those responsible for operations or the management of line or operating departments, functions, and systems must foster teamwork and work together in a collaborative fashion—both inside and outside their own area of responsibility. Without a team effort and collaborative work process, important work flows and processes will break down and be less than optimal. Moreover, patient safety, quality, and service will suffer when there is a lack of intra- and inter-departmental and service teamwork and collaboration. Healthcare leaders must always be on the lookout for this (monitoring), and take corrective action as needed when identified (controlling)—working together as a leadership team. Clearly, this is one of many areas where leaders must model the way with teamwork and collaboration to set the example for employees to follow.

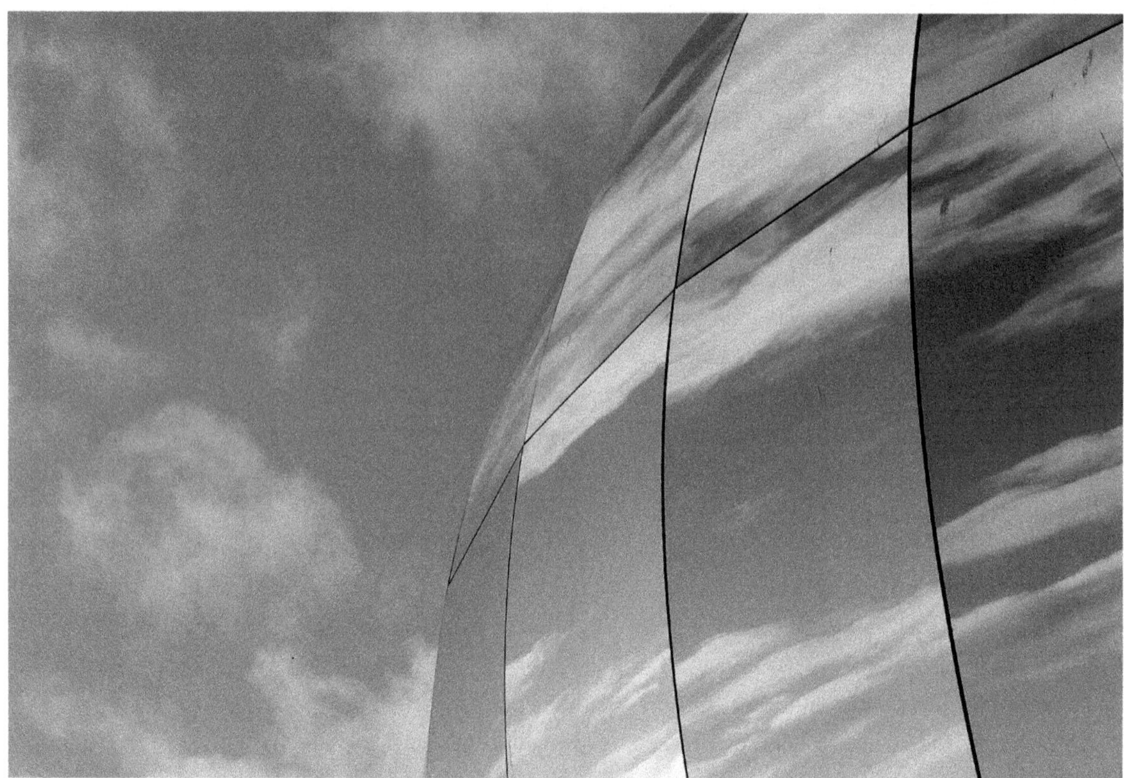

FIGURE 5.1 Sky and Building

A HEALTHCARE ORGANIZATION IS A REFLECTION OF ITS LEADERSHIP

Every organization is a reflection of the leadership philosophy, style, and culture that is fostered by its leadership. This is no different with healthcare. Most healthcare organizations take on the persona of the CEO and senior leadership team that establish and drive the organizational culture and how business is conducted on a daily basis. Just like in the sport of football, which many in the U.S. consider the ultimate team sport, the team becomes a reflection of its coach. How hard does the team practice? How well prepared is the team for its games? Does every player on the team know his role, has he trained properly, and is he ready to effectively execute in a game situation? What's the game plan, how effective will strategies be, how well understood are the strategies and game plan by each member of the team, is the team psychologically motivated and prepared to deal with "big game" situations, does the team work together in synchronicity and support one another, does the coach care about the players, and how does he demonstrate this to them and others? Just like a football team, the healthcare team is a reflection of its leadership.

THE ROLE OF HEALTHCARE LEADERSHIP

The role of healthcare leadership in any health service organization is extremely vital to the overall performance and success of the organization. The overall goal of leadership in a healthcare organization is about providing the vision; direction; organization; design; structure; resources, including personnel; and organizational culture/climate for caregivers and supportive personnel to be as efficient and effective as possible. Healthcare leadership is responsible for establishing priorities, points of emphasis, and a game plan for daily operations and activities of the organization and its people. This role is both broad and general in scope but much more detailed and refined in its implementation and execution at the worksite level.

An illustration of this would be if the healthcare organization's goal is to achieve patient satisfaction at the 80th percentile in the respective data base the organization uses. How does this overall goal relate to an individual nursing unit—like a medical unit—or to a service department, such as food and nutritional services? The respective department manager and/or supervisors in the medical unit, as well as food and nutritional services, must translate how the overall goal for patient satisfaction relates to their individual department and work they do. In addition, this must be communicated so that employees understand how the overall goal for patient satisfaction also relates with other priorities, policies, procedures, and practices to be followed and applied.

SIMPLIFY THE COMPLEX

The US healthcare system is the largest and most advanced healthcare system in the world: it's also the most complex. For example, it is estimated there are well over thirty thousand rules, regulations, and standards in the Medicare program alone! Regulations affect documentation and coding, billing and collection, reimbursement structures and payment models, cost reporting, and much more, all of which are constantly changing. There are advancing medical technologies; new medicines and chemotherapy agents; new surgical equipment and supplies; and a cadre of medical, surgical, and ancillary specialists highly trained in their own respective clinical areas who are practicing their professions based on highly specialized, sophisticated knowledge and training while speaking languages of their own; and the list goes on. Healthcare is complex—and it's a healthcare leader's job to help simplify the complex. Why?

Healthcare leaders—especially those in executive roles—are in a position to see, know, and understand the "bigger picture." This includes trends and changes in the external environment that impact the organization; how the organization fits into its environment and relates to other organizations and providers; and how the different services, functions, and departments of the hospital or health services organization relate to, interconnect with, and support one another in the organization and other organizations in the community. Moreover, the healthcare leader's role is to help educate others in the organization about external and internal factors—ones that are complex and not easy to understand—so that others can understand: in other words, to simplify the complex. All this takes effective communication from the healthcare leader to foster understanding, acceptance, and support from others.

Communication fosters understanding.
Understanding fosters acceptance.
Acceptance fosters support.

Simplifying the complex also includes a healthcare leader's articulation and explanation of organizational priorities, goals, strategies, benchmarks, market data, competitive forces, regulatory requirements, policies and procedures, reimbursement, rate-setting strategies, and even financial statements. For example, how does cost shifting impact the hospital's strategy toward managed-care negotiations and contracting, setting rates, reimbursement, and the generation of net revenue? Why are the practices and policies within the organization's risk management plan and program so important? How does the work of each employee support the mission of the organization? Why is the organization going exclusively with a high-deductible health plan for the employer-sponsored group health plan it offers its employees? How can the hospital afford to open a new physician practice in a growing but remote location in the service area but not purchase new hospital beds for the medical/surgical nursing unit this year?

Simplifying the complex is more art than science. It is a leadership philosophy, style, and skill that leaders can learn. Using examples, illustrations, and stories that people can relate to can be effective in simplifying the complex. The ability to summarize key concepts and points clearly and succinctly is important. Sometimes the leader's goal is to help people step back and see the big picture—a critical skill that can be very effective at the right time. Sometimes it is being analytical and using a few pieces of data to help provide context and perspective on a topic. Being cognizant of the importance of simplification, working to understand people and their views and perspectives, and practicing communication skills in order to be articulate in both speaking and writing all help a leader demonstrate this important approach and skill.

FIVE KEY ATTRIBUTES OF LEADERSHIP

ENGAGING AND MOTIVATING EMPLOYEES ARE CRITICAL OBLIGATIONS OF HEALTHCARE LEADERS

Strong, effective, high-performing executive leadership is essential in healthcare organizations today given the dynamic healthcare environment and the evolving role of consumerism. Expectations of all stakeholders for improved operating performance and outcomes in all areas continue to increase.

Five attributes for fostering high-performing leadership—accountability, engagement, communication, vision, and embodiment of the critical intangibles of being a leader—can help executive leaders drive organizational performance (including financial performance, customer-service and quality outcomes, volume or business growth, internal and external reputation, employee engagement, and other measures) to higher levels.

ACCOUNTABILITY

At the executive level, accountability means being transparent, sharing organizational goals and priorities, and reporting the progress toward those goals. Accountable leaders open themselves up to public evaluation and scrutiny. A leader who models these behaviors will contribute to a culture of accountability across the organization.

A culture of accountability starts with the CEO but also includes department managers and supervisors who hold themselves as well as their employees accountable for both effort and performance. Employees are continually comparing their treatment by leadership with the treatment their colleagues receive, and they are motivated when they perceive they are being treated fairly (and discouraged when they perceive their treatment to be unfair or unequitable). When a manager or supervisor doesn't hold an employee accountable in a fair or consistent manner, other employees see the discrepancy and can become disenchanted and demotivated.

ENGAGEMENT

Good leaders at every level make fostering employee engagement a primary goal. Although *management* is about getting work accomplished through others, *leadership* (one of the four basic functions of management) is about motivating and inspiring others to work hard to achieve organizational goals. Disengaged employees typically give effort commensurate with only the minimum standards and expectations. Countless factors can contribute to employees' level of engagement and satisfaction in their work environment and employment relationship, including the three discussed below.

Recognition and appreciation. Leadership's ability to foster employee feelings of being wanted and appreciated clearly plays into engagement. Leaders can enhance employee engagement and spur productivity just by making rounds, attending regularly scheduled departmental staff meetings, or conducting open employee meetings. Engaging in these activities lets employees know their leaders are paying attention. Conversely, when employees don't feel wanted or appreciated, they are much more apt to "quit on the job" and meet only the minimum standards required to maintain their employment. Moreover, when employees become disengaged, they detract from the organization's mission, vision, values, goals, and priorities. This attitude of disengagement can spread throughout the organization, affecting the effort and performance of other employees, the organization's image and reputation, and the ability to attract and retain high-performing employees.

Inquisitive environment. An effective leader invites employees to be innovative and creative and discusses and implements their ideas for improving the organization's operations and working environment.

Collaboration and teamwork should be valued, and new and different ideas welcomed and appreciated. A leader should consistently convey an openness to consider new ideas and suggestions; otherwise, new ideas and suggestions will not be forthcoming. Unfortunately, executive leaders often create an environment that, instead of fostering new or different ideas, stops them from being presented, discussed, or evaluated and thus prevents them from gaining any traction. If a leader responds to a suggestion with the comment, "That will never work," he or she will promptly shut down dialogue about the matter. The result is a real reluctance of employees to bring new ideas or creative solutions forward.

Participatory leadership. Just as important as listening to employee suggestions is actively seeking them. As a rule, employees want to be involved in problem solving and decision making in matters that affect their job, their work, and their working environment. Effective leaders work collaboratively and openly with employees, utilizing their skills, experience, and critical thinking. To engage employees, leaders should take the following steps:

- Seek input and create dialogue around employee suggestions for improvement, solutions to problems, and new ideas.
- Consider that input within the decision-making process.
- Strive to implement employee ideas into the workplace to the extent possible.

Participatory leadership is a way to recognize that there is no monopoly on good ideas and that people doing the work often have the best ideas about how to make their work more efficient and effective. A leader whose leadership is not participatory creates an environment where employees can become aloof, disinterested, and disengaged because they don't believe the leader cares about them or values their input or opinions.

COMMUNICATION

Action at every level of an organization must begin with communication. Effective communication is a powerful force that includes active listening along with clearly spoken and written communication.

The most powerful component of leadership communication is listening to employees. *How are things going? What other help, support, or resources do you need to get the job done efficiently and effectively? What do we need to change or improve?* When leaders ask these and similar questions while paying attention to employees in a positive, constructive manner, employees feel valued and appreciated. When leaders listen to their employees, they build trust, leading to a stronger level of engagement and a stronger employment relationship. Conversely, failing to pay attention or listen to employees is detrimental to the supervisor-subordinate relationship, to the employment relationship overall, and to employee engagement. Research shows one of the top reasons why an employee leaves an organization is the relationship with their immediate supervisor, which is directly affected by leadership communication.[a]

One of the most effective ways leaders can engage with employees is to engage with them in their work space. Making rounds and interacting with employees in their work area is a visual display that the leader cares about employees and their work and an opportunity for leaders and employees to communicate directly. Furthermore, this action can help a leader see with his or her own eyes problems and opportunities for improvement the leader may otherwise not see.

VISION

A leader without vision typically defaults to a transactional style of leadership—one that is predominantly about directing the daily tasks and functions to be accomplished. Transactional leadership is effective and even necessary in health care: Leaders should understand the operational business functions and processes, be familiar with the skills of employees, and be able to effectively assign tasks and teams to accomplish the work. However, leaders also should be able to establish strategies, goals, and objectives based on internal and external changes, trends, and opportunities for improvement, and be able to connect the work of their organization or department to the larger internal and external environment. In other words, a good leader can see the big picture and communicate that vision in a way that enables others to clearly see it, too.

At the corporate level, the vision of leaders involves strategic planning and positioning the organization to optimally serve its consumers. At the department manager or supervisor level, leaders should be able to interpret how the organization's strategic plan relates to the department, service, or function and should be able to develop action plans that are supportive of and in alignment with the organization's strategic initiatives and priorities. This alignment is paramount to ensure the organization and its employees are working in sync with one another.

In the management by objectives approach, the supervisor and subordinate work together on the following steps to ensure alignment:

- Meet to discuss the employee's work objectives
- Collaboratively identify objectives the employee will adopt
- Set action steps for the employee to accomplish the objectives
- Meet at a designated regular interval to discuss employee progress

The basis for this approach helps create alignment with corporate and department goals at the employee level, fosters maximum employee engagement and support, and encourages collaboration, facilitating dialogue with leadership that includes an employee's personal objectives and interests. The joint development of objectives and plans helps put an employee's objectives and interests in alignment with the organization's. When leaders do not take this approach, employees may feel that leadership isn't interested in their ideas, growth, or development; the result can be discord and a feeling that the leader and the employee aren't really in alignment or even on the same team.

CRITICAL INTANGIBLES

Health care may well be the ultimate people business. The most effective healthcare leaders tend to be those who connect with others in ways that make the leader seem human. Critical intangibles of leadership include trusting in others and being trustworthy, having integrity and credibility, and understanding people.

Integrity. Closely linked to trust, the integrity of a leader is always being assessed by employees, and any void here will result in less employee engagement and the giving of employee discretionary effort: that is, the cognitive and emotional desire to go above and beyond the minimum required standards of the job or work being performed. One example is how a leader reacts to mistakes—both his or her own and those made by others. A leader who outwardly demonstrates a desire for strong effort and performance, but also admits when he or she makes a mistake, helps to create a culture where excellence is personified. Employees are much more apt to give higher levels of effort and performance when they believe in the integrity of leadership, and that an occasional mistake made in good faith is acceptable.

Trust. It can be argued that trust of a healthcare leader is everything. When there is a lack of trust in a leader, followers do not believe the leader is genuine or sincere. Followers become hesitant, reluctant, and sometimes even scared to do more than what is specifically asked or expected of them. Furthermore, a lack of trust in leadership can become contagious, and collaboration and teamwork are negatively affected as well, creating a dysfunctional environment.

Emotional intelligence. There is a growing recognition of the importance of emotional intelligence in effective leadership. Understanding people and how they might react to certain situations or events, including new policies, procedures, and priorities, is a vital leadership competency. In addition, emotional intelligence involves a leader's ability to recognize and understand his or her own emotions and typical reactions to certain people, situations, and environments, and to adapt when necessary—for example, by staying calm when highly frustrated or when confronted in a hostile environment. When a leader misinterprets the emotions of others, or his or her own emotional responses—particularly in difficult or crucial situations—negative reactions or outcomes can result and can have a cascading negative effect throughout the organization.

High-performing leadership requires skills and competencies in the critical intangibles of leadership—aspects that can't be quantified or measured. In a people business such as health care, the critical intangibles of leadership play an important role in organizational performance.

Mastery of these key attributes—accountability, engagement, communication, vision, and the critical intangibles—can be difficult, but it is possible for any healthcare leader who takes them to heart. When a leader adopts these practices, the resulting style of leadership will effectively drive organizational performance to a higher level.

NOTE

a. Efron, L., "Six Reasons Your Best Employees Quit You," Forbes, June 24, 2013. Publication Date: Thursday, June 29, 2017

DISCUSSION QUESTIONS

1. Discuss how the leadership role of a healthcare leader compares and contrasts with that of a football coach.
2. Discuss some of the reasons why someone might want to become a healthcare leader.
3. What are the four basic functions of management?
4. Define each of the four basic functions of management.
5. Describe a few of the functions, projects, and management activities that many healthcare leaders get involved in.
6. What does it mean to be a management generalist?
7. Describe what is meant by conceptual skills.

6

Becoming a Healthcare Leader

Becoming a leader is a journey of learning, growing, developing and becoming the best, most effective leader that you can be. A leader's journey is not always a logical, sequential series of progressive steps, but rather one that has twists, turns, and even setbacks. Becoming a leader in a hospital or health service organization is a calling, a gift, a service to mankind, and an opportunity to make a difference for countless people.

What does it mean to be a healthcare leader? What is the path to becoming a healthcare leader? How does a new leader go about developing the knowledge, skills, and abilities he or she can apply to be effective and make a difference?

OBJECTIVES

1. Understand what it means to become a healthcare leader and why becoming a healthcare leader is a journey with no endpoint.
2. Learn lessons from the experiences of several healthcare leaders who have made major contributions to the lives and communities they served.
3. Provide aspiring healthcare leaders with motivation and inspiration to commit to learning, growing, and developing their leadership skills to reach their highest level of contribution to society.

I'LL NEVER FORGET MY FIRST DAY ON THE JOB AS A HOSPITAL CEO

It was the week after the 4th of July holiday in 1989, and I was sitting in the lobby at Charter Hospital of Denver in Lakewood, Colorado, waiting to be introduced as the new hospital CEO. It was early in the morning—around 9:15 a.m. or so—and I was the only person sitting in the hospital lobby, besides the receptionist. The Regional Vice President, Larry Ashley, asked me to wait in the lobby while he went into the hospital to get the current—and soon to be ex—CEO out of a department manager's meeting he was conducting. Larry got the CEO out of the meeting, escorted him to his office, had him collect his personal items and place them in a small box, and escorted him out of the hospital through the lobby right past me. I remember looking at the guy when he walked past and seeing a dumbfounded look on his face, as he was still processing what was happening to him at that time. It was an awkward moment.

I had been sitting in the lobby by myself for no more than 10 minutes, when Larry came back in to the hospital and got me, and we walked into the hospital to the department manager's meeting, where he introduced me as the hospital's new CEO. After having made a very short introduction, Larry turned and left the conference room and out the front door of the hospital to his car—his work at Charter Hospital of Denver for the day was done. My work was just getting started. As I looked around the room at all the managers, I noticed they all had a look of shock and be-wilderment on their faces. It was an awkward moment. What do you say in a situation like this? I was excited about my first opportunity to be a hospital CEO, but a bit anxious and uncertain about how the events of the day had unfolded so far. I said a few words—but I can't even tell you what I said as that part was all a blur to me but here is what I can tell you.

The hospital was a for-profit, 60-bed psychiatric and substance abuse hospital owned and operated by Charter Medical Corporation—a for-profit hospital company. The hospital had been opened for just over a year and was averaging a census of eight patients a day. The hospital was way off plan and budget and was losing a lot of money. My marching orders were clear: turn the hospital's financial performance around quickly.

It was a big challenge, but one that I was eager and excited to tackle. I felt I was ready. But I knew I would have to use and apply many different skills and leadership techniques I had learned in school—while earning both my undergraduate degree in business management and marketing and my graduate degree in health administration. I also knew I would have to rely on many skills and leadership techniques I learned in my administrative residency experience at Community Hospital in Indianapolis, as well as what I had learned in over five years of hospital administrative experience at that point in my career. I would even use a few things I learned through playing team sports.

I worked hard and tried a lot of things to turn the hospital around. I was going to make the most of it. If I were to fail, it would not be because of a lack of effort. I made a lot of mistakes, but I also did a number of things well. Let me summarize my initial actions into three categories:

1. Create and communicate an inspiring vision for the future to paint a clear picture of where we were going and how we were going to get there.
2. Put the right people in the right places and coach and support them while maintaining a high level of accountability.
3. Foster an internal belief based on purpose, the capabilities of our employees and physicians, and myself as the leader. It was a confidence thing. The organization had a defeatist attitude, and that had to change quickly. As Sam Walton, founder of Walmart, once said, "It is amazing what people can achieve if they believe in themselves." Of course, the opposite is also true.

In addition to these three things, I also spent a lot of time on marketing and sales.

As I have already mentioned, I made a lot of mistakes. But I wasn't afraid of making mistakes, and I learned from them. By the way, I had two great views out my two office windows: one window overlooked downtown Denver whose elevation was positioned a bit lower than where the hospital sat in the foothills on the west side, and the other window overlooked the foothills of the Rocky Mountains. It was a postcard-type setting.

About a year later, Charter Medical Corporation transferred me to Charter Hospital of Terre Haute in Terre Haute, Indiana. When I left Charter Hospital of Denver, the hospital had an average daily census (ADC) of 38 patients and was finally making money. That experience was really a defining time for me in the development of my leadership philosophy and leadership style, as well as my overall confidence. It also gave me the opportunity to become a hospital CEO, as well as the confidence to handle other challenging and difficult management situations that would come my way. I believe we can grow the most as leaders when the times are the toughest—not when things are running smoothly. Herm Edwards, past NFL Head Coach and football analyst is quoted as saying ***"You don't build character, because you're successful; you build character because of the hardships you face."***

This turnaround opportunity at Charter Hospital of Denver was a fit for me regarding where I was emotionally as a young leader. At that time in my career, I wanted to make a difference, to earn more money, to advance in my career, and to make a name for myself—at least a name for myself in my own mind. Don't you want to make some type of name for yourself as a leader? Don't you want to leave your mark, that things were better because you were part of the team? Another way to say that is, don't you want to create a significant and lasting leadership legacy as a healthcare administrator? I think most people in this field do. I have always been good at assessing talent and potential and putting the right people in the right places. I was also committed to the patients, the hospital, and the community and the mission of trying to make the situation a win-win for all. I have come to believe there is far more to leadership than what a position can do for you. I challenge you to think of another profession where there is any more opportunity to impact so many other lives in a positive way and help other people reach their goals.

THE LEADERSHIP JOURNEY

Developing your leadership skills, style, effectiveness and performance as a leader is a journey. The journey is more like a long, slow boat ride down the Mississippi River than a fast drive down the interstate. Take a moment to reflect on your journey to date as a leader—no matter where you are in your career—and think about how you got started. Think about whether your journey has been smooth or a bit rocky so far. Think about whether your journey has been a straight or circuitous route. Think about the obstacles and setbacks you have encountered and the successes and failures you've experienced. Think about your dreams. Think about the shallow water, bad weather or other peril you may have encountered in your journey down the winding river of becoming a leader. And, think about the contributions, achievements, and successes you've had—whatever they have been.

It stands to reason, as a river boat captain, the more you navigate unchartered or unsafe waters, the more experienced you become, and the better boat captain you are. If you were flying in an airplane through a thunderstorm, do you want your pilot to have flown through hundreds of thunderstorms, maybe made a few mistakes or two, lived to fly another day, and learned from his experience? Experience can be a great teacher if we are willing to learn the lesson and apply it in the future. And, it is the same for your journey in becoming a healthcare leader.

BECOMING A HEALTHCARE LEADER

When asked what's your philosophy or model for leadership, Sam Odle states ***"In my career I've just found that I've just done it. It wasn't like I had a conscious plan. But in retrospect, in thinking back on it, I think as a leader I felt like I was always teaching, negotiating, learning, and becoming. That was sort of the order of the day or how things worked. Once I became more mature, I was no longer a 'command and control' kind of leader. I realized you got things done through other people, you didn't get a lot done by ordering people around because there's no way for you to know everything that needs to be done."***

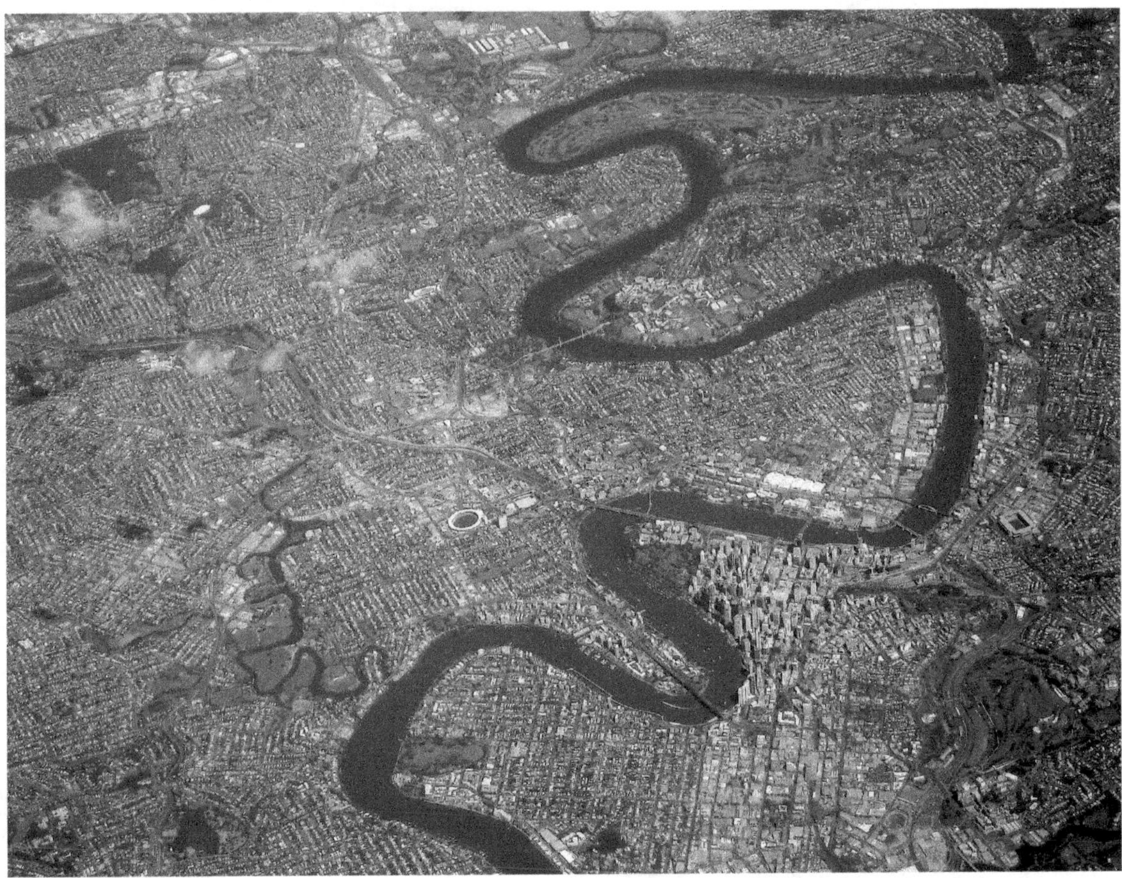

FIGURE 6.1 Brisbane River

Sam's model for leadership can be narrowed down into four things: ***1) "Teaching people what the objectives were, and making sure they understood those 2) Negotiating, because sometimes people may not want to accomplish those objectives, or they may want to go in a different direction 3) And you have to always be learning, because you have to listen to other people and be willing to change your mind and your ideas 4) And by doing those things repetitively, over and over again, then you're becoming the leader that you are"***

Here are three key questions for reflection at any point during your leadership journey:

1. Are you becoming the leader you want to be?
2. What are you doing to become the leader that you want to be?
3. How are you evaluating and assessing yourself as a leader?

Becoming–suitable; appropriate. Any process of change. Any change from a lower level of potentiality to the higher level of actuality. (Dictionary .com) Becoming a leader is about reaching a higher level of your potential. Ideally, becoming a leader is about reaching your highest level of potential, so you can make the greatest contribution possible to the people you serve; to the communities you serve; and to the profession in which you practice as a healthcare leader.

Management–getting work done through others. Leadership is motivating and inspiring others to work hard and achieve individual, team, department, and organizational goals. Leadership is one of the four basic functions of management, along with planning, organizing, and controlling.

Becoming a healthcare leader is about reaching a higher level of your potential.

Healthcare leaders who are effective:

- Lead by example
- Hold themselves and others accountable
- Lead using intangible skills of leadership
- Create a working environment of learning and discovery
- Facilitate the creation of the organizational culture
- Support, coach, and develop others
- Create the vision and the game plan for achieving it
- Motivate and inspire others
- Listen, interpret, understand, and communicate effectively
- Positively impact the lives around them

Why become a healthcare leader? Typically, there is no fame or glory. You probably won't get rich. There is a lot of hard work and long hours. You are responsible for the acts and omissions of others. There are a lot of "politics" to deal with. And, a healthcare leadership position usually comes with a high amount of stress and pressure to perform. The short answer to why anyone should become a healthcare leader–is because a career as a healthcare leader can be worth it.

Take a moment to reflect on your own career choices.

What are you telling others about a career in leadership? Think about it for a moment. The answer to this question may reveal a lot about who you are, how you see yourself as a healthcare leader, and the distinctions you make about your work, about leadership, and its impact on those around you.

I chose/am choosing a career in healthcare leadership because ...
The person most influential in my decision was ...
I believed this career would provide ...
How I feel about my decision now ...
If I could start all over again, I would ...
What I am telling others about a career in healthcare leadership is ...

Healthcare leadership is a possibility. In other words, healthcare leadership can provide the leader with the opportunity to self-actualize by reaching his highest level of potential, in addition to helping others do the same. Maslow's Hierarchy of Needs is a famous need theory found in many writings on management. This theory states that people seek to fulfill lower-order needs before higher-order needs. Once lower-order needs have been satisfied, the person then may seek to fulfill one or more higher order needs. Maslow maintained the highest-order need a person may have is to achieve self-actualization, reaching your own potential at the very highest level. Healthcare leadership provides leaders with the opportunity to self-actualize. Healthcare leadership also provides leaders with the opportunity to support others in their quest for self-actualization, as well.

Leadership is a journey of learning and discovery. It is a process that sometimes boils down to using the Scientific Method—trying a different approach to see if it works.

Leaders who are not reaching out to constantly learn, grow, and develop, tend to stay static in their leadership effectiveness and performance. A leader has to be willing step out of his comfort zone sometimes in order to experience growth and development as a healthcare leader.

What can your healthcare leadership make possible? Take a moment and write down two or three things you believe that your leadership in healthcare can make possible. Don't think about the challenges and obstacles; think about the opportunities and possibilities.

CONNECTING WITH FOLLOWERS

A healthcare leader must first connect with others in the organization before he can expect others to follow him. It has been said that people don't care about what the leader knows until they first know the leader cares about them. Leadership is about influencing others. A leader's followers first must have an emotional bond, connection, or relationship with the healthcare leader before the leader can expect them to be open and receptive to the leader's philosophy and ideas, to be willing to identify with and support a leader's vision for change, or to work hard (individually and collectively as a team) to achieve new goals and objectives identified by the leader.

John Maxwell calls this the "law of connection." Maxwell says a leader must first touch the hearts of others before he can ask for their hands. A leader can't move people to action until he first connects with their hearts. Followers won't buy in to a leader's vision until they first buy in to the leader. A good leader works hard all the time to connect with the hearts of followers and to show them he genuinely cares. This involves communication that is open, transparent, and sincere. Being authentic and knowing the people in the organization is essential for this emotional connection between leader and follower to occur. It is about credibility and practicing what the leader preaches. It is also about going to where the employees are—at the worksite level. Maxwell says, "To lead yourself, use your head: to lead others, use your heart."

An important point to note here: followers are always watching leaders. Does the leader's action match his words? Also, employees will gravitate toward emulating what they see the leader do. If the leader is always punctual, on time, and working extra hours, then employees will be much more apt to do the same. Maxwell says there is nothing more compelling or convincing than when a leader teaches what is right and then models that action and behavior. This is leadership by example—a very powerful form of leadership.

HIRING A MANAGER

What do companies look for in managers? According to Chuck Williams in the book *Effective Management*, companies look for four basic skills or traits in a leader. Technical skills are those skills that involve the specialized knowledge needed to get the work done, or the ability to apply the specialized procedures, techniques, and knowledge required to get the job done. Human skills are also referred to as interpersonal skills or those skills related to a manager's ability to work with people, which include skills such as listening, communicating, and providing feedback that enables people to have effective working relationships with others. Conceptual skills are the ability to see the organization as a whole, understand how the different parts affect each other, and comprehend how the overall organization fits within and is affected by the larger environment. Motivation to manage is the interest, desire, and psychological readiness for a manager to want to lead and manage.

Technical Skills	Human Skills
Conceptual Skills	Motivation to Manage

Healthcare leaders require the use of different leadership skills at different levels of responsibility in a health service organization: the higher in the chain of command, the greater the importance on human skills, conceptual skills, and motivational skills. The chain of command is the vertical line of authority that clarifies who reports to whom through the organization. These are major categories of skills that can also be referred to as critical intangibles of leadership. We'll discuss more on this topic in a later chapter.

Becoming a new healthcare leader is exciting, challenging, and even nerve-racking at times. Common mistakes that early career leaders make include trying to exert authority and be the "boss." Moreover, it is certainly an adjustment for most first-time healthcare leaders to make with respect to the workload, problems and challenges that must be dealt with, and everything involving the management, supervision, and leadership of people. But, experience can teach the new leader about his role and what is important. Most leaders typically go through a learning period or transition where they realize that being a leader isn't about telling others what to do, but rather creating an environment where people want to work hard to achieve organizational goals. Below is a table from *Effective Management* that summarizes some of the changes in beliefs managers will go through in their own perception about their job as a leader or manager.

Manager's Initial Expectations	After Six Months as a Manager	After a Year as a Manager
• Be the boss • Formal authority • Manage tasks • Job is not managing people	• Initial expectations were wrong • Fast pace • Heavy workload • Job is problem-solving and troubleshooting	• No longer "doer" • Communication, listening, positive reinforcement • Learning to adapt and control stress • Job is people development

Below is a list of the common mistakes that many healthcare managers—particularly early on in their leadership careers—make. Some of these mistakes are driven by the leader's feeling he needs—or at least be perceived as knowing everything.

1. Insensitive to others
2. Cold, aloof, and arrogant
3. Betrayal of trust
4. Overly ambitious
5. Specific performance problems with business
6. Over-manages: unable to delegate or build a team
7. Unable to staff effectively
8. Unable to think strategically
9. Unable to adapt to boss with different style
10. Over-dependent on advocate or mentor

Becoming a healthcare leader is challenging enough, but consider some the challenges in healthcare that leaders must confront.

- A sluggish economy
- Skilled healthcare workforce shortages
- Increasing operating expenses
- Increasing laws and regulations
- Increasing global competition
- Increasing consumerism
- Declining reimbursement on a per-unit basis
- Rapidly evolving medical technology
- Distracted employees
- Mounting pressures and profitability
- Growing public scrutiny of health service organization business practices

As a healthcare leader, how can you deal with so many different problems and the knowledge and expertise that it takes to do so?

Sam Odle says as a healthcare leader ***"You don't have to know everything. You can't know everything. The leader can't somehow be insecure about not knowing everything. They should be willing to ask questions, and create an environment that encourages questions to be asked—even by the people around them. I've seen a lot of times when you have your team together, and if one person is really enthusiastic about something, then everybody feels like 'Well, I don't want to question that idea because then when my idea comes up and maybe that person will support my idea.' But you don't want that because you don't necessarily get the best decision-making out of that."*** The leader wants ***"to create an environment where people do question each other, and the person being questioned doesn't see it as a threat to them personally. Rather, they see it as helping them to refine their idea and get the best execution of it. The leader has to demonstrate that by asking questions, and encouraging others to ask questions as well."***

MOVING UP

It's easy sometimes for a younger healthcare leader to become anxious to move up into higher levels of leadership responsibility: sometimes too anxious. Clearly, it is important for any healthcare leader to be ready and prepared to succeed before taking a step up in the ranks of leadership. Like the old adage, "*The top will be waiting when you get there.*" Vince Caponi's advice to aspiring healthcare leaders is to "***Love where you're at. The first job I had in healthcare was the Director of Medical Records. I had no clue what I was doing. It was the training ground for me (to become a healthcare leader). The hospital CEO said 'you're gonna get in there and you're gonna run a department and you're gonna find out about it.' Now I have a college degree at this time, and I'm working on a graduate degree. I signed up for a correspondence course*** *to become an accredited record technician. And the thought was how can you lead anybody if you don't understand their job? I had a lot of great people making great suggestions to me on how you learn. So I got out of my office and set up an office in the medical records department: which is kind of a bullpen thing and you have people all around. When times got really tight I would file charts; I helped set up the files for dictation for the physicians; I taught a medical terminology course. Thank God I had Latin in high school and in college. What this demonstrates is there is no job beneath you. A young graduate from a master in health administration program (typically) has great training but not much experience."*

> What this demonstrates is there is no job beneath you. Love where you're at.

Vince goes on to talk about volunteering for projects or tasks that can give you—as a young healthcare administrator—the opportunity to learn and gain experience. He says when you have the opportunity "*Take the deeper dive. The other thing is people in healthcare love to teach. If you have a young man or woman who wants to learn, they will teach. And they love talking about what they do. Now I did go into pathology one time to see an autopsy and once was enough. What I am saying is wherever you are at, there is opportunity to learn but only if you have your eyes open to learn.* [Sometimes] *we have preconceived notions and we don't take the time to learn. But it is also an opportunity to meet some great people. And when you start talking about medical records and Joint Commission (because you've been there, done that) you get some great credence from employees who say he knows what he is talking about. And I speak of it with great joy.*"

> Wherever you are at, there is an opportunity to learn but only if you have your eyes open to learn.

CREATING AN INQUISITIVE ENVIRONMENT

Mr. Odle goes on to talk about a healthcare leader creating an inquisitive environment, and says that ***"When people's questions are answered, and they have a better understanding of what is being suggested, or recommended, or the direction you are trying to go in, they become bought into it, and they are going to be more effective and helpful in the execution of it. However, if it is sort of the 'silent' by-in where everybody says 'Oh yeah. Go ahead. OK. Do it.' What they're really saying is 'Yeah, if you can get it done go ahead—but I'm not helping.' For example, you start the project and it flounders, it doesn't***

get done on time, and it doesn't get done to the level of effectiveness that you think it should be because only that one person was 'rolling that rock up the hill'. The other people react by saying 'I said okay, but I didn't say I was going to do it!' You see that a lot, especially with management teams."

SEEKING OUT ACCEPTANCE

As a young leader or new leader in a health service organization, it is important to seek out acceptance within the organization—to fit into the culture and environment that exists and has existed: long before you as a new leader showed up on the scene. Ken Stella says it this way. ***"I think it is important when you're young and first starting that you are seeking out acceptance."*** A new leader, who is perceived as not fitting in, will also quickly be perceived as not having what it takes to be effective and get the job done.

CREATING CHANGE WITH A SHARED VISION

Sam Odle talks about the importance of vision as it relates to leadership being able to create positive change in a hospital or health service organization. Mr. Odle states that "***You have to be able to define a future state that is better than where you currently are. The status quo is very powerful: this is the way we do things around here, so people are very comfortable [with the status quo]. So if you want them to move to another level of performance, you [(the leader)] have to define a vision—a future state—that is compelling and better than what they [(employees)] have today. Then people will start to move forward with that. But if you have a vision, and no one else shares it, then it might as well be a nightmare because you [(the leader)] are going to try and get there but these other people [(employees)] don't share your vision and they're not marching or following you. So you have to have vision, and to define it, and you have to be able to build shared vision. That's where you [(the leader)] explain the 'why' and allow people to ask questions and help to improve upon that vision if they have suggestions. [It's about] creating vision, and then building shared vision."***

DEVELOPING YOUR LEADERSHIP STYLE

Developing your leadership style is inherently part of the journey to becoming a healthcare leader. Healthcare organizations are people serving people. Leadership style is how the leader generally behaves toward followers. Healthcare is the ultimate people business. As a healthcare leader, your interpersonal skills are paramount. Getting work done through other people, in a way that motivates and inspires them to work hard and perform at a high level, takes an effective leadership style. But what constitutes an effective leadership style?

This section explores the following six components to developing your style as a healthcare leader:

- Authenticity builds credibility
- Learning through experience
- Outside insight
- Failure versus success
- Communication
- Critical leadership intangibles

AUTHENTICITY BUILDS CREDIBILITY

One thing I never imagined would be tested of me so much by others in the organization where I was working was my authenticity, honesty, and credibility. The actions and words of a leader are tested every day: not from time to time, but all the time. Employees can spot a leader being inauthentic or phony from a mile away. Leaders have to consistently be authentic to establish and maintain the credibility they need with staff in order to be trusted and to lead them. It has been said many times, but it is true in healthcare leadership: you have to always be true to yourself, and let this authenticity touch those around you.

> **The actions and words of a leader are tested every day: not from time to time, but all the time.**

Being the authentic "you" doesn't just mean when in the physical presence of others, but in the different environments in which you work. These environments include telephone conversations; email messages; text messages; team functions and activities; meetings; interactions directly with employees, physicians, trustees, patients or family members, and guests; interactions directly with members of the community; social settings; and even family settings.

LEARNING THROUGH EXPERIENCE

Experience can be a wonderful teacher. Unfortunately, the lesson isn't learned until after you've had the experience. Learning through your own experiences is neither a given nor automatic: it takes thoughtful reflection, analysis, and a willingness to look at the experience through your own eyes, as well as those of others. All of us as human beings have "blind spots"—those characteristics, mannerisms, idiosyncrasies, or quirks that we don't even realize we have. Being self-aware and using the technique of self-reflection is critical to developing your leadership style and skills. In other words, we have our own 'already always way' of thinking, perceiving, acting, and doing. Self-reflection, unfortunately, goes against the grain of our current culture. Our culture says that if you aren't multitasking, then you aren't being productive.

My advice is to find a quiet space in your world where you can think and reflect about experiences you've had; who you are; who you want to become as a leader; what you are learning; what changes you can make in your leadership style to be more effective; and how others may be perceiving you; things you can try and do differently to improve. What's working well for you? What hasn't worked as well for you? One method I've used in my career is to make three lists: 1) what things do I need to stop doing? 2) what things do I need to start doing? 3) what things should I continue doing? You can use this method to seek feedback from others and gain their perspective on areas you might improve in. Using this technique by seeking input from others is one way to solicit what I call outside insight.

OUTSIDE INSIGHT

Outside insight is a phrase I first heard from my friend Stefan Speligene, an advertising executive who recently formed his own agency in Nashville, Tennessee, called Roux. Stefan used the phrase to characterize how many clients would come to him—an outsider to their company—to gain the insight they needed about their company in order to create a more effective marketing function or advertising campaign for them. It can be true about healthcare leaders, as well; many times it is the insight they gain through outside people or experiences outside them that can provide the most meaningful and insightful knowledge. In this context, outside insight is the valuable information we must seek to help us see and understand what we don't know or don't see about ourselves. In a larger context, outside insight is valuable information that someone gives us that helps us discover and learn something we previously didn't know that we didn't know. Here's an example:

One day while working as the chief operating officer at Union Hospital in Terre Haute, Indiana, I was facilitating one of the weekly Hospital Council meetings of the senior management team. I had placed an agenda item first at that morning's meeting that I thought would be a slam- dunk. It was anything but that. I had come to the meeting having done my homework and worked with every person on the senior management team to develop a simple action plan to change the annual employee recognition dinner that had survived for over 15 years. Although the annual recognition dinner was good, it was also boring, and I was hearing the complaints loud and clear about the desire to change it. So I set out to do just that. The Vice President of Human Resources, Mike, who reported directly to me, had created the current employee recognition program format, so I knew I would first need his cooperation and support if we were to make a change. After several meetings with Mike, we had an action plan developed. From there, I discussed ideas and suggestions for changing the annual employee recognition dinner with each member of the senior management team. The new plan had the full support of everyone, or at least I thought so.

So, the proposed new employee recognition dinner was on the agenda first thing at the weekly Hospital Council meeting. I distributed a one-page action plan with various steps outlined for the new proposed employee recognition dinner. I had just started making my informal presentation, when the objections came

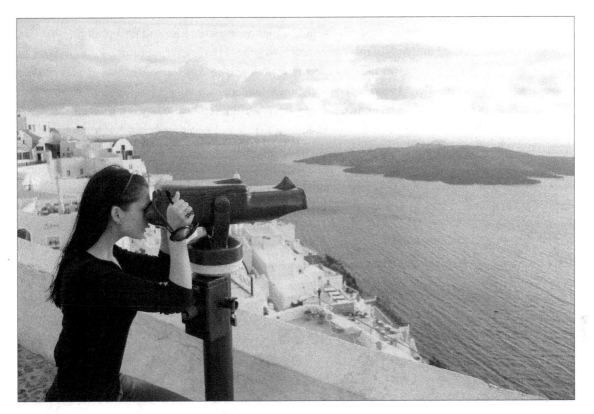

FIGURE 6.2 Girl Looking Through Binoculars

forward, principally from Mike, but also from the hospital CFO. The conversation escalated, and before you knew it, things were a bit heated. As I looked around the room, I realized it was two against one (me being the one) and no one else other than my two opponents were saying anything. Ever had the feeling like you were standing on an island all by yourself? Now, I always prided myself in keeping my cool under the most stressful of circumstances; however, that morning I didn't. I lost my cool, ripped the one page action plan into two pieces allowing the shredded document to fall to the table, and said "***OK then, we aren't changing anything. We'll continue to have the same employee recognition dinner that we've always had. Next topic. What else do you want to talk about***?" You could have heard a pin drop at that moment, and there were several chins that had dropped and almost hit the table. We moved on to several other topics, and then ended the meeting.

Not only had I realized what I had done, but I was embarrassed. I had lost my cool, acted rather childish in ripping the paper, and was less than professional in my behavior. Sure, I felt like I might have been set up; however, there were no excuses for my behavior. I immediately went around and met individually with each senior management person who was in that meeting and apologized for my behavior. Moreover, I promised they would not see that type of behavior again for me. Each of them told me the same thing: they should have said something during the meeting in support of the proposal we had discussed previously, in addition to not worrying about my behavior, as they didn't find it offensive. Then, I met with Bob Meissel,

MD, hospital Medical Director. Bob was my mentor. I highly respected him and his opinions. That day, Bob gave me some outside insight—in this case tough love—that I have never forgotten. He looked me in the eyes and said, "***Steve, if you want to be an effective leader, you need to learn how to deal with conflict in group settings.***" My reaction? I was shocked and dumbfounded. I couldn't believe it, but Bob was right. I did need to learn how to deal with conflict in group settings if I was going to be as effective of a leader as I could be! And, this was the first time I had ever known that fact; I never really saw it until Bob told me in no uncertain terms. Bob gave me the outside insight I needed.

Well, I took Bob's advice to heart. I made a commitment to myself and over the next 12 months worked to develop my skills in being able to manage conflict in group settings. I learned that sometimes allowing conflict to occur is necessary in order to foster constructive dialogue that brings about a sense of engagement, ownership, and consensus—not out-of-control conflict, but constructive conflict. But here's the real point of this story. Bob gave me the needed outside insight, about something that I didn't know and never saw in myself. He made me aware of a leadership "blind spot" that was holding me back from being a more effective leader.

FAILURE VERSUS SUCCESS

In his book *Failing Forward*, John C. Maxwell talks about the important role failure plays in a person's learning, growth, and development—and ultimately in their success. Maxwell emphasizes five key points in his book, highlighted below:

- Failure is not an event
- Failure is not objective
- Failure is usually not fatal
- Failure is not final
- Failure is part of success

Albert Einstein is quoted as saying "***If you haven't made any mistakes, you probably haven't done much.***" Sam Odle talks about being afraid of failure and how that fear can prevent you from being successful. Mr. Odle states "***I think I made mistakes along the way. Fortunately, I was given the opportunity to recover from those [mistakes]. Not all of my negotiations went well: some of them went off track and had to be re-established or fixed along the way. One thing you try to do is to forget your failures: you learn whatever the lesson is, but you forget the real act. If you are afraid of failure, then you won't succeed because it will make you timid; it will make you less likely to take risks; less likely to expand your scope of responsibility. You won't take on new challenges because [you will say to yourself] I've never done that before so I might fail. You freeze yourself out of success. I think you have to look at it as not that you don't have fear, but you have to overcome that [fear]. Again, [you have to] look at the importance of the work you are doing and what result you hope to achieve along the way.***"

In some ways, success and failure are inextricably linked. In becoming a healthcare leader, we typically must first experience some type of failure before we will experience success. We must be willing to try—even if that means risk failure. When we fail, no-matter how we define a situation, experience, or event as a failure, we must learn the lesson and apply that learning into our leadership philosophy and style so that we do it differently—and with success—the next time.

Many times it can boil down to how we actually define success and failure. What we perceive as a failure may be perceived by others as just something we haven't succeeded at—yet.

When we fail, no matter how we define a situation, experience or event as a failure, we must learn the lesson and apply that learning into our leadership philosophy and style so that we do it differently and with success the next time.

COMMUNICATION

Learning to communicate effectively with people at all levels of the healthcare organization is vital to becoming an effective leader. Communication is the process of transmitting information from one person or place to another. An important point about leadership communication is the impact it has on two critical elements: the organizational culture and the emotional feelings of followers. With respect to the organizational culture, what leaders say and how they say it can have a tremendous impact on the organizational culture—the values, beliefs, and attitudes of the employees and other internal stakeholders.

Organizational culture is the unwritten shared understanding about what is important, what is expected, how things are to be done, what is permitted or tolerated, and what gets recognized and rewarded. The organizational culture is the invisible hand that is always at work, shaping and molding the actions and behaviors of employees. Leadership communication has a significant impact on the organization's culture, and should be carefully crafted by the sender. However, leadership communication should always be made clear; crafted in terms that receivers will understand; honest, forthright, and authentic; and consistent. Given the bombardment of information that employees typically receive through various means, including social media on a daily basis, important messages from leadership will need to be repeated multiple times through different mediums in order for it to be effectively received and understood. A mistake commonly made by healthcare leaders is to communicate an important message to employees once or twice and assume the message was effectively received and understood by employees. It is important for healthcare leaders to follow-up on communication they sent to be sure it was effectively received and understood by the receiver.

The organizational culture is the invisible hand that is always at work.

With respect to the emotions of followers, leadership communication can have a tremendous impact—both of a positive or negative nature—on employees. Employees can react emotionally and be inspired, motivated, engaged, or even intrinsically more connected to the organization from leadership communication they interpret and perceive as positive. Employees can react emotionally and be uninspired, demotivated, disengaged, or even intrinsically less connected to the organization from leadership communication they interpret and perceive as negative. Therefore, the emotional connection that employees have with an organization can be enhanced by leadership communication that is inspiring, motivating, authentic, sincere, realistically optimistic, and engaging. For a leader to be as effective as possible, he must have a high level of emotional intelligence and use it effectively when communicating with employees individually and collectively in teams or groups.

Survival-Oriented	Possibility-Oriented
• Complaints	Commitments
• Blaming	Responsibility
• Criticism	Appreciation
• Unsolved Problems	Intentions
• Trivial	Crucial
• Annoyed	Enthusiastic
• Dejected	Gladness
• Confused	Hopeful
• Disgusted	Joyful
• Frustrated	Relieved
• Ignored	Compassion
• Tired	Delighted
• Anxious	Excited
• Contempt	Humorous
• Fear	Prideful
• Anger	Satisfied
• Doubt	Courageous
• Depressed	Inspired
• Guilty	Optimism
• Indifferent	Grateful
• Manipulated	Fascinated
• Concerned	Creative
• Sad	

What's your contribution to the organization's culture?

CRITICAL INTANGIBLES OF LEADERSHIP

Healthcare leadership is complex, multi-faceted, Healthcare leadership and involves both tangible or content skills, and intangible skills, qualities, and characteristics. The tangible/content skills include areas such as management science, economics, finance, accounting, personnel management, health law, information technology, and the like. The intangible skills, qualities, and characteristics (the intangibles)—which, by definition, are hard to define or quantify—involve areas such as the following;

Promise-keeping	Caring	Encouraging
Honesty	Charisma	Principled
Trustworthy	Understanding	Accountable
Consistency	Emotional intelligence	Moral
Personable	Hard-working	Inspiring

According to the Encarta World Dictionary, the word *critical* means crucial, extremely important, or essential. The word *intangible* means hard to describe of define, unquantifiable quality, or asset. Many of the leadership intangibles are critical to leadership effectiveness as they help to motivate and inspire others to work hard to achieve organizational goals. By definition, the critical intangibles of leadership are unquantifiable qualities or characteristics of a leader that are crucial to motivating and inspiring others in a workplace setting. Moreover, the critical intangibles determine a leader's effectiveness in tapping into the discretionary effort that employees have to give and engendering them to provide their maximum effort and performance. The critical intangibles of leadership create the working environment, which in turn, impacts the level of employee satisfaction and emotional connection to their work, their colleagues, the organization, and of course, leadership. The critical intangibles of leadership also impact the level of motivation and engagement for employees to give their best. Lieutenant General Omar Nelson Bradley, Commander in Chief of the U.S. Army forces at D-Day on the beaches of France in 1944 is quoted as saying "*Leadership is intangible, and therefore, no weapon ever designed can replace it.*"

According to Tom Atchison, the intangibles of leadership can contribute up to 65 percent of organizational performance.

QUESTIONS THAT ASSESS FOR THE CRITICAL INTANGIBLES OF LEADERSHIP

As a leader ...

- Are you believable?
- Are you trustworthy? Do followers trust what you say as the truth?

- Will you admit when you make a mistake or blame others?
- Do you treat others as highly respected and valuable or as people who can just be replaced?
- Are you fair, consistent, and predictable in your actions and behaviors?
- Do you model the type of actions and behaviors that set the pace for others to follow?
- Are you interested in the learning, growth, and development of others?
- Do you help support, coach, teach, and mentor others?
- Do you provide opportunities for other to contribute and succeed?
- Do you use your power and authority for the good of others and the organization or yourself?
- Are you willing to do what you ask of others?
- Do you help others identify, interpret, and understand internal and external factors, forces, and trends that are impacting the organization and its future?
- Are you transparent in all your dealings with people?
- Do you encourage others and recognized their efforts and performance?

Below are a few questions for a healthcare organization and its leadership to consider as it relates to critical intangibles.

As an organization, how do leaders responsible for hiring, evaluating, leading, and promoting other leaders ...

- Identify critical intangibles of leadership?
- Recruit for critical intangibles of leadership?
- Evaluate for critical intangibles of leadership?
- Recognize and reward for critical intangibles of leadership?
- Cultivate the critical intangibles of leadership in themselves and other leaders?
- Promote by including the critical intangibles of leadership?

QUESTIONS EMPLOYEES ALWAYS HAVE

This section will discuss the concept of questions that employees always ask—or at least have—about the organization; about their position and the work they do; how they are treated; their direct supervisor; and leadership of the organization overall.

Every employee comes to work every day with questions, and many of those questions get answered throughout the course of their shift. Most of the time, these are questions that employees don't verbalize; however, sometimes they will verbalize these questions—and the employee's answer to these questions—to coworkers.

Regardless of whether questions are verbalized or not, these are questions that employees answer for themselves—sometimes on a conscious level and, other times, sub-consciously. Below, find a sample of the types of questions referred to in this context.

- Do I like my job and the work I do?
- Does my direct supervisor, and the management team as a whole, care about me as a person?
- Does my direct supervisor, and the management team as a whole, care about my growth and development?
- Does my direct supervisor, and the management team as a whole, really want my ideas and suggestions?
- Are my efforts and performance recognized, appreciated, and appropriately rewarded?
- Are my efforts and performance recognized, appreciated, and appropriately rewarded in a way that is fair and equitable with other employees?
- Does the work I do make a difference?
- Does my work contribute to the organization's mission?
- Does this organization have a promising future, and will I be part of it?

It is the leadership of a healthcare organization that helps answers these, as well as other similar questions, that all employees have. The organizational culture, which is largely established by leadership, along with a healthcare leader's management style, directly impact how employees will answer these and other important questions that impact everything. Becoming an effective healthcare leader means being able to see and understand the perspectives and viewpoints of other people in the organization, including directly supervised employees. Developing a management style that will foster a positive response to these and other important questions that employees have about their job, about the work they do, about you as a leader, and about the health service organization, is part of becoming an effective healthcare leader. It starts with being cognizant of the fact that your words, actions, and behaviors have a strong influence on how employees feel they are being treated, feel the organization is operated, and feel about whether they are a good fit or not in the culture and working environment. In large part, we're talking about a direct and significant impact on employee morale, engagement, and retention.

As promulgated in the book The 7 Habits of Highly Effective People written by Stephen R. Covey, ***"You can buy a person's hand, but you can't buy his heart. His heart is where his enthusiasm, his loyalty is. You can buy his back, but you can't buy his brain. That's where his creativity is, his ingenuity, and his resourcefulness. Treat employees like volunteers. They volunteer their best parts—their hearts and their minds."***

REFLECTION ON YOUR LEADERSHIP STYLE

As mentioned previously, becoming an effective healthcare leader includes taking time to reflect on your leadership style, experiences, and lessons you are learning. Below is a sample of questions a leader can use to help reflect upon lessons learned and areas for improvement.

- How am I tapping into the discretionary effort of each employee?
- How am I deciding on what to delegate to whom?

- How do I assess talent and potential in others?
- What am I doing to get top effort and performance from my staff?
- What am I doing to recognize and reward effort, initiative, and performance?
- What am I doing to help my staff reach their potential?
- What makes me motivating and inspiring, so other people want to follow me?
- Who do I look to for guidance, support, and mentorship?
- Who am I modeling my leadership style after?
- Am I becoming the healthcare leader that I want to be?

DISCUSSION QUESTIONS

1. What makes a leader motivating and inspiring to others?
2. Compare and contrast the tangible/content skills with the critical intangibles of leadership.
3. How do the critical intangibles of leadership impact the working environment and employee's level of satisfaction, motivation, and engagement?
4. How can the fear of failure prevent a leader from being successful?
5. What were the four things that, in retrospect, Sam Odle says he was doing as a leader?
6. What is outside insight, and describe one way in which a healthcare leader can access outside insight.
7. Describe what is meant by leadership creating an inquisitive environment, and why this is so important in creating a positive working culture.
8. As a leader, learning through your experience is not a given. Describe how a leader can effectively learn from his/her experiences.
9. Describe outside insight and the ways a healthcare leader can tap into outside insight.
10. Describe how leadership communication can have an emotional impact on followers.

FIGURE CREDITS

7

Scientific Management and Theory

Scientific management is the study of management activities based on theory and research. The Scientific Method of inquiry is a formal five-step process of research that includes: 1) observation and description, 2) hypothesis formulation, 3) data gathering, 4) data analysis, 5) findings and conclusions. Below is a brief summary of several researchers and various management theories that have had significant implications for healthcare leadership.

Abraham Maslow (1908–1970)—Created Maslow's Hierarchy of Needs, a theory of psychological health predicated on fulfilling innate human needs in priority, culminating in self-actualization. Human beings must first satisfy lower-order needs before higher order needs come into play.

Physiological (food and water)
↓
Safety (physical and economic)
↓
Belongingness (friendship, love, social interaction)
↓
Esteem (achievement and recognition)
↓
Self-actualization (realizing your full potential)

Chester Barnard (1886–1961)—Focused on the role of the person in the organization. He proposed that the manager's role was to communicate with workers and encourage them to recognize the common goals of the organization and their performance.

David McClelland (1917–1998)—His need theory contended that three dominant needs—the need for achievement, power, and affiliation—underpin human motivation. McClelland believed that the relative importance of each need varies among individuals and cultures.

Douglas McGregor (1906–1964)—Formulated two assumptions about workers, Theory X (employees naturally dislike work and responsibility and must be controlled) and Theory Y (employees seek responsibility and will be self-directed and committed if the job is satisfying).

Frank Gilbreth (1868–1924) and Lillian Gilbreth (1878–1972)—They believed that cooperation from workers was key to realizing efficiencies in the workplace. They filmed workers and work to identify strategies for reducing time, effort, and worker fatigue.

Frederick Herzberg (1923–2000)—Established a management theory known by two names: the motivation-hygiene theory and the two-factor theory. This theory states there are certain factors in the workplace that cause job satisfaction (motivators), while a separate set of factors cause dissatisfaction (hygiene factors). Herzberg theorized that job satisfaction and job dissatisfaction act independently of each other.

Frederick W. Taylor (1856–1915)—Introduced time and management studies to design the work to promote production efficiency. Taylor's four principles were:

1. Develop a science (process) for each element of an individual's work.
2. Scientifically (systematically) select and train, teach, and develop workers.
3. Cooperate with workers to make sure work guidelines are followed.
4. Divide work and responsibilities between management and workers.

Hawthorne Effect—Summary description given to a variety of management research studies conducted at the Bell Telephone Plant in Hawthorne, Illinois. The crux of this theory states that worker productivity and performance is elevated when management pays more attention to the workers.

Henri Fayol (1841–1925)—Fayol proposed workers should be supervised by a single person and managers had five functions: plan, organize, command, coordinate activities, and control performance (which has evolved to plan, organize, lead, and control).

Henry Gantt (1861–1919)—Created the Gantt chart, a tool that aids the planning and controlling of specific work projects.

Mary Parker Follett (1868–1933)—Addressed the issue of management and worker relations, and its importance with regard to organizational performance.

Max Weber (1864–1920)—Believed that rational principles guide the organization of bureaucracies. Weber believed activity is based on authority relations, which are characterized by a division of labor, a defined hierarchy, and rules and regulations. Jobs consist of well-defined tasks, and authority is based on workers' position in the organization.

Peter Drucker (1909–2005)—Authored 39 books, including *The Practice of Management*. Drucker is commonly referred to as the man who invented management. Three famous quotes from Drucker include: 1) ***"The most important thing in communication is to hear what isn't being said;"*** 2) ***"We now accept the fact that learning is a lifelong process of keeping abreast of change. And the most pressing task is to teach people how to learn;" and*** 3) ***"Long-range planning does not deal with future decisions, but with the future of present decisions."***

Robert Rosenthal, PhD (1964)—Empirical research in 1964 set the stage for the identification of a motivational concept called the "Pygmalion Effect"—that expectations bring self-fulfilling prophecies.

Victor Vroom (1932)—Vroom's expectancy theory states that employee's motivation is an outcome of how much an individual wants a reward (valence), the assessment that the likelihood that the effort will lead to expected performance (expectancy) and the belief that the performance will lead to reward (instrumentality).

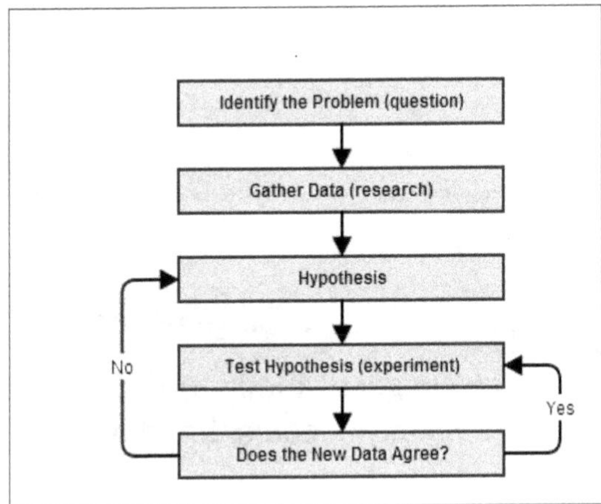

FIGURE 7.1 The Scientific Method

*The above information was summarized from Essential Techniques For Healthcare Managers by Leigh W. Cellucci and Carla Wiggins except for Hawthorne Effect, Peter Drucker and Robert Rosenthal.

SCIENTIFIC MANAGEMENT AND THEORY

There is an old saying: "The difference between theory and practice is in theory it works in practice; but in practice it doesn't." So why study theory at all if doesn't work in practice? The truth is most theories have some relevance in practice. Some theories have a fundamental application that is universal, while others don't. What is important for a healthcare leader is to distinguish the environment, circumstances, and situations in which certain theories have relevance and should be applied.

Moreover, for a healthcare leader, it is not just knowing what theory should be applied (given the environment, circumstances, and situation) but *how* it should be applied. Management science and related theories are predicated on research involving both quantitative and qualitative analysis (determining what works), while the application in practice is about how the science or theory is implemented. Herein lies the differentiation: knowing what to do (knowledge) versus knowing how to do it (application). A healthcare leader needs both skills sets: quantitative and qualitative. The qualitative skills, which cannot be underestimated, can also be referred to as the critical intangibles.

DISCUSSION QUESTIONS

1. How can the Hawthorne Effect be applied through management by walking around (MBWA)?
2. Which of Douglas McGregor's theories would be espoused by a leader whose leadership style could be described as a controlling, micromanager?
3. Use Herzberg's Two-Factor Theory to describe the role money plays in employee motivation.
4. What is the underlying premise of the Pygmalion Effect?
5. Use Herzberg's Two-Factor Theory to explain the role the work itself has in employee motivation.
6. What did Abraham Maslow call a person's highest level of potential?
7. The man considered the inventor of management, Peter Drucker, said "The most important thing in communication is to hear ___________________". Complete this sentence.
8. What did Victor Vroom's Expectancy Theory say?
9. What did Peter Drucker say about teaching and learning?
10. What did Frederick Herzberg say about the connection between job satisfaction and job dissatisfaction?

FIGURE CREDIT

Figure 7.1: Copyright © Michael Fullerton (CC BY-SA 4.0) at http://commons.wikimedia.org/wiki/File:The_Scientific_Method_Blue.png?uselang=csb.

8

Healthcare Leadership: Breaking it Down

Leadership is a fairly complex and complicated discipline. Leadership in the healthcare industry takes on even more complexity and complication that involve the highly-technical and specialty nature of health services, along with regulation, financing, payment, and the growing expectations of stakeholders. What do healthcare leaders do on a daily basis? What does it mean to be an effective healthcare leader in this complex and complicated environment? Healthcare leadership effectiveness can be viewed from both a theoretical and practical framework, as well as from tangible and intangible applications. There are countless aspects that are involved in leadership and most aspects of leadership have some degree of importance for overall leadership effectiveness.

OBJECTIVES

1. Recognize and appreciate the critical role played by the intangibles of leadership.
2. Learn about a framework for viewing the employment relationship through the questions that all employees ask (and answer).
3. Understand the important role played by the department head in a health service organization.

WHAT IS GOOD LEADERSHIP?

What is good leadership? What does a hospital or healthcare leader try to do on a daily or ongoing basis? Good leadership requires so many different things. However, it starts with defining the real purpose or mission of the organization—why it exists and what we want to accomplish—and excellent communication about that mission and goals. The mission and goals must be made very clear, and again, well-communicated and understood

Mr. Allen Hicks was a great mentor to me and so many other hospital and health service administrators during his career. "Mr. Hicks" as everyone called him really led by example. He modeled the way for everyone to follow. He was very smart, and understood people and could relate to them so well. He could anticipate and accurately predict how his board, the medical staff, employees, and even patients would react to something in advance. Mr. Hicks was a great communicator, and spoke in the same "language" as whoever he was addressing never speaking at a level the audience didn't understand no matter who he was speaking with. He was a great storyteller. And Mr. Hicks was always very genuine and sincere.

BEING AUTHENTIC

Being authentic in any environment whether that is on the telephone, in person, via email or text; in a board meeting, medical staff meeting, employee meeting, or management team meeting; at a Rotary Club meeting, service organization functions, or just in the community is critical for any healthcare administrator. Are you really who we think you are? Are you consistent? Can you be trusted? Are you genuine? Are you honest and reliable? If not, people will notice and as a leader you will lose credibility.

LEADERSHIP ATTRIBUTES AND THEIR ANTONYMS

A multitude of different attributes are integral to effective, high-performing leadership. Some of these attributes involve competencies that are quantitative or tangible in nature, such as financial skills, analytical skills, writing skills, speaking skills, etc. The tangible skills of leadership are the ones taught in school or other didactic-based educational programs. Other attributes or competencies are qualitative in nature. The leadership attributes in the following list are qualitative in nature and could also be referred to as **critical intangibles of leadership**. Below, please find a few key definitions (from Dictionary.com):

Attribute – a quality or feature regarded as a characteristic or inherent part of someone or something.

Critical – of decisive importance with respect to the outcome; crucial.

Intangibles – not tangible; incapable of being perceived by the sense of touch, as incorporeal or immaterial things; impalpable.

Leadership – motivating and inspiring others to work hard to achieve organizational goals. An act or instance of leading; guidance; direction.

Review the list of leadership attributes and their antonyms. As you review the list, **please reflect** upon the various adjectives and descriptions that describe important leadership attributes and their antonyms and which may apply to you.

- What have I observed about these leadership attributes and their antonyms in other leaders and people? What effect do these have on me, and how do I typically react?
- In what settings or environments do these critical intangibles show up for me?
- In what settings or environments do the antonyms of these critical intangibles show up for me?
- What aspects of self-awareness and emotional intelligence will help me bring out more of the critical intangibles?
- What steps can I take to heighten my own awareness of when the antonyms of these critical intangibles tend to show up for me?
- How do I incorporate learning through experience and self-reflection into my own leadership philosophy and style going forward?

Leadership Attributes	Antonyms
• Inspiring	Uncharismatic
• High energy	Lethargic
• Accountable	Others blamed
• Responsible	Excuses
• Trustworthy	Untrustworthy
• Credibility	Not always believable
• Empathetic listener: present	Distracted
• Inquisitive	Self-absorbed
• Open to new ideas	Closed-minded
• Appreciative	Takes people for granted
• People-centered	Task- or self-centered
• Understanding	Uncaring/uninterested
• Follow-through	Unorganized/drops the ball
• Self-motivated	Unmotivated
• Enthusiastic	Burned-out
• Optimistic	Negative
• Visionary	Status quo
• Encouraging	Self-absorbed
• Affirming	Doesn't care
• Supportive	Unsupportive
• Role model	Do as I say, not as I do
• Clarity	Ambiguous & confusing
• Teamwork	Silos & individualism
• Planner	Reactionary
• Change agent	Status quo good enough
• Autonomy	Micromanager
• Results-oriented	Task-oriented
• Mission-driven	Self-serving
• Authentic	Phony
• Delegator	Autocratic

TANGIBLE VERSUS INTANGIBLE LEADERSHIP SKILLS

David Handel states that *"One has to assume you [(the leader)] have a certain level of content skills, or the tangibles. That is sort of a given. That doesn't mean you have to be a content expert in everything, but it means you have to have a certain level of content expertise. I think the intangible is what you do and how you do it. What kind of a role model do you serve for the people that work with you? To me it is about emphasizing values, integrity, doing the right thing. The intangible is creating an environment, or being part of creating an environment that people are happy in; they feel it is professionally rewarding and challenging; that it is an open environment where people can say what they feel and think; that you really focus on a team environment. I occasionally call healthcare administration a team sport as it (is about) teams coming together. But you need to create, or be part of creating an environment, where people will be comfortable with that. It is really modeling by what you do that you are open to hearing people's opinions. It doesn't matter if they agree with you or not. What is your opinion? Why do you think that? It is also creating an environment where you try to reach consensus. Consensus doesn't mean that if there are 15 people in the room that every one of the 15 say 'Yes, I agree.' But basically there is pretty good unanimity that is the right way to go. Then it is moving forward with it. Deciding something, taking action, and then holding people accountable. To me the intangible is that people look at you and what you do."*

Vince Caponi states that *"We need the content skills that our physicians and nurses and CPAs and IT people have. But just because you are a good basketball player doesn't mean you are a good coach. That's played itself out many times in a lot of professional sports. Just because you weren't a good athlete, doesn't mean you can't be a fabulous coach. It is a different set of skills. If you think about a coach who creates that milieu in order for people to do their best work, they are not hitting the ball, they are not passing the ball, they are not shooting the ball: what they are doing is seeing what your [(the player)] skills and abilities and gifts are. They are almost like the leader of a symphony pulling everyone together in harmony to accomplish whatever strategy or goal we may have. The intangibility is that you [(the leader)] get the big picture. You are able to take something that is very complex and make it as simple as you possibly can. You have to be a good recognizer of talent. Sometime as a leader it is when to put yourself into play, and when not to put yourself into play. It is knowing when to take the lead, and when to get out of the way and let people go ahead and do that. The (effective leader) knows when the difference is: it may be called street sense or intuition. It is some of that reflection time. (As leaders) I don't think we reflect enough. As humans, we have the ability to reflect, and we have the ability to change. You have to seek out everybody's opinion. And then you have to (communicate) back to people and say 'let me tell you what I've heard, and let me tell you how I think that lines up. The leader then has to decide. That is what a leader does."*

Ed Abel talks about David Windley as a great healthcare leader, saying, *"He preferred to give credit to other folks. When we were successful, he would typically push whoever was part of whatever was going on as being responsible. I think that unselfishness has continued to pervade the organization"* and is handed down to others who are continuing that same leadership style and legacy.

One of a healthcare leader's primary opportunities, as well as responsibilities, is to help develop those around him to be more effective, perform at a higher level, and advance in their own respective career.

One of a healthcare leader's primary opportunities, as well as responsibilities, is to help develop those around him to be more effective, perform at higher levels, and advance in their own respective careers. The book by John Maxwell, *Developing the Leaders Around You*, talks about this important aspect of leadership. Most healthcare leaders are in a position to teach, coach, and mentor others around them and to help others to advance in their careers. A first step is for the healthcare leader to learn and understand the goals, objectives, and passion a co-worker might have about his or her job and career. As a leader, developing those around you pays dividends, not only in terms of impacting the recipient's own effectiveness and performance and overall organizational performance, but it also helps model the way for others to follow. Ed Abel states that "***Peoples leadership styles, to the extent they are advancing the people around them, the likelihood for their success is going to be far greater.***"

When asked about great healthcare leaders and their philosophies and style, Ed Abel states that ***"For the most part they are typically hands-on. They don't delegate the big decisions to other folks, they are part of it. They know what's going on in their hospital (or health service organization). I don't think they micromanage, but they want to understand the facts and what is going on. If somebody is managing [the situation] well, then the leader will typically stand back and really have a hands-off approach. They typically are people with a little bit of personality, and can deal well with other people and enjoy working with other people. And they typically are smart."*** Think about what Mr. Abel is saying, as well as what he is not saying, about this topic. Primarily, he is talking about a healthcare leader's philosophy and style—or the intangibles of leadership, not whether he is an expert in a technical or clinical area.

THE CREDIBILITY AND TRUST OF A HEALTHCARE LEADER MEANS EVERYTHING

Ed Abel states that ***"To me the absolute most important intangible of leadership is honesty/trust. You can't lead if people don't believe what you are saying or they don't trust you. Everything that follows that is double, and triple, or quadruple checked if they don't believe you. A leader can have all the vision in the world, but if they don't trust you and what you are saying, the organization will have a difficult time. I think you could look at a number of different healthcare leaders that have survived without having some other intangible besides trust. One of the books I keep in my office is a book titled*** **The Economics of Trust.** ***The author breaks down that if we could trust everything that is given to us we*** *wouldn't have to double-check it. He talks about the fact that so much of our systems are built around the fact we aren't sure if that's right or not. If you could eliminate this [(we aren't sure if many things are right or not)] how much more productive our society would be. If you can't believe what the hospital CEO is telling you, how are you going to ever get to the next step? I can't describe in enough detail the number of conversations I've had with someone who says 'We'll this is what he said, but we aren't sure what he meant.' They aren't saying they didn't understand the question, they are saying we don't believe it. So how can a leader lead in that kind of a vacuum? It's impossible. With just about any leader who has worked for any significant amount of time, there are going to be certain things that somebody is going to say 'We're not sure he is being totally honest.' There's the truth and then there is the whole truth: which is what is said when a witness is sworn into a court of law to testify. Sometimes people have their days when maybe they don't tell the whole truth, or they hedge a little bit on the facts. That's when you see people lose their effectiveness. Ultimately there is a price to pay for that. That attribute I will tell people early in their career: honesty is something that nobody can take away from you, as a leader you have to give it up. If you can stay true to that as a leader, you are going to be fine. If you don't, there are going to be consequences. Nobody can make you tell a lie. Nobody can make you be dishonest. Only you give that up."*

Honesty is something that nobody can take away from you, as a leader you have to give it up.

LEADERSHIP STYLE MATTERS

How a leader acts, and the style in which he interacts with others, conducts business, and performs his or her job as a healthcare leader, matters; it matters a lot. Why? Again, management is about getting work done through others and providing leadership to motivate and inspire others to work hard to achieve organizational goals. The leadership style a leader employs has a strong and direct impact on the motivational level or psychological readiness of employees and others.

The leadership style a leader employs has a strong and direct impact on the motivational level or psychological readiness of employees and others.

For example, if the subordinate perceives the leader is not interested, caring, or supportive of efforts to improve or enhance patient satisfaction or the patient's experience, then the subordinate probably won't either. Sometimes the employee will perceive such a situation with his manager through the leader's communication, both verbal and non-verbal. Dr. Albert Mehrabian, author of *Silent Messages*, conducted several studies on nonverbal communication. He found that 7 percent of any message is conveyed through words, 38 percent through certain vocal elements, and 55 percent through nonverbal elements (facial expressions, gestures, posture, etc.) (www.nonverbalgroup.com). Therefore, communication is partly the words used (what is said), voice tone and inflection (how it is said), and face and body gestures (what the sender's affect is when it is said) broken into the following percentages:

Communication is:

Actual words used	7%
Voice tone and inflection	38%
Face and body	55%

These statistics about communication have significant implications for leaders, especially as it relates to employees' ongoing assessment of whether the leader "walks the walk" or really means or believes what he says and follows his own words. In other words, is there a credibility gap between what the leader says and what he really means, believes, or does? This point is about substance as much as it is style; however, don't overlook or underestimate the impact that style plays in this leadership communication process.

Leadership style also goes a long way in the process of employees answering the many questions they have about their leaders and if they care or can be trusted; if their work is important and is valued; and whether the organization has a bright future and the employee will be part of it. For example, leadership style goes a long way toward creating the impressions, perceptions, and beliefs an employee forms about questions they have, such as, **"Does my supervisor really care about me as a person?"**

QUESTIONS EMPLOYEES ASK (AND ANSWER FOR THEMSELVES)

For most employees, leadership represents and is the voice of the company. Leaders represent the values, expectations, and standards of the organization and what is important and expected of them on a daily basis. The supervisor–subordinate relationship is one of vital importance in the relationship an employee enjoys (or doesn't enjoy) throughout his employment tenure. The supervisor–subordinate relationship, particularly how it is perceived by the subordinate employee, impacts everything in the relationship. The supervisor—subordinate relationship is the foundation for the employee's motivational level and psychological readiness to work hard, give his or her best, collaborate with others, be productive, perform at a high level, and be satisfied with the work and the employment relationship. A framework for this employment relationship can be described as the questions all employees, at all levels in the organization, have

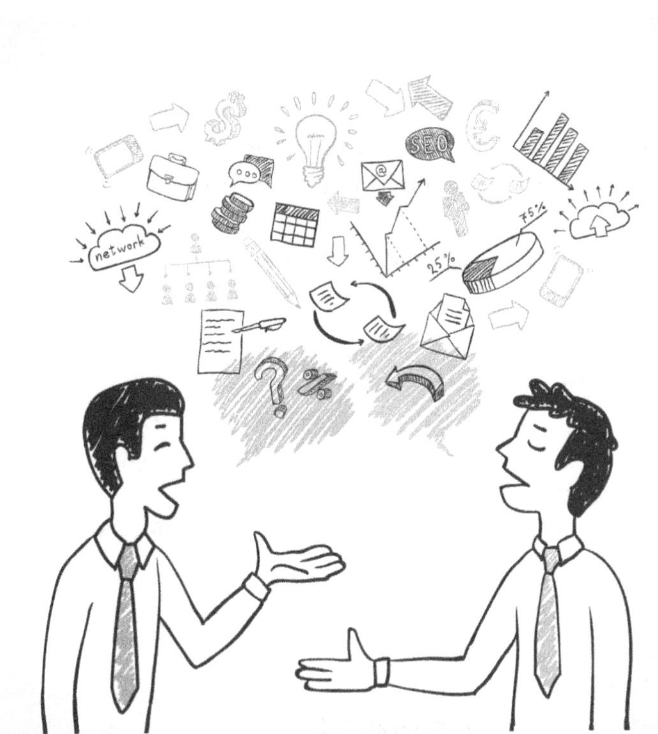

FIGURE 8.1 Business communication

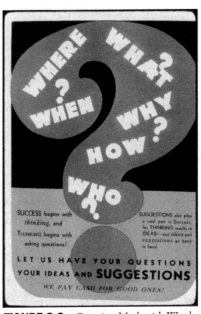

FIGURE 8.2 Question Mark with Words
Office of Emergency Management, War Production Board, "Question Mark with Words," http://commons.wikimedia.org/wiki/File:Where,_When,_Who,_What,_Why,_How%5E_-_NARA_-_534144.jpg. Copyright in the Public Domain.

about their status in the employment relationship. As briefly discussed in a previous chapter but expanded upon here, employees have questions about the organization, their boss, executive leadership, the management team, their position, and their work. How employees think about these questions and the answers will reveal a lot about how they feel in their employment relationship, the level of engagement experienced and discretionary effort given, and their overall level of satisfaction.

- Do I feel a sense of connection with the organization and its purpose?
- Do I like my job and the work I do?
- Do I look forward to coming to work?
- Does the work I do make a difference?
- Does my work connect with my passion?
- How does my job and the work I do fit into the organization's mission and vision?
- Will management position this organization to be strategically competitive in the future?
- Does management care about me as a person, or am I just a number?
- Does management care about my growth and development?
- What opportunities will I have to learn, grow, and develop in this job?
- Will this organization remain financially viable and stable in the future?

- Does the organization have a bright future, and will I be part of it?
- Is my performance appreciated, recognized, or even rewarded?
- If I give more effort in my job, will my boss or anyone notice?
- Will I be considered for other opportunities that may arise at work?
- Does my boss really know who I am as a person and what I am passionate about?
- Does management want my ideas and suggestions? Will management use my good ideas and suggestions?
- Does management really care about the clients, customers, and community?
- Do I trust and believe what management says?
- Will management keep the promises it makes?
- Is the working environment supportive, constructive and productive?
- Can I have fun at work?
- Are employment policies applied and enforced fairly and consistently?
- Do I have input into my immediate work environment?
- Do I have an opportunity to contribute to policies, procedures, and decisions that affect my work and performance?
- Will management support me if I make a mistake in good faith?
- Does management care about/operate with a high regard for ethics?
- Are expectations clear, reasonable, and fair?
- Am I regularly kept informed of important activities, changes, and plans?
- Am I paid fairly compared to others?
- Am I allowed the autonomy to be creative, apply my skills and abilities, and maximize my contributions?
- Does leadership motivate and inspire me to work hard and give my best?

A leader's style of leadership is a primary contributing factor that influences how an employee answers these questions for himself. Sure, there are numerous other factors and variables at work influencing an employee's perceptions of his or her employment relationship and the many factors that contribute to and help determine that relationship; however, there is none more significant or impactful than the supervisor–subordinate relationship. The questions above only represent some of the more common ones that employees—at all levels and in all positions—ask. You may be asking "To whom do they ask these questions to?" The answer is themselves, but these questions are also commonly discussed with co-workers, colleagues, family, and friends. Sometimes these conversations aren't based on questions but the answers to these questions such as "***My boss assigned that project I was interested in completing to someone else. I don't think I have a future here, because I don't get a chance to grow in my current role, so why should I ever think they will consider me for advancement***?" Or "***My boss is quick to point out a mistake when I make one, but seldom recognizes the good work I do. I don't think he likes me.***"

Leaders should think about how employees view their employment relationship and answer these and other questions they ask for themselves. Looking at the employment relationship through the eyes of employees can provide a leader with greater insight into how they are being perceived as a leader and what aspects of their leadership style are being viewed positively or negatively.

MANAGEMENT BY WANDERING AROUND (MBWA)

The visibility of leaders within the organization and with employees is another critical element for leadership effectiveness. Visibility is especially important at the senior leadership level. Most employees want to have a positive relationship with their direct supervisor, as well as other top leaders in the organization. It is incumbent on leaders to take the initiative to foster and develop relationships with employees. It starts with leaders getting out in the organization to meet, interact with, and observe employees in action and take a genuine interest in them—who they are, what they are passionate about, and what work they do. How can leaders effectively motivate and inspire employees when they don't really even know them?

When asked about MBWA, Dr. Judy Monroe states that ***"Employees love that. I think it is a great [leadership] strategy. Certainly I think employees, for the most part, like it when leaders are out-and-about and they can have informal chats with them, and leaders show interest in their work. However, with the move in many organizations to tele-work, that's becoming a more challenging strategy. I've had many days when I realized I have a few minutes and go walking around only to find that folks aren't here because they are tele-working that day."***

MBWA, also referred to as administrative rounding in the hospital or health service organization, should be conducted with a purpose or agenda set ahead of time. The purpose and agenda could be just to interact with employees in order to get to know them better and observe the work they are doing. Other strategic purposes for rounding can include inquiring about good ideas and suggestions employees might have about their working environment, patient safety, patient care, cost containment, service delivery, policies and procedures, or other business or clinical areas; looking into communication practices and the effectiveness of communication within the department and throughout the organization, including what is being discussed at staff meetings, what employees know about the strategic plan, etc.; and insight about physician practices, clinical performance and results being attained, and projects being implemented. MBWA can also be used to disseminate important information about organizational priorities, new policies and procedures, progress being made on key organizational initiatives, and other happenings. Below is a list of questions that can serve as an example or guide for interacting with employees during administrative rounding.

COMMUNICATION

- What are some of the topics being discussed in your staff meetings?
- Are your opinions, input, or suggestions being sought out and listened to by management?
- What methods and sources do you find the most effective in learning about what is happening in the organization?

PATIENT SATISFACTION

- What are the goals and objectives for patient satisfaction in this department?
- What is the plan and what are the steps being taken to increase patient satisfaction and achieve the overall customer service goals and objectives of the department?
- What suggestions do you have to improve our customer service delivery?

STRATEGY

- What do you know about the organization's strategic goals and initiatives?
- Are organizational strategies discussed in staff meetings?
- How do the organizational strategic goals and initiatives relate to the work being done in your department?

DEPARTMENTAL GOALS AND OBJECTIVES

- What are the goals and objectives of this department?
- How are the goals and objectives monitored and reported on and what progress is being made towards goal achievement?
- Do employees have individual goals and objectives in their respective jobs that support the departmental goals and objectives?

POLICY

- What organizational policies do you like the most and the least and why?
- Are there any organizational policies and procedures that detract from your ability to be efficient and effective in your job?
- What departmental policies and procedures would you like to see changed and why?

EXTERNAL FORCES

- How do you see healthcare reform impacting the organization or your job?
- What external regulations have the biggest impact on your job, and how do you deal with those?
- What is the competition doing that we aren't?

PARTICIPATORY LEADERSHIP

Participatory leadership is a leadership style in which the leader consults with employees for their suggestions and input before making decisions. Employees want to be consulted and involved in problem solving and decision making in those matters that affect them and the work they do. Dr. Monroe talks about participatory leadership as being "***One that is really critical. You [(the leader)] are going to kick yourself if you don't do it as well as possible. This happens at all levels. An example here at CDC is we have 'winnable battles'. When I arrived here at CDC I learned we had these 6 winnable battles, and certainly I was going to embrace those as the Deputy Director of the agency and it's my job to carry forth the agency priorities. But what I found was folks were disgruntled both within CDC and outside CDC because they had not been engaged in the process of developing and selecting what those areas of priority would be. My first few weeks at CDC included doing a lot of 'smoothing over' and helping to heal those bad feelings that people had because they hadn't been engaged [in the process]. Once we got past it, then people really began to embrace it and carry it forth. Now it's actually been a really positive thing, but that had been a hard lesson learned for the agency. It would have been a whole lot better to have done that engagement [by getting employees involved in the selection and decision process for the 6 areas for the winnable battles] within CDC and out to our partners as well. And the thing I've found is that, honestly, it doesn't take that much. I think that leaders sometimes don't get that input for fear it's going to take too long and they just need to make an executive decision. What I have found is that if you (the leader) reach out and get that input: 1) it doesn't have to be a big, long, laborious process. Folks are so happy they are being asked that it just takes you a long way, and 2) then when you do have to make the executive decisions—clearly when you are running an organization of any size, clearly the day will come when sometimes an executive decision has to be made—those decisions are going to be much better accepted because employees know your usual pattern is to get input. They will recognize that boy; this is one that an executive decision just had to be made.***"

EMOTIONAL INTELLIGENCE

Emotional intelligence, or EQ, is the ability to recognize one's own strengths and weaknesses, see the linkage between feelings and behaviors, manage impulsive feelings and distressing emotions, be attentive to emotional cues, show sensitivity and respect for others, be an open communicator, and be able to handle conflict, difficult people, and tense situations effectively.

Ed Abel says a leader's emotional intelligence is about "***Trying to stay balanced and not let your own emotions dictate the issue can sometimes be pretty difficult. You can get excited about things. And sometimes when you get excited you can say something pretty stupid. The number one thing that is important when you are trying to have a pretty candid discussion is to make sure you understand what, if they are available, the facts are. Because if you don't understand, and you are trying to consult, or move to a position in some area, and you say something that isn't aligned with or misrepresents the facts, it is going to throw a monkey wrench into things. I've seen it where somebody says something pretty stupid and it***

quickly raises the temperature in the room pretty quickly and all of a sudden there is no collaboration. It becomes us vs. them and finger-pointing and it can escalate pretty quickly if people don't understand what they are talking about. Having said that, I am not afraid to say something to get people to talk about a topic and get the real issues on the table. All too often people don't want to give you what their real position on a topic is, so they will talk around the edges. The quicker you can get to the heart of the issue, the sooner you'll get to a resolution on the matter.

"The healthcare leaders I've seen having the most competency with emotional intelligence, I can't ever remember seeing them lose their temper, in any public or private meeting. That's a pretty tough thing to do and a key attribute for a leader who is going to be in a public position. And the opposite is true when these leaders would hear things that were said by others that were stupid. In a very kind way, go through and dissect it and say 'Is this really what we want to do?' That's a talent a lot of leaders don't have. To be able to bring somebody back to seeing the impact of what they are saying and re-evaluating if it was the right thing to say or not. I've seen healthcare leaders with a high EQ do that very professionally and very effectively."

REACHING OUT FOR ADVICE ON TOUGH DECISIONS

As Sam Odle states that, as a healthcare leader, ***"You don't have to know everything. You can't know everything."*** Dr. Monroe states that ***"When you are up against some tough decisions and tough challenges, one lesson I've learned is when I forget I can phone a friend. You can send out a lifeline with that. There are times when just stopping and realizing you need more data; realizing there are experts out there and you can just pick the phone up, or access the paper they've written, or whatever. Sometimes you will kick yourself if you haven't done your homework."***

DON'T MISS THE BIG PICTURE

Conceptual skills are a leader's comprehension of the overall organization and how it fits within the larger environment; it is the ability to see the organization as a whole, understand how the different parts affect each other, and recognize how the organization fits into or is affected by its environment. Dr. Monroe states that ***"I've learned along the way that if you've got your head down and you get too buried in the details with your head down you are going to miss the big picture. That can be a hard lesson sometimes. Especially in leadership, you've got to make sure you are scanning the whole picture and don't go down the rabbit hole."***

In addition, it is the leader's responsibility to help others around him see and understand the big picture, as well. Many times during conversations, people get too focused—and sometimes too concerned—with the details and lose sight of the more important bigger picture of what the objective is or what is being accomplished. Seeing the bigger picture can help put things—including the details—into their proper context and perspective. Many times, just taking a step back to recognize and acknowledge the bigger picture and its importance can facilitate teamwork and collaboration, as well as working together toward goal achievement.

WHAT A LEADERSHIP TEAM NEEDS FROM THE CEO

What does a leadership team need from the top leader in a healthcare organization? What's important to vice presidents, department heads, front-line supervisors, or even employees, physicians, or board members? As the hospital CEO, what do these internal stakeholders need from you; what do they want from you; what do they look for from you? Above everything, internal stakeholders need a leader who they can trust and who is consistent. People in an organization don't want to always be guessing how a leader will act, what he will say, or what actions he might take. Predictable leaders provide a sense of trust and certainty that is critical to creating a positive organizational culture. Obviously, a leader needs to possess knowledge and competencies in a variety of healthcare and business subject matters, along with wisdom that is developed through experience. But consistency and predictability are vital.

In today's fast-pace working environment, it is difficult to plan for and focus on the longer term. Much of what a healthcare leader typically deals with are day-to-day problems and challenges. However, decisions need to be placed into their proper context. Some decisions have much longer-term implications than others. Sometimes a decision will set a precedent; therefore, for consistency purposes, one decision may mandate that other similar decisions should follow suite or be consistent with it. One thing that Mr. Hicks would say to those young administrators that he mentored was "If you make decisions like you are going to be there for 20 or 25 years, you might just be there for 20 or 25 years. But if you make decisions for that month's or that quarter's financial statement, you are going to be shortsighted in your perspective and leadership and lose sight of the long term. The short-term approach can create turnover and cause you to have or want to leave your position.

AUTHENTIC OPTIMISM

Previously in this chapter, we discussed the importance of honesty, credibility, and authenticity of a leader. Leaders who aren't authentic are quickly seen as posers—phonies—and are not believable. Posers have no credibility. Leaders must stand behind their word, promises, and commitments. And, leaders need to be authentically optimistic. What does that mean?

Optimism, just like negativity, can be contagious. Optimism can be infectious and spread, but only if it is genuine and authentic. In other words, optimism must be backed up and supported by the facts surrounding the situation. In management terminology there must be a legitimate business case for the optimism. The optimistic view or position must also be believed by the leader—it can't be phony or contrived. It's like the old adage ***"Whether you believe you can or can't, you are correct."*** If the leader doesn't believe in himself, his employees, or the team's ability to achieve a goal, complete a project, or complete a task successfully, then guess what? He is usually right.

Who wants to work for a leader who isn't authentically optimistic about what he is doing, about what can be accomplished or achieved, and the organization or team's ability to perform and get the job done? Most people don't. Why? It's demotivating. It saps energy. Again, the optimism must be authentic for it to be motivating and effective—and authentic optimism can be very motivating and encouraging.

LEADERS AS ENCOURAGERS

Think about someone in your life who made an impact on you. Someone who showed confidence in you, believed in you, trusted you, or encouraged you. Maybe that person showed more confidence or belief in you than you did in yourself at that moment when you needed their encouragement to move forward. When you think of that person, think of both the simplicity of their actions and the magnitude of the impact their encouragement had on you. That person and their impact will stay with you forever, because it made a difference. Healthcare leaders have this same opportunity on a daily basis with those around them. Again, any encouragement given to others must be genuine and authentic, not phony or contrived to be effective. It is a matter of credibility and believability.

Great leaders are encouragers: they encourage others to work hard to give more, to strive for more, to work together as a team, and to believe in themselves.

Great leaders are encouragers: they encourage others to work hard, to give more, to strive for more, to work together as a team, and to believe in themselves. There are countless opportunities in health service leadership to be an authentic encourager of others. As a leader, look for the opportunities and situations where your encouragement is needed. Put yourself in the situations of others and think about how they might feel about a problem, task, or challenge they are faced with. Do they need encouragement? If so, be the first in line to recognize and provide the encouragement they need to move forward with conviction and optimism.

There are countless opportunities in health service leadership to be an authentic encourager of others. As a leader, look for the opportunities and situations where your encouragement is needed.

BALANCING CONFLICTING INCENTIVES

Healthcare leaders are increasingly being forced to balance conflicting incentives, such as increasing quality of care and service delivery with cost containment. A common phrase used in the industry for this is ***"doing more with less,"*** as the expectations increase for improved operating performance in all areas at all levels while doing so with reduced reimbursement on a per-unit basis. In other words, improved financial performance cannot come at the expense of lower quality of care or service to patients. At the same time, health service organizations are competing for critical healthcare manpower, such as licensed therapists, registered nurses, licensed technologist, physicians, ancillary professionals, and other staff. Therefore, issues of recruitment, retention, morale, satisfaction, motivation, employment relationship, and engagement are important as well. This is quite the balancing act for healthcare leaders. Changes and improvements can't be made in one area at the expense of others, or sub-optimization will occur. Sub-optimization is performance improvement in one part of an organization, but only at the expense of decreased performance in another part.

SIMPLIFYING THE COMPLEX

There are many, many aspects of healthcare that are complex: off-pump cardiovascular surgical procedures; powerful new drugs and medicines like tissue plasminogen activator—a clot busting drug used to treat stroke; advanced clinical and therapeutic technologies like computed tomography, magnetic resonance imaging, or radiation therapy; surgical procedures, like neurosurgery or maternal-fetal surgery; billing, tracking, and follow-up computer software systems used with third party accounts; and electronic health records. The list goes on as the complexity and interconnectedness of many elements create an increasingly challenging environment, and one that is sometimes hard to understand. Add to this the changing incentives, regulations, and competitive dynamics brought on by healthcare reform, along with the increasing anxiety that sweeping change and uncertainty have created. Healthcare is a very complex, dynamic environment and, many times, it requires a more simplified explanation for others to really understand what is happening and the impact and ramifications of change.

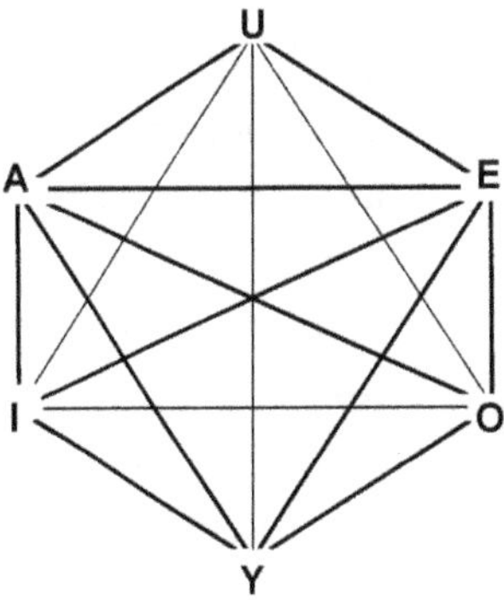

FIGURE 8.3 Hexagon
Greg Bard, "Hexagon with Vowels," http://commons.wikimedia.org/wiki/File:Logical-hexagon.png. Copyright in the Public Domain.

It is a healthcare leader's responsibility to understand these complexities and their impact well enough to articulate these is a way that others can relate to and understand. This includes the organization's strategy and approach to dealing with the complexity and change that is occurring and why. If employees don't understand the impact of external forces and changes on the organization, they won't understand the organization's strategies and actions to address them. As Albert Einstein said, "***If you can't explain it simply, you don't understand it well enough***" www.brainyquotes.com.

MOTIVATING AND INSPIRING

At its most basic fundamental level, leadership is motivating and inspiring others to work hard to attain organizational goals. As a healthcare leader, what attributes do you possess that are motivating and inspiring to others? What attributes can you develop that will make you more motivating and inspiring than you currently are? What attributes and characteristics do you have that will compel others to follow you? What attributes and characteristics can you develop that will compel others to follow you? Ultimately, who a healthcare leader is (as a person, at his or her core) and what he or she does (his or her actions, words, and leadership style) is what makes him or her motivating and inspiring. Ken Stella says that motivation is "***An absolute requirement in a service industry***" like healthcare. Ken goes on to say "***I think motivation, whether it's individual, team, or organizational—it just has to be a constant.***"

Effective leaders are motivating and inspiring. But what makes someone motivating and inspiring? There are probably an infinite number of possible factors or reasons why someone is motivating and inspiring. A leader's style must be congruent or compatible with who he or she is as a person and his or her values and what he or she believes. A leader needs to be aware of and cognizant of his or her effectiveness in motivating and inspiring others and assess this on an ongoing basis.

QUESTIONS FOR ASSESSMENT AND REFLECTION

- What attributes make me motivating and inspiring as a leader?
- How can I use or apply my attributes in more or different ways that would make me more motivating and inspiring?
- What actions can I take to develop my attributes, so they are more motivating and inspiring to others in my capacity as a leader?
- What behaviors am I not displaying or actions am I not taking that would elevate my level of effectiveness in motivating or inspiring others?
- How much of my time, attention, and focus in spent in efforts to motivate and inspire others?
- What should I stop doing that is counterproductive to fostering motivation and inspiration?
- What should I continue doing that is productive and effective to fostering motivation and inspiration that I might do more of?

THE ROLE OF THE DEPARTMENT/MANAGER

In a hospital's organizational structure, as well as in other health service organizations, the leader with 24/7 management responsibility at the department or service level typically carries the title of Department Head or Department Manager. It is common for the department head to function at and be considered a middle manager in the organization's leadership hierarchy, organizational chart, or chain of command. The organizational hierarchy refers to the levels of authority in the organization. The organizational chart depicts the formal structure, chain of command, formal authority relationships, and patterns of communication within the organization. The chain of command is the vertical line of authority that clarifies who reports to whom throughout the organization. The level of authority concerns one's hierarchical level in an organization (*Leadership: Enhancing The Lessons Of Experience*, by Richard L. Hughes, Robert C. Ginnett and Gordon J. Curphy).

When an organization has a centralized decision making culture, most or all decisions are made by one person or just a few at the very top of the organizational chart. When an organization has a decentralized decision making culture, most decisions are being dispensed and made at the lowest levels in the organization. The scope of responsibility of a department head can vary immensely, particularly given the organizations and department's size and complexity. The department head may be responsible for only one or two employees and a small operating budget that may not consist of more than department salaries, wages, and benefits to being responsible for literally hundreds of employees, thousands of dollars of supplies and other resources, and an operating expense budget from $10 million to $25 million or more. In a large, tertiary care hospital, a department head of a high revenue–generating department may be responsible for net revenue of $50 million to $100 million or more. This compares to a critical access hospital (CAH) of 25 beds that has a total net revenue budget of $25 million. Many factors and variables impact the scope of a department head's management responsibilities, not just the size of the organization or department being managed.

In a typical community hospital, the department head is the level of management where the "*Rubber meets the road*" for the implementation and enforcement of policies and procedures; translation of the corporate vision, strategies, goals, priorities, and projects at the department level so that employees understand what these mean; communication about other internal and external changes, factors, and forces, what it all means, and how it affects employees in their respective work and roles; and the expectations, standards, and requirements of the department and organization. Another important role played by a department head, given their position as middle management between the front line and top management, is to provide the communication and insight for top-level management to hear and learn about what is happening at the work-site level with employees, patients, physicians, families, volunteers, suppliers, vendors, etc.

What's working well and where do opportunities for improvement exist; reports on implementation of policies and procedures, clinical quality and service protocols and initiatives; updates and progress reports on projects, working relationships, and morale; budget variances and action steps being taken to achieve budgets; ideas on how to grow the business, improve working conditions, the environment of care, equipment, or service utilization or issues; and more. High-performing organizations have top management that provide needed resources, direction, support, communication, and autonomy to their department heads, so they can be efficient and effective, and hold them accountable for their efforts and performance. Autonomy is the degree to which a job gives workers the discretion, freedom, and independence to decide how and when to accomplish the job. Training, coaching, and mentoring of department heads by appropriate top management can pay dividends for both departmental and overall leadership effectiveness and performance.

Department heads tend to have a high level of technical or clinical knowledge, skill, and ability in their respective department or service area that can be a great asset to the organization, even outside the purview of the department or service. Department heads typically function as the "Chief Business Officer" or "Chief Clinical Officer" for their respective department or service. They are actively involved in the human resource processes of hiring, training, evaluating, promoting, firing, and assigning roles and tasks to staff. With 24/7 responsibility for staffing, department heads have an enormous impact on quality, service, productivity, and other matters of operational service and performance. These middle managers are also typically in the best position in the organization to discover, learn, or identify new and innovative techniques, technologies, or processes and procedures that can elevate or streamline operations; create new efficiencies; reduce costs; or delivery safer, more improved patient care and service. Again, in a typical hospital or health service organization, the department head level is where the "rubber meets the road."

DISCUSSION QUESTIONS

1. How do you define good leadership?
2. What does it mean for a healthcare leader to be authentic?
3. Describe the difference between tangible and intangible leadership skills.
4. Describe the role leadership style plays in a healthcare leader's overall
5. effectiveness.
6. Why does the trust of a leader matter?
7. List two or three questions a healthcare leader might ask employees when conducting administrative rounds? Why?
8. Describe why the position of department head is where the "rubber meets the road" in most hospital or health service organizations. What is the difference between line authority and staff authority?
9. What is the definition of leadership?
10. What is the chain-of-command?

FIGURE CREDITS

Figure 8.1: Office of Emergency Management, War Production Board, "Question Mark with Words," http://commons.wikimedia.org/wiki/File:Where,_When,_Who,_What,_Why,_How%5E_-_NARA_-_534144.jpg. Copyright in the Public Domain.

Figure 8.2: Greg Bard, "Hexagon with Vowels," http://commons.wikimedia.org/wiki/File:Logical-hexagon.png. Copyright in the Public Domain.

9

Building a Collaborative Team Culture

The heart of teamwork and collaboration is trust. A trusting relationship between coworkers, and with leadership is an essential foundational ingredient necessary for employees to be open with their opinions and suggestions; to be vulnerable and trusting—letting others really get to know them on a personal level; and to be vulnerable and trusting in extending themselves—even going out of their way—to help and assist others in various ways that are outside the boundaries of their own role and responsibilities. A culture of trust manifests in employees helping, assisting, guiding, and supporting one another to benefit each other, patients, their care and service, and the organization as a whole.

The heart of teamwork and collaboration is trust.

Healthcare may be the ultimate people business. The delivery of healthcare service is about people caring for and helping people. In a typical hospital or other health service organization involved with the delivery of direct patient care, there is an impressive diversity of clinical and non-clinical staff involved in the delivery of care to the patient. Whether it is a physician, nurse, therapist, or technician involved in delivering patient care directly to the patient, or a maintenance worker, switchboard operator, patient account representative, or administrator involved in creating and fostering the environment of care and the supportive services necessary in the overall care delivery, the role of collaboration in the delivery of patient care is vital. It is healthcare leadership's role and responsibility to build a collaborative team culture to foster and promote organizational efficiency and effectiveness. For the highest level of quality care, patient outcomes, patient safety and comfort, patient experience and satisfaction, and efficiency and effectiveness overall, clinical and non-clinical staff must all be working together as a cohesive team.

OBJECTIVES

1. Define collaboration and the important elements that go into creating it in a healthcare organization.
2. Outline 10 steps healthcare leaders can take to build a collaborative team culture.
3. Highlight several management theories that apply in building a collaborative team culture.

THE PATIENT AND FAMILY'S VIEW OF COLLABORATION AND TEAMWORK

Patients and families judge the care and service we deliver, and rate their experience—and their providers and caregivers—from the central standpoint of how their needs and expectations were met and how they were cared for as human beings. Moreover, patients and families expect the treatment team of caregivers to work together as a team. When patients and families detect a lack of teamwork and collaboration on the part of the treatment team, it raises concerns about the care and treatment they may receive—many times making them feel anxious, nervous, unsure, and vulnerable. In other words, teamwork and collaboration are major factors that impact not only the efficiency and effectiveness of the care, treatment, and service provided, but the overall caring environment, including patient satisfaction.

TEAMWORK

Teamwork and collaboration go hand-in-hand. In hospitals and other health service organizations involved in direct patient care, much of the delivery of care, as well as supportive work behind the scenes, is done in teams. Team diversity is always present, which includes the variances or differences in ability, experience, personality, or any other factor or characteristic of a team. There are five stages recognized in forming a team: forming, storming, norming, performing, and adjourning.

Forming—the first stage of teamwork, during which members are given their charge or the purpose of the team.

Storming—the second stage of teamwork, during which team members learn about one another. This stage is characterized by conflict and emotional issues that may inhibit a team's progress.

Norming—the third stage of teamwork, during which team members agree upon working styles, conflict is reduced, and group cohesiveness emerges.

Performing—the fourth stage of teamwork, during which team members are engaged in the work and purpose of the team.

Adjourning—the final stage of teamwork, during which team members review outcomes and successes and individuals disengage from the team.

Please note: although this model denotes a sequence to team formation and the different stages, there usually isn't anything linear about the process. Moreover, teams can experience multiple stages of teamwork at any given time.

There are different types of teams that can be formed and operated in the workplace setting. Here is a list and definitions of the primary types of teams.

Cross-functional team—a team composed of employees from different functional areas of the organization.

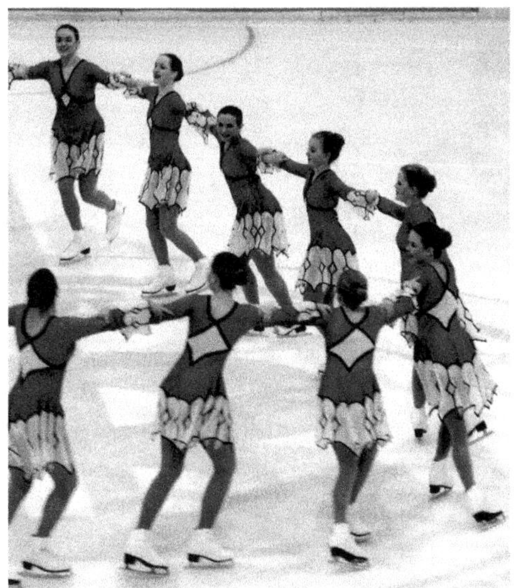

FIGURE 9.1 Ice Skaters in Purple

Interdisciplinary team—a team of people who represent different disciplines working together to accomplish a common goal.

Employee involvement team—a team that provides advice or makes suggestions to management concerning specific issues.

Project team—a team created to complete a specific, one-time project or task within a limited time.

Self-managing team—a team that manages and controls all the major tasks of producing a product or service.

Semi-autonomous work group—a group that has the authority to make decisions and solve problems related to the major tasks of producing a product or service.

Traditional work group—a group composed of two or more people who work together to achieve a shared goal.

Virtual team—a team composed of geographically and/or organizationally dispersed coworkers who use telecommunications and information technologies to accomplish an organizational task.

Work team—a small number of people with complementary skills who hold themselves mutually accountable for pursuing a common purpose, achieving performance goals, and improving interdependent work processes.

Unfortunately in healthcare, just like in other industries, there are some employees who engage in social loafing from time to time. Social loafing is behavior in which team members withhold their efforts and fail to perform their share of the work. Team leaders must work to prevent social loafing and address it, should it occur; otherwise, it can create a negative downward spiral on the rest of the team. Another possible negative phenomenon that can occur in teams or groups is groupthink—where there is unmerited conformity to group values, ethics, ideas, and decisions that can lead to negative outcomes. Healthcare leaders need to be cognizant of groupthink as they can unknowingly instigate it in a team or group environment just based upon their position of authority. An illustration for this would be when a healthcare leader is quick to state his idea or position in a setting where he really wants to solicit the ideas and opinions of the team members and promote dialogue. Depending on the working environment and organizational culture, a healthcare leader stating a strong idea or opinion quickly can quash the input from other employees. Why? Who wants to openly oppose their boss or other leader in a group setting? Is it safe to do so? If not, this could lead to groupthink.

COLLABORATION

The word ***collaborate*** is defined as *working with others; working with another person or group in order to achieve something* (Encarta World Dictionary). As it relates to the delivery of direct patient care, collaboration refers to the level of support and assistance individual employees provide to one another in a timely, professional, efficient, and effective manner when completing the various tasks, functions, and work processes involved in the clinical and administrative delivery of patient care.

Collaboration is about working together in a synergistic fashion to provide safe, complete, thorough, high-quality care delivered in a manner that fosters respect, dignity, mutual trust, empathy, and compassion for coworkers and patients alike. Collaboration is about promoting cohesiveness or the extent to which team members are attracted to a team and motivated to remain with it and work together with others. So, what creates a collaborative work environment?

Collaboration is based on relationships and trust. Knowing the person/people you are working with on a personal level, and having strong, valued, trusting relationships are key ingredients for collaboration.

Collaboration is based upon relationships and trust.

A working environment of trust is essential for employees to have confidence in one-another, as well as the organization and its leadership. Trust and confidence are both essential ingredients for employees to readily rely on one another; support and assist one another; anticipate actions that can be taken to enhance workflow efficiency and effectiveness, and make someone's job easier; and to work collaboratively as a team.

Work processes in health service organizations can be highly specialized; highly technical; use specialized technology; be labor-intensive; include a division of work processes, work flows, functions, and procedures; and be provided by a workforce that is diverse in a multitude of ways. This type of division in work functions and assignments requires a high amount of interconnectedness among all staff for efficiency and effectiveness to be realized in these dependent work relationships. Moreover, collaboration and teamwork require staff to be dependable: that is, able to be trusted to act in the way required or expected. Examples of how caregivers are dependent on each other include: nurse-dependent upon the physician's orders and communication; physician-dependent upon the nursing assessment and patient monitoring; radiologist-dependent upon accurate film images produced by the x-ray technologist; clinical staff-dependent upon having available medical supplies needed; patient account representative-dependent upon physician's final diagnosis; and administrator-dependent upon all staff. The employees and providers in a health service organization—including leadership—are all dependent upon one another to provide the best care and service possible to patients. Therefore, it can be stated that ***collaboration impacts everything.***

For patients, collaboration impacts quality, safety, and service. For families, collaboration impacts the overall patient and family experience. For physicians, collaboration impacts their ability to diagnose and treat efficiently and effectively. For coworkers, collaboration impacts their ability to perform in an efficient and effective manner. And for leaders, collaboration impacts all critical success factors of organizational performance. The level of collaboration in an organization results from the organizational culture that fosters collaboration.

WORKFORCE DIVERSITY

The typical workforce in a health service organization is diverse. Diversity can be based on a variety of characteristics, such as education, sociocultural status, income, age, race, culture, values, beliefs, and experience. While workforce diversity can be a real strength for a health service organization, given the diversity of patients and other stakeholders the organization serves, it can also be a challenge in terms of staff collaboration. Effectively understanding, relating to, and trusting people who are different in one or more ways can sometimes take diversity and cultural sensitivity training to promote and foster collaboration. Diversity training should be offered using qualified trainers who can teach and educate employees about diversity sensitivity as it relates to serving patients and families, as well as working with other employees.

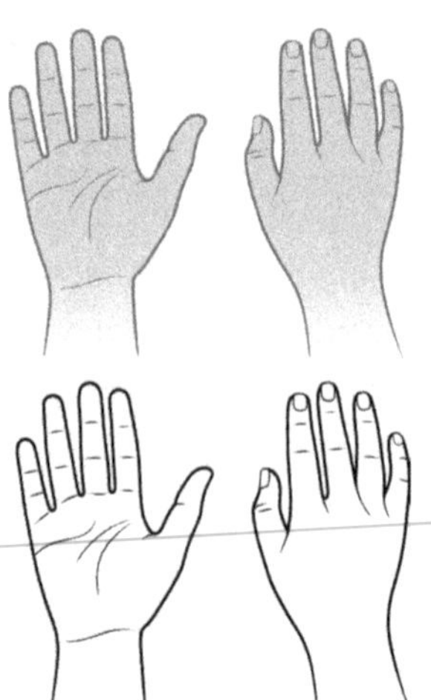

FIGURE 9.2 Invisible Hand

ORGANIZATIONAL CULTURE

Organizational culture can be defined as the values, beliefs, and attitudes of the employees and providers in a health service organization. The culture is how things are done, what is expected, and what is important. The culture is the invisible hand that is always at work shaping expectations about everything.

The culture is the invisible hand that is always at work shaping expectations about everything.

Without question, leadership has the most influence and impact on organizational culture. Every organization is designed by its leadership to produce its resulting culture, results, and performance.

Building a cohesive team and fostering a culture of collaboration involves a multitude of factors, all of which can be impacted by leadership. At the core of collaboration lies the follower's motivation to collaborate.

Fostering a culture of collaboration is more about creating a climate that motivates and inspires follower's to collaborate—it's a feeling thing.

Motivation is the set of forces that initiates, directs, and makes people persist in their efforts to accomplish a goal or affect the direction, intensity, and persistence of voluntary behavior. Fostering a culture of collaboration is more about creating a climate that motivates and inspires follower's to collaborate—it's a feeling thing.

COLLABORATION'S IMPACT

Collaboration impacts the working environment and critical success factors of a healthcare organization, such as quality outcomes; service delivery; productivity, discretionary effort, and financial performance; employee satisfaction; physician satisfaction; problem-solving; and even recruitment and retention. Collaboration impacts everything. With collaboration, much can be achieved. Without collaboration, a lower level of results and performance are sure to be realized.

Some of the sounds of collaboration include: Can I help you ... ? What do you think about ... ? How do you think we should ... ? Have you thought about ... ? What if we ... ? Is there anything else you need from me? I appreciate your willingness to ... I thought you would like me to assist in ...

HARDWIRING FOR A COLLABORATIVE CULTURE

Hardwiring collaboration in a health service organization means to imbed the expectations and standards for collaboration in various structures of daily operations, including new employee orientation, job descriptions, performance appraisals, meeting agendas, ongoing training, management by walking around (MBWA) agenda, and more. For collaboration to thrive, it must be expected, discussed, measured, monitored, evaluated, reported on, reinforced, celebrated, and planned for.

THE FIVE DYSFUNCTIONS OF A TEAM

In his best-selling book *The Five Dysfunctions of a Team*, Patrick Lencioni outlines five key dysfunctions inherent in poorly performing teams: inattention to results, avoidance of accountability, lack of commitment, fear of conflict, and absent of trust.

10 STEPS LEADERS CAN TAKE TO ENHANCE TEAMWORK AND COLLABORATION

1. **Build trust**—An absence of trust creates a working environment where weaknesses and mistakes are concealed; employees hesitate to ask for help or provide constructive feedback; hesitate to offer help outside their own job or area of responsibility; and fail to recognize and tap into one another's skills and experience.

   As previously stated, trust is the foundation of teamwork and collaboration and can be developed and fostered by the following leadership actions:

   - Modeling the way by being personable, vulnerable, open, and honest, as well as supportive of employee mistakes made in good faith.
   - Acknowledging your own mistakes and failures and creating a culture of honesty and transparency.
   - Paying attention to employees, recognizing their effort in performance, and offering support and advice for improvements at the individual employee level.
   - Cultivating a decentralized, participatory leadership style and process.
   - Teambuilding through internal and external activities. Simple ideas can be the most effective—such as leadership hosting an employee luncheon with an open agenda for employees to discuss whatever issues are on their minds.

2. **Mastering conflict**—constructive conflict among team members requires trust, along with engaged employees who feel comfortable offering their own insight and perspective. It is about creating an inquisitive environment for various perspectives to be shared through constructive dialogue. A culture of constructive conflict can be developed and fostered by leadership creating expectations and norms for constructive conflict to occur.
3. **Commitment for achievement**—commitment for achievement requires clear understanding, goal clarity, and emotional ownership/buy-in. Commitment for achievement requires leadership to help all employees understand and feel a strong connection with the work they do and how it impacts the organization's mission, vision, and goals. Employees need to clearly understand and see how the work they do contributes to the work done by others and the overall achievement of organizational

goals. Leadership also needs to be very clear about a select number of very important goals for the organization; articulate why these goals are crucial to patient care, the employees, and the organization's mission; the game plan for goal achievement; and the role each employee plays in that process.

4. **Fostering accountability**—a culture that lacks accountability can be deflating and demoralizing to employees. When employees see colleagues not being held accountable for effort and performance, they will simply perceive that leadership doesn't care or isn't serious about results.

When employees see colleagues not being held accountable for effort and performance, they will simply perceive that leadership doesn't care or isn't serious about results.

Credibility and trust of leadership is directly impacted by leadership's willingness and ability to hold employees accountable for effort and performance, including their efforts and performance in working together as a team in a collaborative environment. Clarity around goals and actions to achieve these goals; ongoing reporting on progress being made towards goal achievement; and efforts to get back on track, as needed, including education, training, and coaching, are imperative.

5. **Results-driven leadership**—a constant, consistent, ongoing focus by leadership on results achievement is paramount. Team initiatives should be prioritized and made highly visible. A balanced scorecard at the corporate level, with clarity of alignment of various scorecard key performance indicators (KPIs) at the team level, is important. Moreover, ongoing clarity and reporting around team achievement and how it supports corporate goal attainment is important for feedback and affirmation.
6. **Visibility**—it has often been said that people don't care what you know—as the leader—until they first know you care. One important way to show you care is to be visible in the follower's work area, even pitch-in and help out when needed. Follows want to know their leaders as people, and most want to feel there is a personal relationship at some level. Management-by-walking-around, a phrase coined by Peter Drucker, applies here.
7. **Communication**—effective leadership communication should be a constant, open, ongoing process through various mediums, including face-to-face. It is incumbent upon leadership to explain and foster understanding about the external factors impacting the organization and the organization's response.
8. **Employee Recognition**—what gets recognized gets reinforced; what gets reinforced gets repeated. When leadership, at all levels, recognizes employees for their efforts and performance—extending their genuine, sincere appreciation—employees will be more motivated to work hard, give their best, and collaborate with others.
9. **Employee Engagement**—engaged employees are far more apt to work hard, give their best, and collaborate with others. There are many important ingredients that go into creating an engaged workforce, but none more important than creating alignment between the organization's mission, vision, strategies, and goals and the important work performed by each individual employee. This alignment

must be clearly seen, understood and connected with by the employee; however, it is imperative that leaders at all levels help employees see and make this important connection, as many don't see it clearly or feel a strong connection with it.

10. **Leading By Example**—whether we realize it or not, as leaders we are always modeling the way for others to follow. Leaders set the expectations by what they do and say. While leadership is responsible for the written rules of the organization, they are also pivotal in setting the "unwritten" rules that apply in the organization as well. Followers typically take their cue on what to do; how to act; what's expected; what's permitted; and what's tolerated from leadership. Expectations about teamwork and collaboration are generally not exceptions to this rule.

MANAGEMENT THEORIES APPLIED TO COLLABORATION

Expectancy Theory—suggests that a follower's motivation to collaborate is partly a function of the perceived consequences (positive and negative) that are derived as a result.

The Pygmalion Effect—suggests that creating a working climate with clear, well-understood expectations for collaboration at all levels will create a self-fulfilling prophecy of collaboration.

The Hawthorne Effect—suggests that fostering a working climate for collaboration takes leaders paying attention to followers—including through direct observation and personal interaction.

Servant Leadership Theory—suggests that collaboration may be enhanced when leaders set the example by looking for ways to support followers in their efforts to collaborate with others, and clear obstacles and hindrances that may be in the way for collaboration to occur.

Path Goal Theory—suggests four different leadership styles should be used individually with employees to foster collaboration, depending upon the employee's readiness (job readiness includes job knowledge, skills, abilities, and experience; and psychological readiness or willingness and motivational level to do the job). This theory suggests that one size does not fit all as it relates to the management and leadership of followers. Therefore, to foster a culture of collaboration at the highest level, this theory suggests that different leadership styles need to be used by leaders with follower's based on their level of job readiness and psychological readiness. Simply put, some employees may not have the experience working in a cohesive, team environment and collaborating with their colleagues while other followers may not have the willingness or motivation (yet) to do so without leadership support, direction, and encouragement.

1. **Directive Leadership**—a leadership style in which the leader lets employees know precisely what is expected of them, gives them specific guidelines for performing tasks, schedules work, sets standards of performance, and makes sure that people follow standard rules and regulations.
2. **Supportive Leadership**—a leadership style in which the leader is friendly and approachable, shows concern for employees and their welfare, treats them as equals, and creates a friendly climate.
3. **Participative Leadership**—a leadership style in which the leader consults with employees for their suggestions and input before making decisions.
4. **Achievement-Oriented Leadership**—a leadership style in which the leader sets challenging goals, has high expectations of employees, and displays confidence that employees will assume responsibility and put forth extraordinary effort.

Healthcare organizations where collaboration is strong and consistently part and parcel with how work processes are completed are, in general, more efficient, are more effective, and provide higher levels of quality patient care and service. The delivery of healthcare services to patients takes a high level of collaboration, given the tremendous division of labor; highly specialized areas of medicine, surgery, diagnostics, and therapeutics requiring special clinical knowledge, skills, and expertise; support areas, such as purchasing, credentialing, patient accounts, environmental, or central sterile supply; and administrative areas. It takes all these functions and more and the staff in these areas working together in a collaborative fashion to render the very best quality care and service to patients. It is leadership that creates the organizational culture and working environment for collaboration to thrive.

DISCUSSION QUESTIONS

1. Identify one management theory discussed in this chapter and how it applies to collaboration.
2. Describe one or two steps leaders can take to foster collaboration.
3. What lies at the heart of collaboration?
4. Describe what collaboration impacts in a healthcare organization.
5. What is the Path–Goal Theory, and what are the four types of leadership-styles under this theory?
6. What does hardwiring for collaboration mean?
7. What are the five stages of teamwork?
8. Define collaboration.
9. How do most employees view management when they don't hold other employees accountable for effort and performance?
10. What is groupthink?

FIGURE CREDITS

10

Putting Motivational Theory into Practice

Motivation is what makes people move, act, respond, and take action. Motivation is the fuel that drives action. Without motivation, action is either not taken at all or taken without as much energy, intent, or purpose. Why do hospital or health service organization trustees volunteer their time and energy without compensation? Why do hospital volunteers give their time and energy without compensation? Why do caregivers and physicians care for people with infectious diseases, come in when called during their off shift without hesitating or work weekends and holidays? Why do many healthcare leaders work countless extra hours and give of their time and energy to multiple community organizations and initiatives? For starters, these people are committed and motivated to make a difference in their service to others—including countless people they don't know or have never met before in their lives.

OBJECTIVES

1. Appreciate the important role motivation plays in employee and organizational performance.
2. Learn about 10 motivational theories and concepts plus feedback and some of their applications in healthcare leadership.
3. Identify a few motivational theories and techniques that you can incorporate into your leadership style.

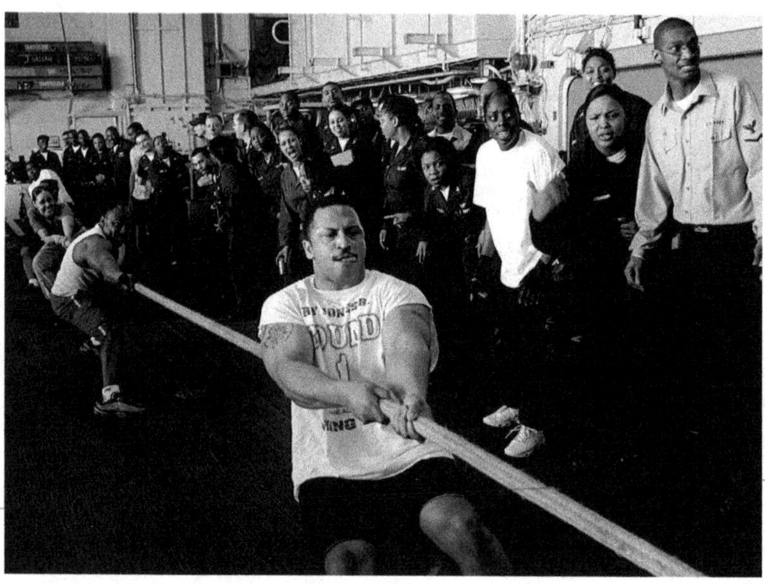

FIGURE 10.1 Navy Tug-of-War

U.S. Navy, "Navy Tug-of-War," http://commons.wikimedia.org/wiki/File:US_Navy_030329-N-1512S-008_Yeoman_2nd_Class_Christopher_Chatman_from_Baton_Rouge,_La.,_leads_the_ship%5Ersquo,s_Administrative_Office_Tug-of-War_team.jpg. Copyright in the Public Domain.

According to Ken Stella, *"Motivation is an absolute requirement in a service industry. I think motivation whether it's individual, team or organization is just a constant. The way you really have power as a leader is through the employees. The more successful you are in motivating your workforce, the more success you'll have in implementing your plan."* Sam Odle says, *"Leaders have to be able to motivate staff. It doesn't always have to be a heroic leadership style. But [leaders] have to be able to motivate, and to use motivational theory to get people to act."*

Mr. Odle also talks about being motivated and *"getting inspired by thinking about the work you are doing is important. It really was when you stop and think about providing a secure, safe place to work where people can count on it, whether they are the person receiving healthcare or delivering it. I used to tell our directors all the time the reason we have to be good stewards of our resources is because we want to be an ongoing concern. We want our employees to know we are financially secure, and they know that paycheck is going to be there every two weeks. It's not just about building a bigger health system, or getting more patients, it really is about making the community a better place."*

What is motivation? Motivation is the set of forces that initiates, directs, and makes people persist in their efforts to accomplish a task or a goal. According to Dalton E. McFarland, "***Motivation is the way in which urges, desires, aspirations, striving order needs direct, control or explain the behavior of a human being.***" The origin of the word *motivation* comes from the Latin word "motivus," which means "serving to move". Thus, motivation stands for movement.

Motivation of people involves four key areas of science and their application through the function of leadership: psychology—study of the human mind and mental status; sociology—study of behavior of individuals and groups in society; human behavior—how humans act and behave; and emotional intelligence—an individual leader's skill and ability to perceive, express, understand, reason, and regulate emotion.

Human behavior suggests the following:

People go where ..... *they are wanted*	Recruitment
People stay where ..... ***they are appreciated***	**Retention**
People excel when ..... ***they are motivated***	**Performance**

Have you ever stopped and reflected on exactly what motivates you? A prerequisite for any leader is to know what motivates him or her and to use positive motivation methods, techniques, and activities for his or her own self-motivation in his or her healthcare leadership role. Although many healthcare leaders have an innate motivation to manage and lead, all leaders will experience moments in their career when they must call on inspirational experiences, sayings, or beliefs to give them the motivation they need to address a difficult challenge; confront a difficult but necessary personnel issue; or tackle a conflict that can no longer be left unresolved.

What role does motivation play in the workplace? The role of motivational leadership is to develop and intensify in every member of the organization the desire to work hard, work efficiently, and perform at a high level to be effective. Leadership is motivating and inspiring others to work hard to achieve organizational goals; therefore, motivational leadership is central to leadership in general.

Leadership can be divided into two general categories: transactional leadership, which is leadership provided in daily activities, processes, procedures, and workflow, and transformational leadership, which generates awareness and acceptance of the group's purpose and mission and gets employees to see beyond their own needs and self-interests for the good of the team, organization, and patients and other customers served.

One point to ponder is this: a health service organization is always perfectly designed to produce the results it is producing. If it has quality problems, cost problems, or productivity problems, then the behaviors associated with these outcomes are being reinforced. This is not conjecture. This is the cold, hard reality of human behavior (*Leadership: Enhancing the Lessons of Experience*).

According to research, the number one reason people leave an organization is limited recognition and praise. The number one reason people stay with an organization is a promise of long-term employment (USA Today, February 10, 1998).

TABLE 10.1: Why People Leave an Organization

Limited recognition and praise	34%
Compensation	29%
Limited authority	13%
Personality conflicts	8%
Other	16%

TABLE 10.2: Why People Stay in an Organization

Promise of long-term employment	82%
Training and education support	78%
Hires/keeps hard-working people	76%
Encourages fun and collegiality	74%
Job evaluation based on innovation	72%

So, a key question for healthcare leaders to ponder is this: how can I motivate employees in a way that taps into the discretionary effort that every employee has to give? Management is getting work done through others. Therefore, healthcare managers are concerned with getting the greatest amount of effort and performance every employee has to give—individually and collectively as members of the healthcare team. Therefore, motivational leadership is concerned with the initiation, direction, and persistence of effort being made by employees. Initiation of effort is concerned with the choices people make about **how much effort** to put forth in their jobs. Direction of effort is concerned with the choices people make in deciding **where to put forth effort** in their jobs. Persistence of effort is concerned with the choices that people make about **how long they will put forth effort** in their jobs before reducing or eliminating those efforts.

Creating highly motivated and satisfied followers depends, most of all, on understanding others. As discussed in the beginning of this chapter, motivation involves the fields of psychology, sociology, human behavior, and emotional intelligence. Understanding people and what motivates them is clearly an important skill that any healthcare administrator must develop. Moreover, healthcare leaders should go out of their way to make sure people at all levels of the organization understand the "why" as it relates to decisions being made. Informing and educating others to better understand why policies, procedures and decisions are being implemented or made as they are in critical to gaining the understanding, acceptance and support an organization needs at all levels.

According to *Leadership: Enhancing The Lessons of Experience*, research shows that most people believe they could give as much as 15 to 20 percent more effort at work than they currently do or reduce their effort at work by 15 to 20 percent, and nobody, including their own boss, would notice the difference!

This is a startling point about how some managers just aren't paying attention to the work, effort, and performance of their employees and/or aren't acknowledging or recognizing their efforts.

The need to motivate caregivers and other employees in healthcare also includes physicians. According to a recent article in the USA Today, "***Nearly half of doctors report symptoms of burnout. The Mayo Clinic (Rochester, Minnesota) reports nearly 1 in 2 or almost 46% of the nation's doctors already suffer a symptom of burnout.***" Participants of an assessment of physician burnout completed a 22-item Maslach Burnout Inventory questionnaire, considered the gold standard for measuring burnout. Issues examined were emotional exhaustion, depersonalization (treating patients as objects rather than human beings), and low sense of personal accomplishment. The article goes on to say "***It's the physicians on the frontline of care who are at the greatest risk.***" Again, this startling point has implications for the quality of care and service that a physician may provide to his patients, as well as his productivity and longevity in the medical profession.

How relevant is motivational theory in its application in healthcare leadership today? Motivational theory is very relevant—maybe more critical than at any point in the history of healthcare. Motivational theories and concepts we will explore in the remainder of this chapter include the following:

- Pygmalion Effect
- Hawthorne Effect
- Need Theory
- Equity Theory
- Expectancy Theory
- Theory X and Y
- Reinforcement Theory
- Goal-Setting Theory
- Two-Factory Theory
- Empowerment
- Feedback

PYGMALION EFFECT

Robert Rosenthal, PhD, conducted empirical research in 1964 that set the stage for the identification of the motivational concept called the "Pygmalion effect," or Rosenthal effect, which involves the idea that expectations can bring about self-fulfilling prophecies.

The Pygmalion effect is what psychologists consider a form of self-fulfilling prophecy. It is a theory showing that people will often end up behaving in the way that others had expected them to when the person has been repeatedly exposed to others expectations about them. This effect can be both positive and negative. (http://www.youtube.com/watch?v=EjbL7zW-Wig)

In Dr. Rosenthal's classic 1964 study, elementary school teachers were told that, on the basis of psychological tests, some of their students were designated as "intellectual bloomers" or "late bloomers." Furthermore, even though they hadn't shown any academic success, those late bloomers were expected to bloom and show an intellectual growth spurt during the school year. In actuality, the students were randomly given the designation of intellectual bloomers. In a very short time, those teachers began to treat those children differently; those children began to think of themselves differently; and as a result, those children performed significantly better than the other students. These students were transformed by their teacher's positive expectations.

The Pygmalion effect has been documented to improve employee performance, as published on April 18, 2009 by Ronald E. Riggio, Ph.D. in Cutting-Edge Leadership 27 (Psychology Today) in an article titled "*Pygmalion Leadership: The Power of Positive Expectations.*"

As a leader, simply holding positive expectations about team members' performance can actually lead to better team performance. Research has clearly shown the power of holding positive expectations of others. In other words, we typically get the outcomes that we expect. This is what is known as the "self-fulfilling prophecy," or the "Pygmalion effect," named after George Bernard Shaw's play in which Professor Henry Higgins transforms a common flower seller, Eliza Doolittle, into a lady, because he believed that it would happen (you may be more likely to be more familiar with the musical version, *My Fair Lady*).

The power of the Pygmalion effect, first captured by psychologist Robert Rosenthal, in his study of elementary school children, has been well documented as a simple and effective way to boost performance in the classroom, the workplace, the military, and healthcare.

What are the implications for leading work groups? Tel Aviv University professor, Dov Eden, has demonstrated the Pygmalion effect in all sorts of work groups, across all sectors and industries. If supervisors or managers hold positive expectations about the performance of those they lead—for instance believing that they can solve a challenging problem—performance improves. On the other hand, if the leader holds negative expectations—expectations that the group will fail—it leads to performance declines (the dreaded Golem effect).

As Dov Eden says, **"it sounds so simple; it seems too good to be true."** A recent meta-analysis (a statistical analysis that combines the results of studies) found that Pygmalion leadership training was a very effective leadership development intervention.

As an employee, does it make a difference if your direct supervisor believes you are a high performer or a low performer? The answer in most cases is probably "Yes."

THE HAWTHORNE EFFECT

This phrase was coined in 1950 by Henry A. Landsberger when analyzing earlier experiments from 1924 to 1932 at the Hawthorne Works Plant outside of Chicago, Illinois. This plant was owned and operated by the Western Electric Company. Hawthorne Works had commissioned a number of different studies to see what the effects would be on worker productivity and performance. Researchers spent five years measuring how different variables affected group and individual productivity. Different variables were introduced into the work environment. Some of the variables were: giving 5-minute breaks and then changing to 10 minute breaks; providing food during breaks; shortening the workday by 30 minutes; and other similar variables. What came out of these different studies was the fact that worker productivity and performance improved in response to being observed. In other words, when managers and researchers paid attention to their employees, the productivity of those employees improved.

Although there was some debate—and even skepticism on the part of some researchers—about how the studies were conducted, or even the results thereof, the Hawthorne Effect has real, practical application for healthcare. It is important for healthcare leaders to pay attention to healthcare workers. Most healthcare workers want to have some kind of relationship with their management; know that the work they do is appreciated by management; and feel a sense of connection with management. Clearly, creating this type of working environment and positive relationship with employees takes healthcare leaders paying attention to the people who are providing the care and doing the work. And, recognizing employees for their hard work, efforts and contribution is a key part of the paying attention process.

Ken Stella states that he ***"Always tried to make sure that somebody close to that spouse [would know how hard the employee was working]. Surprisingly you'd have no idea how many times that individual would look back and say to me "I really appreciate that and I am glad you noticed it, or realized it." The spouse is coming home telling their partner "Man this is what I'm doing" and so now there's recognition." Ken goes on to say, "You can also do that sometimes through a written letter to the house addressed to the employee. Just a letter of commendation that says 'I haven't seen you but I want you to know I've been getting good reports that you are really working hard.' They might even show that to their kids and say "See what you get if you work hard in school."***

NEED THEORY

Need theory assumes that all people have basic needs, and leaders can motivate followers by helping them satisfy their needs. Abraham Maslow created the hierarchy of needs, a theory of psychological health predicated on filling innate human needs in priority, culminating with self-actualization. This theory suggests that human beings first work to satisfy lower order needs before higher order needs come into play.

In general, need theory suggests the following:

- People are motivated by unmet needs.
- Once a need is met, it no longer motivates.
- Lower order needs must first be met before higher order needs motivate.

David McClelland proposed a need theory that featured three dominant needs that underpin human behavior—the need for achievement, power, and affiliation. McClelland believed that the relative importance of each need varies among individuals and cultures.

Need theory suggests healthcare managers should first look to satisfy lower-order needs of the workforce, and then look toward opportunities to assist and support employees in satisfying higher-order needs. It also suggests that some things leaders might think are insignificant are actually important. A simple example of this is making refreshments conveniently available to employees in their work area. If an employee is thinking about getting a cup of coffee, water, or soft drink, but nothing is available or convenient, this can impact that employee's productivity as they may be more motivated by the basic need of thirst than the work they are performing.

EQUITY THEORY

Equity theory assumes that people value fairness in the leader–follower exchange relationship. In other words, employees will pay close attention to how they are treated, particularly in relationship to how others are treated around them. Equity theory suggests that employees are motivated when they perceive they are being treated fairly, particularly in comparison to others. Employees will make comparisons on a variety of factors, including the demands of the job; pay and benefits; application of policy; job opportunities, including tasks and assignments; and recognition, rewards, and promotions. Fair and equitable treatment of employees has both legal ramifications and practical application in regard to creating an environment that is motivating to employees. How are the different positions slotted on the company's pay grade, and does it accurately reflect the knowledge, skills, and abilities required to perform each respective job? Are policies and procedures being applied fairly and consistently? Are all employees being recognized fairly and consistently for their work and performance?

EXPECTANCY THEORY

Victor Vroom's expectancy theory is concerned with clarifying the links between what people do and the rewards or outcomes they will obtain as a result. This theory suggests that employee motivation is an outcome of how much an individual wants a reward (valence); the assessment of how likely the effort will lead to expected performance (expectancy); and the belief that the performance will lead to the reward (instrumentality). Expectancy theory assumes two things: motivated performance by an employee is the result of a conscious decision and choice that employee is making, and people do what they believe provides them the best, highest, or surest rewards. This theory suggests that employees are motivated when they believe their expectations will be met, the rewards for their work are viewed as attractive and desirable, they see a direct link between their effort on the job and the resulting performance or outcome, and they believe their own performance will result in the reward.

There are two different kinds of rewards. One kind of reward is an extrinsic reward, which is tangible, visible to others, and given to employees contingent on the performance of specific tasks, behaviors, assignments, or achievements. Extrinsic rewards are typically controlled and allocated by leaders. Examples of extrinsic rewards can include pay increases, bonuses, company car, bigger or nicer office, tickets to a movie or restaurant, and even a promotion. Organizations typically use extrinsic rewards as motivators. However, another motivational theory that will be discussed in this chapter is the two-factor theory. This theory suggests that extrinsic rewards would be classified as hygiene factors and not real motivators.

Another kind of reward is an intrinsic reward, which is a natural reward associated with performing a task, activity or assignment for its own sake. Many believe that serving others and the satisfaction of knowing you contributed to the betterment of someone's life is the type of intrinsic motivator that compelled most caregivers and other healthcare employees, including healthcare leaders, to get into healthcare. Examples of intrinsic rewards can include the feeling of gratification or satisfaction in doing a good job;

a sense of responsibility; the opportunity to do work that is interesting, challenging, and meaningful; and a sense of accomplishment. Again, the two-factor theory suggests that intrinsic rewards are the true motivators. Therefore, healthcare leaders should pay more attention to the intrinsic factors of the work employees do, as they are more motivating than those of an extrinsic nature.

REINFORCEMENT THEORY

Reinforcement theory explains motivation in terms of the antecedents and consequences of behavior. This theory is also referred to as behavioral modification theory. Many times, the delivery of healthcare services provides caregivers with the reinforcement that their work and efforts in caring for patients makes a difference. In general, reinforcement theory suggests that employee behaviors are a function of their consequences. A common belief in management that has been long-held by many in the field is to reinforce, recognize, and reward behavior that you want repeated. Moreover, don't let negative employee behaviors go by without being appropriately addressed. Why? Because negative employee behaviors that are tolerated and permitted are tacitly reinforced as acceptable and will, therefore, be repeated, as well.

Don't let negative employee behaviors go by without being appropriately addressed. Why? Because negative employee behaviors that are tolerated and permitted are tacitly reinforced as acceptable, and will, therefore, be repeated.

Ken Stella says that ***"You have to know when to be firm so a management team recognizes that you're serious. And you'll need to push a team to complete a project. There comes a time in all leadership when you have to realize it's time to love em', and you back it down a little bit. "***

Positive reinforcement strengthens the frequency of behavior that is desired through recognition, appreciation, and reward. Positive reinforcement is desirable at any level of healthcare leadership. Mr. Stella says ***"Let's say you are having a conversion of an accounting system, and everyone works from 6:00 pm on a Friday night until 6:00 am Monday morning converting to a new data processing system."*** You celebrate by "***having a party when it's done. There are those kinds of short term celebrations that you have as well.***"

GOAL-SETTING THEORY

Author Brian Tracy says that "***Goals are the fuel in the furnace of achievement.***" Goal-setting theory is concerned with setting goals and bolstering one's belief about their own ability for task accomplishment and goal achievement. Goal setting theory suggests that healthcare managers need to create an environment of active, ongoing goal-setting achievement. Providing frequent, specific, performance-related feedback from the manager to the employee is important. On an individual employee level, management by objectives, or MBO, is a proven method to establish the development of individual employee goals, in concert with the employee's supervisor or manager, and the development of action steps and tactics to achieve them. MBO has been proven to work and is particularly applicable in a health service organization.

In addition, the use of a balance/corporate scorecard, department-specific objectives, and other key performance indicators have proven to be quite useful in creating both focus and alignment in a health service organization and depicting what strong performance and success look like when attained in a quantifiable way.

Sam Odle states that ***"I used different models throughout my career .... All of them were [some type of] management by objectives. Management by Objectives (MBO) is a fundamental tool that we define what it is that we are going to try and accomplish; tactics that outline what we're going to do; so we don't just accidentally get through the year. There are things we are going to try and accomplish, and there are things that are important to the company. Especially in organizations where there is a lot of autonomy, you have to make sure those MBO's are aligned. That means you have to cascade them from the top. Senior management must decide what are the priorities for the organization: those five or six important areas of emphasis that we want everyone to focus on. Then you cascade down to [determine] how does each leader, each department or each unit, by its objectives help accomplish the overall area of emphasis or pillar? Eventually you can cascade it down to the individual employee level. What does it mean to be employee? If MBO is just an isolated [activity], it [probably] won't get you good performance at all—it may get you confusion." Senior managers must make sure there is alignment around the corporate areas of priority at all levels in the organization. We have to make sure "everybody is rowing the boat in the same direction."***

Setting goals is a form of planning and, typically, includes the creation of tactics or action steps to achieve the desired goal. When setting goals, healthcare leaders should consider the use of SMART goals. SMART is an acronym and stands for specific, measurable, attainable, realistic, and timely or time-specific goals. SMART goals are appropriate for corporate goals, department or service goals, and individual goals.

TWO-FACTOR/HYGIENE THEORY

Established by Frederick Herzberg, this theory is known by two different names: the two-factor theory or the hygiene theory. This theory provides direction on how to bolster employee motivation satisfaction through the use of motivators, and how to minimize employee demotivation and dissatisfaction through the use of hygiene factors. Hygiene factors relate to the environment in which an employee performs his job, including pay and benefits. Although hygiene factors are not strong contributors to job satisfaction, they can significantly contribute to job dissatisfaction if they are perceived negatively. Motivation factors, on the other hand, relate to the nature of the work itself and the way the employee performs his job. Motivation factors include interesting and challenging work that provides fulfillment and satisfaction that an employee receives from doing the work itself. If the motivational factors are strong, employees will be motivated to work hard and give their best.

Herzberg theorized that job satisfaction and job dissatisfaction act independently of each other. Moreover, contributors to job satisfaction are necessary in order to motivate an employee to higher levels of performance.

THEORY X AND Y

Douglas McGregor formulated two assumptions about workers. Theory X suggests that employees naturally dislike work and responsibility and must be controlled. Theory Y suggests that employees seek responsibility and will be self-directed and committed if the job is satisfying. It has long been believed that theory Y is more pertinent and applicable in managing people in today's modern society. Although this theory may not be universally applied throughout the world of healthcare management, it has relevance, particularly as it relates to a leader's own belief about employees and his own style of leadership. For example, a healthcare leader who believes in theory Y is much more apt to provide freedom and autonomy that generates a sense of engagement and empowerment with employees in the workplace.

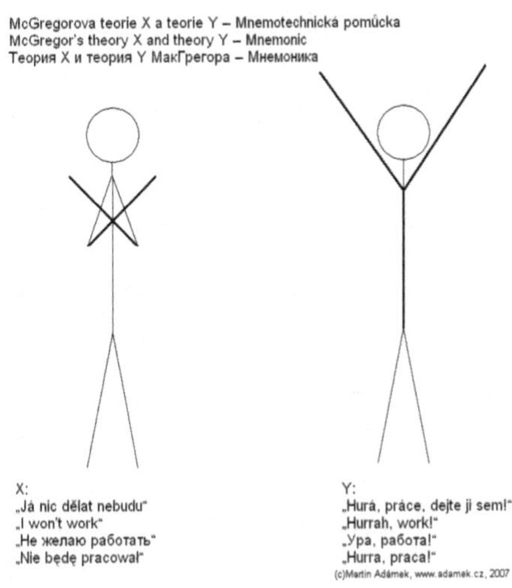
McGregorova teorie X a teorie Y – Mnemotechnická pomůcka
McGregor's theory X and theory Y – Mnemonic
Теория X и теория Y МакГрегора – Мнемоника
X:
„Já nic dělat nebudu"
„I won't work"
„Не желаю работать"
„Nie będę pracował"
Y:
„Hurá, práce, dejte ji sem!"
„Hurrah, work!"
„Ура, работа!"
„Hurra, praca!"
(c)Martin Adámek, www.adamek.cz, 2007

FIGURE 10.2

EMPOWERMENT

Empowerment is a term often used to signify the amount of autonomy or control employees feel towards their work and the work environment. Empowerment is a situational approach having two components: delegating authority and decision-making to the lowest level possible, and allocating and equipping employees with the knowledge, skills, and resources necessary to make and execute the decisions. Empowerment is creating feelings of intrinsic motivation in which employees perceive their work to have impact and meaning and perceive themselves to be competent and capable of self-determination. Empowerment is about giving employees autonomy and latitude in order to increase their level of motivation to work. Empowerment requires managers to look for opportunities to restructure work processes, procedures, and even schedules to provide employees with more latitude with their own work. Moreover, empowerment requires healthcare leaders to continually provide employees with the support and resources they need.

> **Empowerment is creating feelings of intrinsic motivation in which employees perceive their work to have impact and meaning and perceive themselves to be competent and capable of self-determination.**

Frederick Herzberg said ***"If you don't want people to have Mickey Mouse attitudes, then don't give them Mickey Mouse work."*** Sam Odle states that healthcare managers should ***"Give people assignments that stretch their abilities. People only stay in that box if you keep them in that box: you say 'they're really good at that and that's all they can do.' In 80% of the cases, if you give them a chance to get outside of that box—if they are performing well in that box—they will perform well outside the box too. That doesn't mean they won't make mistakes, that they won't stumble, and you'll need to be there to help them understand what things they could do differently to be successful. But constantly giving people the opportunity to get outside the box they're in today, as far as their responsibilities, that is the encouraging thing. Talk is one thing, but actually giving them the opportunity to do the work is more powerful. How you get the results is really important."***

FEEDBACK

Constructive feedback is that which is intended to be helpful, corrective, and/or encouraging. Most employees need some level of encouragement on a routine or periodic basis to help reaffirm the work they are doing and the difference they are making. When managers provide positive feedback and encourage their employees, they are providing the type of support and affirmation that inspires confidence and motivates employees to give their best. Feedback can be both positive and negative. Constructive feedback is typically positive in nature, whereas destructive feedback is negative without any intention of being helpful and almost always causes a negative or defensive reaction in the recipient. Constructive or positive feedback must be timely in order to have the desired impact. For example, an annual performance review is a form of feedback; however, this type of feedback should be a summary of what has already been discussed between the manager and the employee throughout the year.

Judy Monroe, MD says ***"Feedback is the breakfast of champions. I love that quote because I learned long ago when I was the [family practice] residency program director [at St. Vincent's Hospital in Indianapolis, Indiana,] when I went to a conference where they made the distinction between feedback and evaluation. They said the annual evaluation that's really long-term, looking back to see if they met their goals and objectives. Feedback is where the gold is. So if feedback is the breakfast of champions, and you want a champion team, feedback has to be timely—on the spot—because otherwise it becomes an evaluation and you've lost the moment. I am a big believer in the value of feedback. If it's done correctly, then it is a very powerful tool for employee engagement."***

Dr. Monroe goes on to say ***"I don't know if there is anything more powerful than a leader in a top leadership role to admit when they are wrong: humble themselves. That is incredibly powerful. Or [for a leader] to change their own behavior when it hasn't been as productive as it could be. People are very forgiving. It really builds the trust in the leader. "***

Motivating the workforce is really about employee engagement. Employee engagement is the employee's emotional and cognitive motivation, self-efficacy to perform the job, perceived clarity of the organization's vision and the employees specific role in that vision, and the belief employee has the resources to get the job done.

MOTIVATIONAL THEORY	MANAGERS SHOULD . . .
Pygmalion Effect	• Set high but reasonable expectations for self and others. • Outwardly demonstrate trust, confidence and belief in employees. • Reinforce expectations and beliefs about accomplishments that can be achieved.
Hawthorne Effect	• Pay attention to your employees. • Show appreciation to employees for the work they do. • Treat employees like volunteers. • Do not take employees for granted! • Use Management by Walking Around to be visible with employees.
Need Theory	• Ask employees about their needs. • Satisfy lower order needs first. • Expect employee needs to change. • Create opportunities for employee's to satisfy higher-order needs.
Equity Theory	• Validate that decision-making, policies, procedures, etc. are fair and equitable. • Continually monitor the perception of equity. • Correct perceived inequities in the work environment.
Expectancy Theory	• Systematically discover what employees expect from their jobs. • Link rewards to performance. • Set high but attainable performance standards. • Link opportunities to performance.
Reinforcement Theory	• Identify, measure, and evaluate critical performance-related behaviors. • Don't reinforce undesired behaviors. • Administer behavioral consequences when appropriate. • Reinforce desired behaviors. • Provide positive feedback and affirmation to others as appropriate.
Goal-Setting Theory	• Create S.M.A.R.T goals through employee collaboration. • Foster understanding and acceptance of organizational goals through communication. • Use management by objectives. (MBO) • Provide frequent, specific, clear, performance-related feedback. • Continually reinforce goals and their importance.
Two-Factor Theory	• Eliminate dissatisfiers. • Promote motivators/satisfiers. • Look for ways to help foster the growth, development, and performance of employees. • Focus on intrinsic rewards with the work itself.
Theory X & Y	• Identify employees who take initiative, and are responsible and motivated—provide them with autonomy • Identify employees who don't take initiative, appear unmotivated or not very responsible—provide them with greater structure, direction and accountability
Empowerment	• Delegate projects from the beginning and hold employees accountable for results. • Provide freedom and autonomy for employee innovation. • Organize and delegate key functions to self-directed work teams. • Conduct periodic employee meetings: solicit input and implement good ideas. Complete circle of communication. • Treat employees like volunteers.
Feedback	• Continually provide feedback to employees. • Provide positive and negative feedback. • Seek feedback from others on your own performance. • Provide specific, behavior/performance-related feedback.

WHAT LEADERSHIP INTANGIBLES CAN BE USED IN MOTIVATING OTHERS?

Listen to understand needs and expectations.
Delegate to empower others.
Recognize effort and provide positive feedback.
Model behavior you want emulated.
Communicate expectations and encouragement.
Trust employees with key business functions.
Provide opportunities for employees to grow.
Encourage employees to reach their potential.

DISCUSSION QUESTIONS

1. What is motivation?
2. Describe how motivation of employees in a hospital or health service organization matters?
3. How can a healthcare leader motivate employees?
4. What role does motivation play in the workplace?
5. How relevant is motivational theory in its application in healthcare today?
6. Identify one motivational theory and how it can be applied in a healthcare setting.
7. What leadership intangibles can be used in motivating others?
8. What does it mean for employees to be engaged?
9. What is Management By Objectives, and what motivational theory does it support?
10. What is the number one reason people leave an organization?

FIGURE CREDITS

Figure 10.1: U.S. Navy, "Navy Tug-of-War," http://commons.wikimedia.org/wiki/File:US_Navy_030329-N-1512S-008_Yeoman_2nd_Class_Christopher_Chatman_from_Baton_Rouge,_La.,_leads_the_ship%5Ersquo,s_Administrative_Office_Tug-of-War_team.jpg. Copyright in the Public Domain.
Figure 10.2: Copyright © Martin Adámek (CC by 3.0) at http://commons.wikimedia.org/wiki/File:McgregorXY-languages.gif.

11

Fostering a Culture of Accountability

The importance of accountability to be present at all levels of a health service organization is more important today than ever before. The performance expectations that all stakeholders have for a health service organization's performance has and will continue to rise in the future. Consumerism towards the purchase of healthcare services is vibrant and continues to grow as consumers have an increasing number of choices for their healthcare. Growing consumer expectations are for improved, more personable service; higher-quality and better clinical outcomes; a safer environment of care and improved patient safety; use of more effective medicines, procedures, and technologies; and even the expectation that health service organizations need to work harder to reduce their own costs of operations and charges to consumers at the same time. How can these growing consumer and stakeholder expectations be met? Only through an organizational culture that fosters a heightened level of accountability within the health service organization for effort and performance will these growing expectations be met.

OBJECTIVES

1. Appreciate the increasing mandate in healthcare for accountability and understand the vital role accountability plays in producing organizational results and performance.
2. Learn about how healthcare leaders can foster accountability.
3. Discover 10 characteristics that are present in healthcare organizations that have strong cultures of accountability.

David Handel describes the healthcare environment this way: ***"I've never seen the [healthcare] environment where it's more clear what you need to do to be successful as an organization, nor is it more difficult to actually do those things. I can enumerate what a healthcare organization needs to do in just a couple of minutes. Some of those things we've been talking about, in my career, for 40 years. If it was really easy to do we would have done it a long time ago. The other thing that is important is being open to change. Things are going to be a lot different in the future. Most of us will have an inkling of what it [the future] will be. But as you've seen in your career, it's never exactly what you think."***

Mr. Handel goes on to say ***"I can't think of many industries where you can help as many people, or have an impact on as many people, as you can in healthcare. Obviously it is the patients and their families, but it is the staff, and also healthcare has a big impact on communities."***

Accountability in healthcare is no longer optional. The days when healthcare leaders really didn't have to hold their employees, physicians, or even themselves accountable for effort, results, and performance are gone. The expectations—even demands—of all stakeholders continue to increase as it relates to the results and performance of hospitals and other health service organizations. Patients, regulators, payers, visitors, employees, physicians, all internal and external stakeholders want more and better results and performance and expect more and better results and performance. At the same time, the financial incentives under healthcare reform are changing to demand more, as well. In short, the changing environment of healthcare demands accountability—at all levels in healthcare and in healthcare organizations.

Fostering can be defined as encouraging the development of something. Culture is the shared values, beliefs, and attitudes within an organization—or how things are done. Accountability is being responsible for something, such as an action, effort, result, or outcome. Healthcare leaders must encourage the development of a culture that is based on accountability.

Where does a healthcare leader begin in his efforts to foster a culture of accountability? Ken Stella suggests that it starts with the organizational culture and creating the type of family environment that people know you, as a leader, care about them and know what is expected. Ken talks about being an Italian and that "***Family is very much a theme with Italians. One of the things that in my leadership I've always tried to do is create an environment for the staff that I am working with and for, of family. [As a hospital CEO I]*** *really wanted to create this environment for the people that they could be proud of their family—the hospital. They could be proud of the part they played, the role they played, within that family. And wanted them to understand they had a responsibility as part of the family. As an undergraduate [student] I was really going to be a coach. Because of that undergraduate experience of learning, I've always tried to get the highest potential out of a manager. I've always tried to get the highest potential out of a vice president. I've always tried to get people to push themselves and reach a little further. Real defining moments for me have been when others that I have coached or had as part of the family—have achieved. Their achievements have made me feel good. In turn, many of their achievement have made me look good. So I owe many, many thanks to many, many people that have been associated with me and I've been associated with them, because they've helped my career by virtue of my being involved with them."*

Management is getting work done through others. Leadership is motivating and inspiring others to work hard and achieve organizational goals. It, therefore, stands to reason that a healthcare leader's job as a manager and leader is to foster accountability for organizational performance, that is, getting the highest level of effort, productivity, and performance out of each individual employee, each work team, and each department.

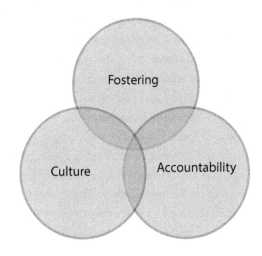

FIGURE 11.1 Fostering Culture Accountability

> **A healthcare leader's job as a manager and leader is to foster accountability for organizational performance, that is, getting the highest level of effort, productivity, and performance out of each individual employee, each work team, and each department.**

Look at a typical healthcare organization's organizational development and business planning cycle. The process begins with an assessment of the purpose of the organization and its vision, followed by how it best fits into the environment and community it serves; what strategies, tactics, and resources are needed to best fulfill the mission, vision, and goals; implementation of actions plans to pursue the mission, vision, and strategies; and a culture of accountability to foster and guide the work and efforts to produce the desired results and performance.

ACCOUNTABILITY

Accountability is essential to performance. Accountability includes the Board of Directors holding management accountable. Accountability includes a leader being self-accountable. Accountability includes leaders holding other leaders accountable. Accountability includes leaders holding employees accountable. So, what is accountability about at its core? Effort and performance.

Ken Stella talks about ***"The way I held people accountable was not to keep them in limbo or hide what they were going to be evaluated on. You are going to be evaluated on the plan that you and I work out for yourself. Your job will be to implement it, but if you need help I'll help you. Then we both will evaluate how well the plan got implemented. And the plan could be anything. The plan could have been in the next 18 months I am going to become an LPN. What are the steps necessary: let's lay them out. Where do you need assistance? My sense of holding people accountable is to pick one or two items. Too many times I think we overload. You have to ratchet it down and say 'these are things I'm really going to look at.'"***

Ex-NFL coach and ESPN football analyst Herm Edwards says that, in football, "***You're either coaching it, or you're letting it happen.***" The same can be said about healthcare leaders and their management: healthcare leaders are either managing it, or they're letting it happen. This is a key point about managing people and processes and about accountability. You are either paying attention to both the effort being made and respective performance being achieved or you aren't. If you aren't paying attention to these, then you are letting it happen. Either way, as a healthcare leader, you are still accountable. Now this is not an endorsement of a micromanagement style—quite the contrary. However, it is a statement saying that fostering accountability is about paying attention to both effort and performance.

Accountability is about a healthcare leader's intention to take action, make good things happen, and get work done through others (management) by motivating and inspiring them to work hard to achieve organizational goals (leadership). It is also about taking responsibility, being responsible, and holding yourself and others accountable for effort and performance. It's not about blaming and complaining about what is happening, but putting forth the effort to make things right. The words and actions of a healthcare leader that has good intentions and takes the responsibility for himself and others is motivating and inspiring. In most cases, employees expect and want to be held accountable. In most cases, employees are de-motivated when neither they nor other employees are held accountable. This situation looks and feels a lot like leadership doesn't care about effort or performance.

A healthcare leader's actions can be seen by others in the organization, and those actions paint the picture in the minds of everyone watching as to his leadership style and character. A healthcare leader's words can be heard by others in the organization, and those words form sounds and impressions in the minds of everyone listening as to his leadership style and character. But, a healthcare leader's actions and words do even more than that. They help create the organizational culture that cascades throughout, providing unwritten guidance, direction, motivation, expectations, and rules. Leaders set the example—with or without intention to do so. Leaders model the way for others to follow. The organizational culture is not what the organization says it does, but what it actually does. An example of this is with regard to change and innovation. Some healthcare leaders talk about promoting change and innovation within their organizations; however, the organizational culture doesn't promote or foster this. . Sometimes leaders talk about wanting to support innovation, but their actions say they aren't willing to. When this occurs, employees are usually quick to figure out this "gap" in leadership credibility. The point here is the culture is what is done, not what leaders say is done. The organizational culture is the invisible hand that is always at work; structuring expectations, guiding actions and behaviors, and encouraging or stymieing effort—depending on the culture. What employee wants to offer his ideas and suggestions for improvements—even when those ideas and suggestions are asked for by management—when he knows those ideas and suggestions won't be given any thought or consideration by management and the request is just "lip service?"

The organizational culture is the invisible hand that is always at work; structuring expectations, guiding actions and behaviors, and encouraging or stymieing effort—depending on the culture.

There are four basic functions of management: planning, organizing, leading, and controlling. Accountability is embedded in the management function of controlling. Controlling is measuring performance and taking action to ensure desired results. Control is a process of establishing standards to achieve organizational goals, comparing actual performance against the standards, and taking corrective action when necessary.

There are two basic requirements of accountability: paying attention to effort and performance with repetition and consistency. Healthcare leaders must pay attention to the effort and performance each subordinate gives and monitor that effort and performance for repetition and consistency. This is the management function of controlling. Moreover, it is the leader's job to provide whatever resources, support, training, coaching, or insight the employee needs in order to be effective in meeting his objectives in an efficient manner. However, a healthcare leader's first job is to provide clarity around the objective: what it is, what it means, why it is important to patients, the department, the organization, co-workers, etc. In chapter 11, Sam Odle is quoted as saying "***Leaders need to make sure they are really clear on whatever the problem or opportunities are they are working on.***" Mr. Odle goes on to say "***It is important that employees clearly understand what the objective is, and why it is important. Clarity and understanding are necessary to engender employee effort and performance on a consistent basis.***"

When asked how he fostered accountability with his staff, Mr. Odle stated "***Throughout my career there were different systems, but all of them were [based upon] Management by Objectives models. Sometimes we called them different things. Making the objectives really clear; letting the person participate in setting the objectives; and then regular intervals of reporting on those objectives. Where the objectives were not being achieved, trying to help the person with tactics or ways they could be achieved. Most of the time if the objectives are clear, and you support the person with suggestions or ideas when they get stumped—and if you're stumped reach out to somebody else to help both of you to figure out a way to do it—about 95 percent of the time, the person wants to do the work and they do it: that's how***

you develop that accountability. But there are sometimes when the person either does not have the skills, or isn't really interested in doing the work. They may want the position but they really aren't interested in doing the work. In those situations I think you have to counsel them out of the organization and let them try something else."

According to Chuck Williams in the book *Effective Management*, there is a 97 percent chance that companies that use MBO will outperform those that don't. MBO works!

LEADERS MODEL THE WAY

Leaders set the example by modeling the way. However, whether leaders are aware they are setting the example and modeling the way or not—they are. Employees are generally aware of the actions and behaviors of their leaders, which sets the expectations for employees about what is expected, how things are actually supposed to be done, and how they, in turn, should behave. For example, if a hospital leader is walking down the hallway in the hospital and walks right past a large piece of paper or trash lying on the floor without picking it up, a statement has been made without any words being spoken: it is acceptable for employees to ignore paper or trash lying in the hallway and not pick up the debris. That is somebody else's job.

If healthcare leaders don't hold themselves accountable for effort and performance and if healthcare leaders don't consistently hold employees accountable for effort and performance, the employees will probably perceive the leader as not believing that accountability is important. If the leader doesn't believe accountability is important, then why should an employee worry about being accountable?

When asked about leading by example or modeling the way and the role it plays in a healthcare organization, Judy Monroe, MD, states "***That one ranks up there at the top. I think that's really powerful.***" Dr. Monroe tells about when she was "***listening to a speaker one time talking about their employees.***" The speaker told a story about a hospital President that had just started at the hospital. ***"The speaker had gotten up in front of the employees and [asked the employees] how many of you have taken the new President home with you? We all had to laugh because when you have a new leader, that new leader is being discussed over the dinner table; that new leader is being discussed over drinks; that new leader is being discussed in lots and lots of circles. People are watching. They are clearly watching. And if the leader does model the way, that's the way you change culture. Here at CDC I, in many ways, was brought in to this particular office to impact change across the agency and out in the field. We were very aware of [the fact] this is what we needed to do: modeling the way.***

"When I first got to CDC, early on there were some communication products we put out that were very atypical for CDC. My staff was pretty nervous. CDC is a scientific organization and for good cause they are very deliberate and things can take a long time sometimes to get done. This is one that I knew it was the right thing. I said we've got to do it. And the result of that is not only did we show the agency a new way of communicating, but also then developed a reputation for getting things done. Folks in the office kind of wear that as a badge of honor. They like being part of an office that is known for getting things done. That came with modeling the way showing this is the way to do it. Dr. Freedon is the leader

of CDC and he bikes to work; he models the way for healthy lifestyles; he climbs 12 flights of stairs [everyday]; he lets people know about his vacations where he biked a hundred miles a day; those kinds of things are a very powerful message."

What is accountability about? Accountability is about creating clear expectations on an individual employee level for things like work effort; quality of work; adherence to policy, procedure, and protocol; compliance; behaviors; values; performance; recognition and reward; and negative consequences. But don't confuse accountability with innovation. Compliance, structure, monitoring, and control must be balanced with freedom, autonomy, and experimentation in order to promote innovation. Moreover, leaders must demonstrate tolerance for failure when genuine and sincere effort is made in the spirit of innovation; otherwise, future innovation will be quashed at the first occurrence when things don't work as planned.

Much of a top healthcare leader's job is to build the organizational culture. Remember the words of ex-NFL coach Herm Edwards: "***You're either coaching it, or you're letting it happen.***" This applies to a healthcare organization's culture and leadership. Leaders are either driving the organizational culture to foster accountability or they are just letting it happen. Typically the "default" position—or just letting it happen—results in a culture dramatically lacking the necessary accountability for performance to thrive and prosper.

10 CHARACTERISTICS OF AN ORGANIZATIONAL CULTURE OF ACCOUNTABILITY

Here are 10 characteristics for a culture of accountability in any healthcare organization, or accountability works best when . . .

1. It permeates the organization at all levels
2. It becomes part of the organizational culture
3. It's hardwired through policies, procedures, practices, and human resource systems
4. It's modeled by the CEO and senior managers
5. It's transparent and discussed regularly
6. It's consistent throughout the organization
7. It's sustainable through turnover and transition
8. Consequences are negative when appropriate, as well as positive
9. The culture fosters learning, creativity and innovation
10. It's spoken as a common language within the organization

Accountability works best when it permeates the organization at all levels—from senior management to middle management to front-line supervisors and employees. When accountability doesn't exist at a certain level of the organization, then effort and performance will break down. This results in a lack of accountability being passed down throughout the chain of command.

As mentioned in this chapter already, accountability either is part of the organizational culture of how things are done, or it isn't.

Hardwiring accountability through policies, procedures, practices, and human resource systems helps to provide the necessary structure, organization, tools, and working conditions for accountability to exist and flourish within the healthcare organization's operations. Healthcare organizations should audit their policies, procedures, practices, and human resource systems to be sure they adequately provide the tools for accountability to be fostered by management.

When accountability is modeled by the CEO and senior managers, it is a powerful message of what is expected. The opposite is true, as well.

Transparency around accountability means it is discussed regularly and openly at all levels. Expectations about accountability are clear. Accountability practices are assessed and monitored by management—primarily on an informal basis—and changes are made for improvement and enhancement, as needed.

Accountability practices are consistently applied by top, middle, and front-line management so that employees at all levels, in all departments, services, and functions experience the same level of accountability. One key point here involves equity theory. Employees will evaluate and assess accountability practices used towards them and their own work effort and performance compared to that of others and ask the question: is it equitable or fair? As an employee, am I being treated fairly and consistently with other employees in relation to accountability? If employee's answer "No" to these types of questions, they perceive inequitable treatment regarding accountability and will feel unfairly treated, mistreated, or even discriminated against. This is not a good situation from several standpoints, including from a legal standpoint and its impact on morale, engagement, productivity, and performance.

Accountability should remain constant and endure the turnover and transition that is inevitable in all organizations. In general, the average length of service for employees working in the same organization has dropped in healthcare, similarly to what has been experienced in other industries. Historically, it was not uncommon for some healthcare employees to work in the same organization for most of their career. Today, in the era of layoffs, downsizing, mergers and acquisitions, the employment relationship has been altered.

Under reinforcement theory, behavior is said to be a function of its consequences. Behaviors followed by positive consequences will occur more frequently, and behaviors followed by negative consequences, or not followed by positive consequences, will occur less frequently. Therefore, accountability must be accompanied by both positive and negative consequences, including reinforcement, as appropriate, for the effort and performance that is generated. For example, if the supervisor and subordinate discuss and agree upon an action plan and a timeframe for the subordinate to complete an important task, and the subordinate doesn't take any action towards completion of the task by the deadline, then some consequence may be appropriate in this situation. The consequence might be anything, from discussion between the supervisor and subordinate with the supervisor asking for an explanation of why no action was taken, a verbal warning issued or other appropriate disciplinary action, or even assignment or re-assignment to other jobs or tasks, if appropriate. If the employee successfully completes the jointly agreed–upon important task by the deadline, then positive reinforcement by the supervisor may be in order. Reinforcement is the process of changing behavior or encouraging it to be repeated by changing the consequences that follow behavior. Positive reinforcement is reinforcement that strengthens behavior by following behaviors with desirable consequences. Positive reinforcement can also assist in motivating the subordinate to persist in his or her efforts. Persistence of effort is about the choices that people make about how long they will put forth effort in their jobs before reducing or eliminating those efforts.

The organizational culture is the invisible hand that is always at work. It structures expectations: what employees believe is expected of them. It also structures expectations about what consequences will be realized or experienced from a given level of employee effort or performance. When an organization is considered a "learning" organization, it is where leader's promote and foster learning and the sharing of knowledge at all levels of the organization through a variety of ways, including on-site training and education sessions; informal coaching and mentoring; seminars and conferences; formal educational programs; and an ongoing scanning or search for best practices, methods, and techniques in both clinical and non-clinical areas. Learning organizations are also typically organizations that embrace innovation. Many times, this looks like research and development striving to discover or learn new ways, using new technologies and new methods, to improve results and performance.

Leadership teams that foster accountability at all levels in their organization speak and promote a common language and style of leadership and work together as a team to consistently promote accountability and what is important. Accountability is discussed on an ongoing basis, and it is monitored and assessed for consistency. Changes are made when gaps and inconsistencies of accountability are identified.

Leaders must also hold themselves accountable in order to demonstrate credibility for accountability through leading by example.

Sam Odle says that ***"One of the traits of a really great organization is that leaders hold themselves accountable and leaders hold others accountable for their performance as well. That comes from making sure the metrics of success around those objectives are real clear. If the objectives are real clear, people want to be successful. But the organizations that struggle are those (in which) the metrics aren't clear. [For example,] we all are going to do better this year. Well what's better? You have to make it real clear. Because if it's not, then people will [be] out there doing things they think are the right things to make it better, but you don't have a common understanding of the objectives and the metrics."***

LEADERS ADMIT WHEN THEY ARE WRONG

Judy Monroe, MD states that ***"I don't know that there is anything more powerful than a leader in a top leadership role to admit when they're wrong and humble themselves. That's incredibly powerful. Or to change their own behavior when it hasn't been as productive as it could be. When I see leaders do that, people are very forgiving. If a leader has started down a path that's not very productive, and could be the demise of the leader either has folks around them of wise enough to alter that behavior; people are not just forgiving but I think that really builds trust in the leader."***

Fostering accountability also requires leaders to be very clear about expectations on an individual employee level for work effort; quality of work; adherence to policy, procedure, and protocols; regulatory compliance; value-based behaviors in line with organizational values; performance; recognition and reward; and negative consequences.

SITUATIONAL AND PATH–GOAL LEADERSHIP

Situational leadership is a contingency leadership theory that states leaders need to adjust their leadership style to match followers' readiness. Worker readiness is the ability and willingness to take responsibility for directing one's own behavior at work. Worker readiness consists of job readiness or the amount of knowledge, skill, ability, and experience an employee has to perform his or her job. Psychological readiness is the self-confidence and motivation an employee has to perform his or her job.

Path—goal leadership is a contingency theory of leadership based on the expectancy theory of motivation that relates several leadership styles to specific employee and situational contingencies. This model highlights four leadership styles and several contingency factors:

1. **Directive Leadership**—A leadership style in which the leader lets employees know precisely what is expected of them, gives them specific guidelines for performing tasks, schedules work, sets standards of performance, and makes sure that people follow standard rules and regulations.
2. **Supportive Leadership**—A leadership style in which the leader is friendly and approachable, shows concern for employees and their welfare, treats them as equals, and creates a friendly climate.
3. **Participative Leadership**—A leadership style in which the leader consults with employees for their suggestions and input before making decisions.
4. **Achievement-Oriented Leadership**—A leadership style in which the leader sets challenging goals, has high expectations of employees, and displays confidence that employees will assume responsibility and put forth extraordinary effort.

LEADING WITH QUESTIONS

Leading with questions is a contingency theory of leadership where the leader fosters discussion with an employee by asking appropriate and insightful questions to lead the conversation, rather than making comments or statements. Leading with questions is appropriate when the leader wants to solicit thoughts, opinions, comments, perspective, insight, or even self-awareness on the part of the employee. An example of when to use this technique would be when the employee's effort or performance isn't meeting the minimum acceptable standards. In this instance, the leader's objective might be to get the employee to acknowledge his or her lack of acceptable effort and performance, identify possible reasons, and identify possible solutions and commit to taking corrective action to get back on track. In a private conversation with the employee the supervisor might ask "***How do you feel your effort and performance has been lately? Has your effort and performance been meeting a level that is acceptable and what is expected and required?***" If the employee doesn't acknowledge they haven't been meeting acceptable standards of performance, the leader might then ask ***"Has your effort and performance remained constant and at the same level over the past year"?*** If the employee still doesn't acknowledge the drop in performance, the leader might ask the employee to ***"Describe the effort and performance that is expected in your position."*** The point here is to get the employee talking by asking questions that will lead the employee to acknowledge his or her effort and performance might have dropped off, so the conversation can then be directed towards what steps the employee can take to get back on track.

Leading with questions can be a powerful technique, if used wisely and appropriately by a healthcare leader. Leading with questions can:

- Solicit the employee's own perspective, expectations, and understanding.
- Be seen as less "bossy" and dictatorial by the employee.
- Promote employee engagement and emotional ownership for their performance.
- Help get the employee's acknowledgement of the situation and even verbal commitment.
- Promote a respectful conversation with an employee during a difficult, crucial conversation.
- Promote clear understanding.
- Promote the employee taking ownership for changing, as people don't typically argue with themselves if they acknowledge the situation and offer possible solutions.

A TRAGIC STORY OF NO ACCOUNTABILITY

The provision of healthcare services can make the difference of life, death, morbidity, and quality of life. Patient safety has increasingly received national attention and scrutiny, particularly since the publishing of the report from the Institute of Medicine (IOM) in 1999 entitled *To Err is Human*. In this report, research was published based upon two prior studies projecting that up to 100,000 patients die each year in hospitals in the U.S. from preventable mistakes. Patient safety in U.S. hospitals today is better than ever in the history of U.S. healthcare, in large part because of the IOM report and the attention it brought to the hospital industry's need to improve patient safety.

The story of Orville Lynn Majors, LPN, and Vermillion County Hospital in Clinton, Indiana, is a tragic story of what can happen when there is an absence of accountability that emanates from the top. This story, which received national attention at the time, took place in a small, rural, Indiana hospital in the early 1980s. Orville Lynn Majors was a licensed practical nurse (LPN) who worked in the hospital's intensive care unit (ICU). The hospital, after running a report that conclusively identified a significant number of deaths in the hospital's ICU, reported the problem to the Indiana State Police. Subsequently, it then became local and then national news, and a firestorm then occurred within the hospital and the small community.

The following story is provided first-hand by Marilyn Custer-Mitchell, the hospital administrator brought in after the horrible story unfolded at Vermillion County Hospital with Orville Lynn Majors, LPN.

BACKGROUND

Mrs. Custer-Mitchell states that, "Vermillion County Hospital, a small hospital back before there was the critical access hospital program or that it was even an option. [The hospital was] in trouble and struggling financially. The hospital had an LPN who was accused at that time of killing several patients, maybe six or seven at the time. [His name was] Orville Lynn Majors. Internally, what I found out later, was they thought something was wrong; they thought something was a problem, and they were doing an investigation. The CEO had asked the Director of Nursing (DON) to investigate."

When asked what prompted the investigation, Marilyn stated *"What we were told by employees, after the fact, was that when a code blue was called employees would say 'Oh, Lynn must be working today.' There was the feeling that Lynn was always around when people were dying."*

NOBODY'S RUN THE REPORT

"The CEO (at the time) had asked somebody in nursing to run a report, or do this study, to determine what nurses—staff person by staff person—were working on each shift when the hospital experienced a patient death to see if there were any trends. The first person [who was assigned the task of running the report or doing the study] didn't want to do it. The DON at the time—a wonderful lady—but if someone didn't want to do something she would say 'OK, don't worry about it.' She usually jumped in and did it. Well [in this situation] she [the DON] didn't do it either. Then the person who was supposed to run the report went on maternity leave, and someone else was going to do it during the maternity leave. She was gone three months on maternity leave and the report wasn't run because they decided to wait until the maternity leave was over and that person was back. So it went probably six months [of time] where this study was supposed to be done and nobody did. And employees would tell us later that when they would hear a code call people would say 'Oh, is Lynn working today?' So culturally they knew something was wrong, but nobody was doing anything about it."

REPORT GETS RUN

So finally, the report was run. What did the report show? *"Mortalities were up, although not significantly. So next they wanted to look at staffing during mortalities. They eventually did that [study], and it was creepy. It was this four week staffing grid that highlighted each person [each nurse that had worked*

during that four week period of time when a mortality had occurred during the four week period]. All the nurses were in the single digits [as to when deaths occurred during a shift they were working] like 4% and 7% of all mortalities, and Lynn was at some astronomical number like 60-some percent or more. There was one other nurse who was at, maybe, 15%."

Marilyn Custer-Mitchell states that ***"Holding people accountable—that is not as much of an intangible as a tangible skill. That became very important there because nobody was being held accountable for anything. No leadership, no anything. So when we started doing that—I am guessing that is part of the reason Judy, the Director of Nursing (DON) at the time—resigned the first day. I had been up and had lunch with her and talked about how are things were working there; what do we need to work on; from her perspective, what are the priorities. And then just talking about that and how she was holding people accountable. She knew we needed to go there, and she was not going to do that. That was not in her nature, and it wasn't going to happen anyway. So my guess is she thought 'I'm going to get out now'. She had been through a nightmare in her role [as DON] trying to hold things together. She was also of the age where she could retire. Holding people accountable became huge. That is why some people decided to leave, and others flourished. The coolest thing about that was we ended up giving lots of people opportunities, either people who worked at Union [the hospital that took over the management of Vermillion County Hospital subsequent to this event] or were there [at Vermillion] and had some leadership potential. We ended up with a lot of turnover at the leadership level. We were able to hire some people, who didn't have any leadership experience, [but we could] help them and train them. So we got to see a lot of people grow and blossom and that was a lot of fun. But gaining people's trust is the hardest thing."***

CONCLUSION

Orville Lynn Majors was found guilty and convicted of murdering six patients while working as an attending LPH in the Vermillion County Hospital ICU between 1993 and 1995; however, it was believed that Majors may have committed dozens or more murders during this time period. It was reported that he may have targeted patients who were demanding, whiny, or disproportionally added to his workload. It was believed that Majors injected high doses of potassium chloride into patients as the means to kill them.

Majors had his nursing license suspended in 1995. The State of Indiana launched a criminal investigation, and Majors was arrested in 1997. A total of 79 witnesses were called to the stand at his trial. Some of the witnesses testified that he hated elderly people, and that he believed some of them "should be gassed."

The judge in the case ruled that the supervisory study that showed the number of deaths rose during the duration of Majors' employment at the hospital was inadmissible as evidence, because Majors was only being tried for six murders. However, other (http://en.wikipedia.org/wiki/Evidence) evidence that was admissible included witnesses who heard Majors refer to elderly patients as "a waste" and other derogatory terms. Additionally, some of the deadly substances that were allegedly used in the murders were found at his house (http://en.wikipedia.org/wiki/Orville_Lynn_Majors–cite_note-NYTimes-5).

In October 1999, Majors was found guilty of murdering six patients and was sentenced to 360 years in prison. Majors is serving his sentence at an Indiana State Prison.

DISCUSSION QUESTIONS

1. Why is accountability no longer optional in healthcare?
2. Identify one or two ways a healthcare leader can drive accountability.
3. Describe the role organizational culture and the working environment play in fostering accountability.
4. What basic function of management is accountability embedded in?
5. Describe what the following quote from ex-NFL coach means and how it applies to healthcare leadership: "You're either coaching it, or you're letting it happen."
6. Identify one or two characteristics of a health service organizational culture where accountability is strong.
7. Describe how healthcare leaders can model the way for accountability
8. What does the phrase organizational development mean?
9. What is meant by the organizational culture being an "invisible hand that is always at work"?
10. Why is it important for the organization's CEO to lead by example when it comes to accountability?

12

Fostering Employee Engagement for Organizational Performance

While management is about getting work done through others, leadership is motivating and inspiring others to work hard to achieve organizational goals. On the surface, the difference may appear subtle—but a deeper investigation reveals a much more profound difference. In comparison, both management and leadership involve the management and supervision of people to complete various jobs, work processes, and related functions. However, in contrast to leadership, management concerns a much broader scope and spectrum of functions, processes, and workflow efficiencies. Leadership has a more central focus on leading and directing people in a motivating and inspiring way: with the central theme being how, as a leader, one can maximize the performance and contributions of employees working individually and collectively in organized teams. Management is the broader domain with leadership as one of its basic functions—along with planning, organizing, and controlling.

OBJECTIVES

1. Understand employee engagement and appreciate how it impacts critical success factors, such as quality outcomes, patient safety, employee productivity, and organizational performance.
2. Learn 10 action steps managers can take to foster employee engagement in a healthcare organization.
3. Inspire you to consider employee engagement a top priority for a healthcare leader.

There are a multitude of actions, behaviors, characteristics, methods, techniques, strategies, tactics, mannerisms, styles, theories, and other intangibles that are involved in leadership and its effective application in practice. One area somewhat recently recognized as a critical aspect of leadership effectiveness is employee engagement. Employee engagement lies at the heart of leadership. Employee engagement is the employee's emotional and cognitive motivation, self-efficacy to perform the job, perceived clarity of the organization's vision and his or her specific role in that vision, and belief that he or she has the resources to get the job done. An engaged employee has both the willingness and the ability to take

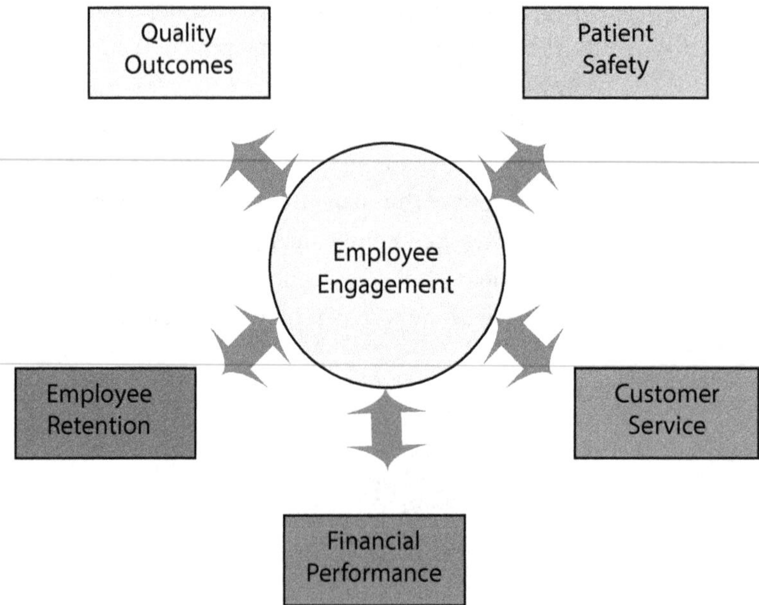

FIGURE 12.1 Employee Engagement

responsibility for directing his or her own behavior at work and completing tasks and assignments (worker readiness). An engaged employee has both components of worker readiness: psychological readiness, which is the motivation to do the work, and job readiness, which is having the requisite skills, knowledge and abilities to do the job. In addition, an engaged employee can clearly see a connection between the work that he does or will be doing and the mission and vision of the organization and is motivated to work hard and contribute to the achievement/attainment of individual, departmental, and organizational goals.

Sam Odle talks about the importance of employee engagement. ***"Employee engagement is vitally important no matter what type of business you are in: whether its healthcare, information technology, building houses or whatever you are doing. If your employees are not really engaged in what they are doing, and they are not as passionate about it as you [(the leader)] are in doing it well, then you are not going to be a high-performing company: it's not going to happen."***

Clearly, the journey of becoming a leader and developing an effective leadership style includes developing the ability to promote and foster employee engagement in the healthcare workplace environment—at all levels in the organization. However, how a healthcare leader defines his or her job—and its critical aspects and priorities—will largely determine how much emphasis the leader places on the function of employee engagement. Again, the process of leadership is motivating and inspiring others to work hard to achieve organizational goals; therefore, fostering employee engagement is virtually synonymous with the definition of leadership. Moreover, a healthcare leader should assess his own performance—in part—by his effectiveness in fostering employee engagement. Furthermore, a healthcare leader should consider developing his skills and abilities to foster employee engagement in order to elevate his overall leadership performance and effectiveness.

> The process of leadership is motivating and inspiring others to work hard to achieve organizational goals: therefore, fostering employee engagement is virtually synonymous with the definition of leadership.

Judy Monroe, MD, says ***"What I have observed, probably everyplace I've been, and most recently here at [Center for Disease Control (CDC)] is ... for real satisfaction on the job, most folks aren't there for the paycheck. The paycheck is necessary and you need that. But they're there for the mission."*** And if they can visualize and see the mission, it helps employees to be engaged.

Dr. Monroe states that ***"Folks want to be involved and they are frustrated if they don't feel they are engaged and have the opportunity to be involved."*** An example is Dr. Monroe's work with the Center for Medicare and Medicaid Innovation and the implementation of the Affordable Care Act. Dr. Monroe goes on to say, "***It became very clear a little anxiety had begun to develop, even among some of my best leaders. The feedback I got was they weren't sure how to help me, because this is cutting-edge work for***

us and they don't know how to help me because I don't know yet what I need. I was on a journey [alone] trying to figure it out. But it really stopped me when I got that feedback. I realized I needed to take some time, sit with the team, and at least make sure they know what I know and help them understand we need their collective wisdom. They also need to know what I know to help them feel like they haven't been left behind. And there are different ways of getting employees engaged."

Dr. Monroe goes on to say that ***"Employees want to be engaged with the leadership. They want to be engaged in the problem solving and see how their work connects to the bigger picture. They need to hear from the leaders."*** Dr. Monroe provides an example of a method she has used at the CDC to get employees involved and engaged that involves scheduling separate one-hour meetings with leaders and the entire staff of each work unit team that reports up to her in the chain of command at the CDC. These were "***No agenda meetings***" says Dr. Monroe ***"where employees would introduce themselves, tell me about their work, and ask me anything."*** Dr. Monroe says these have been ***"The most fabulous meetings."*** Dr. Monroe concludes by saying ***"Employees want to be engaged. They need to be engaged. And if we want the best results we need to engage them and keep looking for creative ways to engage them."***

Healthcare leaders today face a myriad of challenges, including a growing shortage of primary care physicians; increasing responsibility for population health management, including with readmissions; declining reimbursement on a per-unit basis; and increasing public and governmental scrutiny of business practices, to name a few. However, a principle function of any healthcare leader is to foster and promote employee engagement amidst all the challenges faced. So, a key question for leaders is this: how do you get the most return on your organization's largest investment—your people? Clearly employees must be engaged in order to give their best, contribute more of their potential, and perform at a high level.

The central function of any hospital or health service organization that delivers direct patient care is the delivery of that care. And for caregivers to provide great care to patients, a healing, caring environment is required. Caring for patients is a personal interaction between caregiver and patient. Caring is a gift that is given by the caregiver out of compassion and love. Caregiving can be a life-changing experience that creates a lasting impact on both the patient and the caregiver. So, what if a hospital or health service organization's caregivers aren't engaged?

What about proper hand washing? Proper hand washing is one of the most effective ways to prevent 2 million hospital-acquired infections annually. However, research shows that caregivers follow proper hand washing procedures only about 40% of the time. Un-engaged caregivers are much less likely to follow proper procedures, such as for hand washing. Un-engaged employees are much less likely to give their discretionary effort. What is discretionary effort? Discretionary effort is the amount of "extra" effort and performance that every employee has to give. Think of it this way: discretionary effort is the difference between meeting "minimum acceptable standards" of performance and the maximum performance potential an employee has to give. Typically, there is a considerable amount of extra effort and performance, that an employee is capable of giving over and above the minimum acceptable standards or requirements. This difference can be referred to as discretionary effort. So, a leader's job is to tap into the discretionary effort that every employee has to give.

Key leadership questions involved in this critical leadership skill: how do I maximize the effort and performance of employees—working both individually and collectively in organized teams—and how do I tap into the discretionary effort that each employee has to give?

What is discretionary effort? Discretionary effort is the amount of effort and performance an employee is willing, interested, and actually giving through his or her job at any given moment in time—over and above the minimum job requirements. It is discretionary, because it is not automatically given, but rather given freely by the employee. Employee discretionary effort cannot be mandated, regulated, or coerced by leadership. In its most simplest and fundamental form, discretionary effort is two things: effort that can include mental and physical energy that is exerted in order to achieve a purpose and results or performance. How hard an employee tries; how much attention the employee devotes to what he or she is doing; and the results and performance the employee achieves towards the desired results are all part of discretionary effort.

Key leadership question: As a leader, how do I maximize the discretionary effort that every employee has to give?

So, what's at stake in a hospital or other health service organization with regard to leadership's ability to foster a culture of employee engagement? The short answer *is* ***everything's at stake!*** Every critical success factor of the organization is impacted by the level of employee engagement in the organization including quality patient care, patient safety, customer service, employee satisfaction and retention, physician satisfaction, employee problem-solving and innovation, organizational financial performance, and the list goes on. Fostering employee engagement is the way to drive organizational performance. Without employee engagement, organizational performance will suffer.

Sam Odle talks about a couple of common problems healthcare leaders sometimes encounter in creating an environment that is not fostering employee engagement. "***There are two fundamental flaws that sometimes leaders start out with that cause them to create an environment where employees aren't engaged. The first one is this idea that employees can't handle complicated things. That somehow only the boss has the ability to do complicated things and employees can only take orders and do what they've been told to do. The second fundamental flaw is the leader believes that employees show up to work to try and see what they can get away with and do things wrong. Both of these are flaws in leadership philosophy that will create the wrong environment and will create a workplace where employees are not engaged. The way around that is to create an environment where we assume everyone is showing up today to do their best, and as a leader we are supposed to make sure they have the resources so they can***

do the best job—no matter what the work is. In addition, if we can share our vision of what the work outcome is and make sure we make clear the "what" we want to accomplish, then we allow the employee as much freedom as possible to accomplish that "what". So assuming everybody's here trying to do their best, and assuming if I share the vision of what we are trying to accomplish, then those employees will try to get together and work to achieve that outcome and do the best job they can. If you create that kind of environment you are going to have a more engaged workforce."

What does employee engagement look like in a health service organization, and what else can a healthcare leader do to foster employee engagement? One thing employee engagement looks like in a healthcare organization is teamwork. Judy Monroe, MD, talks about conducting teambuilding exercises that help to promote and foster employee engagement. She also talks about giving awards around innovation. An example is when Health and Human Services has put a problem out for employees to try and solve, and we "***open it up for people to be innovative in terms of the solution to that problem and then give prizes to the ones who came up with the ideas. They allow employees to be part of the solution in a more formal way or a fun way, and recognize that. Those are really terrific.*** "

Employee engagement in a health service organization manifests in teamwork, innovation, clinical collaboration, problem-solving, great customer service, a culture of caring in a healing environment, transparency and open communication, high productivity, and intention and responsibility. And it takes leaders modeling the way for others to follow. Dr. Monroe says that leaders modeling the way is a very powerful force for employee engagement. "***People are watching. They are clearly watching. And if the leader does model the way, that is the way you change culture.***"

Ken Stella talks about how a leader's actions have to match their words in order for the leader to truly model the way. Ken gives the example of picking up a piece of paper or trash on the floor. "***If the leader preaches to employees about the need to pick up a piece of paper or trash on the floor or in the elevator when they see it, but the employees never see the leader pick anything up—and they see him walk by it—why should they do it?***"

EMPLOYEE ENGAGEMENT'S TOP 10 LIST

There are many things that go into fostering employee engagement in a healthcare organization. Here is a list of 10 items healthcare leaders should consider in their efforts to foster employee engagement.

1. **Believing is seeing.** If a leader doesn't believe in the importance of employee engagement or how it impacts every single critical success factor in a healthcare organization, they will never see an engaged workforce.
2. **"Good" is the enemy of great.** A level of employee engagement that can be described as "good" can create complacency and satisfaction with the status quo. Eric Mangini, Ex-NFL Coach and football analyst says that "***Success is like a martini: it relaxes you.***" The same can be true in an organization that has "good" employee engagement.

3. **Have a plan.** The old axiom "A goal without a plan is simply a wish" applies here. Leaders should have a plan and spend significant time motivating, inspiring, and creating a culture in a working environment that fosters employee engagement.
4. **Create an environment of learning.** Author John C. Maxwell, in his book entitled *Developing the Leader Around You*, says that "**Recruiting and keeping good people is a leader's most important task.**" He also states "***Grow a leader, and you grow an organization. Great leaders share themselves and what they have learned. Leaders and/or potential leaders multiply their effectiveness. To develop positive, successful people, look for the gold—not the dirt.***" Leadership needs to create an environment for learning, growth, and personal and professional development. People go where they are wanted; stay where they are appreciated; and grow where they learn.

> People go where they are wanted; stay where they are appreciated; and grow where they learn.

Judy Monroe, MD, says that "***Culture eats strategy for lunch. And if it's a strong and productive culture then you have a winner: people want to work there. And if there is an organizational culture that is unproductive or not healthy, it is the job of the leader to change that culture.***"

5. **Treat employees like volunteers.** Author Stephen R. Covey, in his book *The 7 Habits of Highly Effective People*, talks about treating your employees like you want them to treat your best customers. Covey suggests that employees 'volunteer' the best they have to give and it is incumbent on leadership to provide effective leadership to tap into the best each employee has to offer.

   Ken Stella talks about a healthcare leader having to care for the people. "***I did not have any medical skill set that enabled me to help a patient in that hospital. But the people I supervised had all of the skills to care for that patient. The only way I could feel any kind of reward for caring for patients was to have a good team taking care of that patient. So you have to care for the people. You have to care about the employees. And you have to try to motivate them to develop the best skill set they can which is going to then translate to better care for that patient. And it starts by having that employee know you care about them.***"
6. **Help employees see the connection in their work to the organization's mission.** Po Bronson, a freelance writer, says it this way: "***People thrive by focusing on who they really are, and connecting that to work they truly love.***" Judy Monroe, MD, talks about the use of a strategic map and to "***engage your employees in the development of the strategic map—which is really a one-page***" document. Dr. Monroe talks about the strategic map as a one-page document that outlines the organization's mission, vision, and values, along with key strategic initiatives and goals; unit, division, or department objectives that support the corporate or organizational goals and objectives; and more detailed objectives that are rolled out to each of the employees and what they need to do to support the organization. At the bottom of the map are broad values and key points of emphasis that cut across all areas of the

organization and place emphasis for how the work is to be done, such as responsiveness, strategic thinking and collaboration, and stewardship. Dr. Monroe states the strategic map is a ***"Nice way to roll it all up so that, given the work of the day, people know how their work connects to the larger mission."*** Dr. Monroe used this tool at both the Indiana State Department of Health as State Health Commissioner and in her position as Deputy Director at CDC.

7. **Help employees see the bigger picture: provide 'big picture' communication.** Employees aren't typically in a position in the organization to see a lot of the bigger picture, like external forces and how they impact the organization or the different functions, services, and processes of the organization and how they impact each area and fit and work together. These types of conceptual skills require development, and managers need to communicate clearly with employees to assist them in this process. Leader's must take the time to communicate with employees on an ongoing basis about the bigger picture in order to help foster their understanding and why the organization must respond in certain ways to address these forces and changes. Communication fosters understanding, understanding fosters acceptance, and acceptance fosters trust and support. One of the primary ways for healthcare leaders to foster trust and support for changes the organization needs to make is through clear communication.

Communication fosters understanding; understanding fosters acceptance; acceptance fosters trust and support.

Dr. Monroe states that healthcare leaders, in their efforts to foster communication ***"Can never listen too much. You can never go wrong with listening."*** She also talks about the importance of leaders not losing sight of the big picture, as well. ***"I've learned along the way, if you've got your head down and you get too buried in the details you're going to miss the big picture. That can be a hard lesson sometimes. In leadership, you have to be sure you are scanning the whole picture."***

8. **Put the right people in the right places.** Dewey Greene, past Division President with HCA Hospital Company, would talk about putting the best people you could find in key hospital management positions. Mr. Greene says that "***As a hospital CEO, if you don't surround yourself with really good people you will fail—no matter how good you are as a leader.***"
9. **Accountability is mandatory.** Ken Stella states that it is time—maybe long overdue—for hospital and healthcare leaders to be held accountable for what they do: for the decisions they make, as well as the clinical outcomes, service, and overall performance of their organizations. Mr. Stella says that "***Early on, there were the 'mystics of medicine' and*** **[hospitals and their leadership]** ***weren't held as accountable. What gets measured gets improved, and today we have all the measurements. The feeling I have on accountability is drive it down as low into the organization as you can—all the way through the organization. There is individual accountability. There is department accountability. There's section accountability. And then ultimately the overall accountability."***

10. **Focus on leadership's critical intangibles.** In thinking about healthcare leadership, we can divide all of leadership into two major categories of competencies the content knowledge and skills, such as in the areas of financial management, human resources management, information technology, quantitative analysis, scientific management, etc., and the intangibles of leadership. Many believe the heart of leadership is about the intangibles. General Omar Bradley states that ***"Leadership is intangible, and therefore, no weapon ever designed can replace it."*** Tom Atchison, author, speaker, and healthcare consultant maintains that the intangibles of leadership account for as much as 65% of organizational performance. The intangibles of leadership are crucial to being an effective healthcare leader. Healthcare is the ultimate people business, with people taking care of people in what is, many times, one of their greatest times of need. And, leadership is about motivating and inspiring employees to work hard to achieve organizational goals and meet the tangible and intangible needs of the patients and families we serve. The leadership skills it takes to be effective in motivating and inspiring others are primarily intangible, that is, hard to describe or quantify; however, by definition they are critical to organizational performance. A few examples of leadership intangibles include likability, trust, charisma, follow-through, promise-keeping, inspiring, work ethic, heart, and caring.

    Critical intangible of effective leadership includes a myriad of different factors and characteristics too numerous to list; however the following offers a few more examples of what these intangibles can look like in a healthcare setting. Dr. Monroe states that ***"I don't know that there is anything more powerful than a leader in a top leadership role to admit when they're wrong."*** To "***Humble themselves. Or to change their own behavior when it hasn't been as productive as it could be. That's incredibly powerful. People are very forgiving and I think that really builds the trust in the leader.***" When a leader admits when he or she is wrong or changes behavior to a more effective or productive style in some way, the employees then look at the leader as being more human—just like them. Dr. Monroe states, "***And you are going to get more out of those employees if they see the leader is human just like they are.***"

    Management by wandering around, or MBWA, ***"is a great strategy. Employees love that. For the most part, employees do like it when the leader is out and about, showing interest in their work, and they can have some informal chats with them."*** However, with more organizations allowing certain employees to work from home and do tele-work, MBWA is becoming a bit more challenging. However, at the same time, we have to recognize there is value in tele-work, as well.

    Participatory leadership plays a critical role in employee engagement. Participatory leadership is a leadership style in which the leader consults employees for their suggestions and input before making decisions. Dr. Monroe states that "***You're going to kick yourself if you don't do it [get input from others] as much as possible—in all levels of the organization. And the thing I have found is that honestly, it doesn't take that much. I think sometimes leaders don't get that input for fear it's going to take too long, or we just need to make an executive decision. But I have found if you reach-out to get that input: 1) it doesn't have to be a long, laborious process, and folks are happy they are being asked that just take you a long way and 2) then when you have to make the executive decision—and running an organization of any size—the day does come when sometimes an executive decision***

needs to be made, those executive decisions are going to be much better accepted because people know your usual pattern is to get input and recognize this is one where an executive decision had to be made."

Dr. Monroe goes on to state that ***"Another lesson that comes to mind is—and this one has to do with people—wherever you are, be there. And whoever you are with at the time, be with that person. I had a situation one time where I was interviewing a medical student, and I was in the middle of an interview, and the nurse came and said that one of my patients was in [the clinic] and could I come as there was something needed. I thought at that moment I was role modeling, so I chose to interrupt the interview and told him that I would be right back."*** Dr. Monroe left to see what she was needed for and came back and ***"told him a little bit about whatever the clinic scenario was, and then finished the interview. What came back was the medical student did not rank our program [highly] and indicated that I was more concerned with what was going on in the clinic that day than him and the interview. That was a hard lesson. [As leaders,] we've got to realize the impact we have on those around us. And that was the lesson I learned early on: make sure you make time for the person you've bought time for."***

Ken Stella talks about the role administrative promise-keeping plays in employee engagement. Ken states that ***"You have to carry through on what you say. If you promise something you have to deliver. I've never tried to promise [something]. But I tried to say if we're successful, we might have this outcome: but you had to deliver."***

An example that Mr. Stella gives to help foster employee engagement is a simple, yet impactful, one: ***"Do you sit with the employees [in the hospital cafeteria], or do you only sit with the elite? You have to show that you care about them, and you can demonstrate that in a lot of easy ways."***

CONCLUDING REMARKS ON EMPLOYEE ENGAGEMENT

Employees give their best for their own reasons—not management's. The more in-touch healthcare leaders are with employees and their reasons for wanting to give their best effort and performance, the more leaders will be able to tap into the discretionary effort each employee has to give—individually and collectively. Most caregivers want to make a real difference for others and aren't there just for the paycheck. They want to be engaged with leadership to help solve problems and make a difference. Most caregivers will respond to help the organization achieve its mission and vision, but they must be able to clearly see how the important work they do every day contributes to the mission and vision. In a very similar way, many employees don't see how dependent others in the organization are on them and the work and performance they provide. It is leadership's responsibility to help employees clearly see the connection between the work they do every day and how their work impacts others in the organization, including the attainment of the mission and vision.

Most employees want to have a personal connection with leadership and see leaders as real people—as human—with similar needs and desires as them. Leaders must spend time with employees communicating, listening, and getting to know them and what their goals and passions are. Employees can't be required or mandated to give extra effort—their discretionary effort—is only given freely. Treat employees like volunteers, as only they can volunteer to give the best they have to give. Healthcare leaders can evoke the best from an employee only through the critical intangibles of leadership.

> **Employee engagement is not a thinking thing, it is a feeling thing.**

Employee engagement is not a thinking thing, it is a feeling thing. It is about creating a positive organizational culture within the organization, and a positive emotional condition towards the job, work, organization, patients, co-workers, and leadership. Emotional engagement is four times more valuable than rational engagement in driving employee effort and performance. Much of the emotional engagement of an employee is about belonging: do I fit? Is there chemistry in my job and the working environment around me? Am I supported? Do I have ample freedom and autonomy to give my best? Am I valued? Does leadership understand me and am I important to the organization? Are the expectations clear? Is my work meaningful? Is there a purpose to what I do?

Fostering employee engagement takes a lot of effort on the part of healthcare leaders, necessitating them to spend significant time working to foster employee engagement. Sam Walton, the founder of Walmart, said that "***Outstanding leaders go out of their way to boost the self-esteem of their personnel. If people believe in themselves, it's amazing what they can accomplish.***"

Employee engagement is a process: one without an end point. And it is a process that lies at the heart of effective healthcare leadership.

DISCUSSION QUESTIONS

1. What is employee engagement?
2. Why should healthcare executives and leaders be concerned with employee engagement?
3. What is discretionary effort, and why is it important for leaders to foster and tap into employee discretionary effort?
4. Why can employee engagement be considered a critical leadership function?
5. Describe what employee engagement looks like in a healthcare organizational setting?
6. How much of a senior leader's time should be spent fostering employee engagement?
7. What does Dr. Monroe mean when she says "Whenever you are with people, be there."
8. What does it mean to say employee engagement is not a thinking thing, but rather a feeling thing? Please explain.
9. What is participatory leadership, and how can it be applied to foster employee engagement?
10. Describe how employee engagement can be tapped into through management by walking around (MBWA)?

13

The Power of Communication: Leaders are You Listening?

What happens in a hospital or health service organization that doesn't first start somewhere with a conversation? Maybe it's a conversation about organizational goals and priorities. Maybe it's a conversation about a special project or routine procedures and work processes. Maybe it's a conversation about an administrative policy or clinical protocol. Maybe it's a conversation about the working environment, culture, expectations, clinical outcomes, results or performance. Maybe it's a conversation about training, supervising, coaching, or evaluating an employee. Whether it's on a formal or informal basis, nothing occurs without some type of communication to guide, direct, or initiate action.

OBJECTIVES

1. Understand the power of effective leadership communication and its various different forms.
2. Understand some of the important considerations in crafting an effective communication message.
3. Appreciate the power of feedback, what isn't said in a communication message, and a leader's inner conversation.

Open, clear, effective communication from leadership at all levels in an organization is critical. But what exactly is effective communication? Communication involves the crafting and sending of the communication message and the receiving and interpreting of the message.

CRAFTING AN EFFECTIVE COMMUNICATION MESSAGE

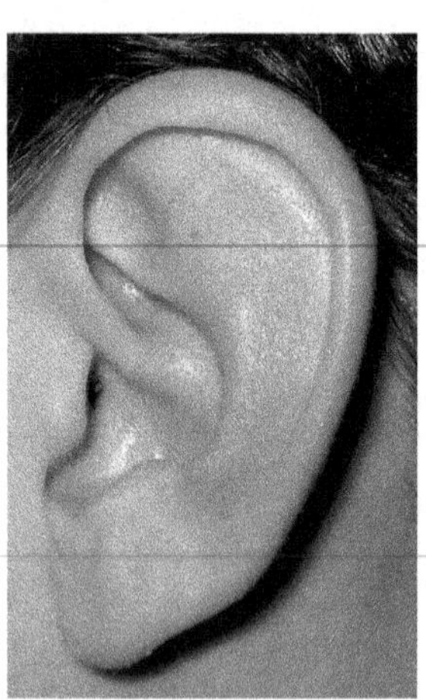

FIGURE 13.1 Human Ear

At the center of communication lies the message—communication that has been spoken, written, or otherwise provided through voice tone, inflection, body language, or other non-verbal cues. So, what is important to consider when crafting the communication message?

- Is the message really clear? Will it truly convey the intended meaning?
- Is it written at the appropriate level of abstraction for the receiver (general information vs. specific details and free of technical terms and jargon)?
- How will the receiver of the message feel when receiving/decoding and interpreting the message? What emotions will the message inspire?
- What are the appropriate communication mediums for the communication to be sent?
- Will repetition of the message be required to be certain the message is actually received and understood by the receiver?

- How should the sender seek feedback from the receiver to validate that a clear understanding of the intended communication message has occurred?

Communication is effective when the desired, intended message is received by the sender (amid all the typical noise and interference), and clearly and easily understood as intended, and delivered in a way that engages the receiver to listen, interpret, and understand the intended meaning of the message desired. Typically, it is important to convey why the message is important to the receiver, along with creating some type of feedback loop back to the sender to ascertain and validate the key messages being sent and received are being correctly interpreted and clearly understood.

Effective communication in an organization is critical, and it relies on leadership's effective communication skills. Leadership must foster and promote clear communication for employees to understand and connect with the organization's mission and vision; organizational goals and priorities; policies, procedures, and work processes; and events, activities, and other important information about the organization and its affairs. Effective communication is also important for employees to receive needed training, direction, and updates, as well as to understand expectations about work performance and results. But, one of the most important elements of leadership communication is effective listening.

One of the most important elements of leadership communication is effective listening.

LEADERS ARE YOU LISTENING?

In order for any leader to effectively manage and lead employees, he/she must have a clear understanding of the attitudes, beliefs, and perspectives of employees individually and collectively. Being in touch and close connection with the workforce takes, among other things, good listening skills on the part of the leader.

Leaders need to continually inquire about and assess many matters on an ongoing basis, including: How is employee morale? Do employees have any issues with the working environment, policies and practices, or care and service delivery? What obstacles do employees perceive are in their way to high performance? What ideas or suggestions do employees have for improving various work processes? What is the level of employee understanding about organizational strategies, goals, and priorities, as well as the impact their individual work has on these? What changes need to be made to improve the working environment? Effective listening provides leaders with the in-depth understanding they need to help assess the current state of the organization and the workforce and lead effectively.

Effective listening is multi-dimensional and takes on many forms and environments. Listening is much more than hearing. The difference between hearing and listening is the attention given to the sender and message by the receiver.

The difference between hearing and listening is the attention given to the sender and message by the receiver.

Sam Odle states, ***"The times that I've been involved in really difficult situations, I've always found that more listening—harder listening, more intently—was really where the solution was to be found. It wasn't in restating my position, or being more firm, or being more direct. It was really in letting the person talk about the differences, and why they wanted that. In listening, that's where the wins are to be found. Our listening skills are probably more important than our verbal skills as a leader."***

Judy Monroe, MD, states, ***"You can never listen too much. You can never go wrong with listening."***

CRITICAL FACTORS FOR EFFECTIVE LEADERSHIP COMMUNICATION

Seek feedback—getting input and feedback from employees about communication practices within the organization is important for leadership to ascertain and understand how effective their leadership communication practices and methods really are. One technique that can be employed is to ask employees individually and collectively about what communication practices should be: 1) stopped, 2) started, or 3) continued.

Listening with an open mind—it seems reasonable to conclude that leaders could not really have their employees' best interest at heart if the leaders aren't, in fact, good listeners. When leaders listen to employees with an open mind and intent to understand, it is evident.

Listening helps build trust, along with a sense of caring and understanding. Responding to an employee by saying *"if I'm hearing you correctly, I think you are saying ..."* sends a powerful message that the leader cares and understands what is being communicated by the employee.

Listening helps build trust, along with a sense of caring and understanding.

Asking the right questions—part of the art of leadership is learning to ask the right questions, to the right people, at the right time. Asking the right question can provide a leader with important information and insight they seek. Asking questions can move the conversation forward and provide more opportunity for the leader to listen and understand.

Body language—a significant percentage of the true meaning of a communication message lies in the body language, voice tone, and inflection of the sender. Leaders should develop their skills in assessing for the important non-verbal cues of communication.

Emotional intelligence—much has been written recently about the significance of a leader's emotional intelligence (EI) in the workplace. A leader's EI involves being in touch with the emotions of others, as well as your own, and managing his emotions in the various environments and situations he faces as a leader. Moreover, leaders should be willing to use their intuition, gut instincts, and feelings to help gauge appropriate communication in difficult situations or crucial conversations.

Being present—in our fast-paced, multitasking world, being present with others has become a major challenge. However, there may be no more powerful form of leadership communication than being truly present—beyond just our physical presence, but with our undistracted mental presence—with others. Making eye contact, acknowledging and recognizing others, listening with intent, and providing feedback along with understanding and support for the efforts and work of others are all part of being present.

There may be no more powerful form of communication than being truly present—beyond just our physical presence, but with our undistracted mental presence—with others.

COMMUNICATION MEDIUMS AND ENVIRONMENTS

There are numerous mediums and environments for communication to occur in any organization. Leaders must be authentic and consistent in their communication style in the various communication mediums and environments they work in.

Email—don't fall into the trap of using text message jargon in business email communication. And, yes, spelling matters.

Meetings—it's important for leaders to distinguish when to provide guidance, direction, and structure in a meeting situation, versus allowing employees space to provide input, feedback, opinions, and ideas. One comment or statement by a leader that is perceived in a negative fashion by employees—as inadvertent as it might seem—can quash suggestions and innovative ideas right in their tracks.

Management by Wandering Around (MBWA)—is a great way for managers to be visible and connect with employees, to listen and observe for how employees interact with one another and work together, identify roadblocks to efficiency or great performance that may exist, and foster direct communication with employees.

Open employee meetings—held on an annual or bi-annual basis, open employee meetings are a great way to foster direct communication with employees. These meetings can include both structured-agenda and open-forum content.

Management meetings—regularly scheduled or special meetings called as needed are important ongoing forums for communication to be exchanged among managers.

Staff meetings—it's good for managers to occasionally attend routine staff meetings to be visible and foster communication directly with employees.

Employee surveys—paying close attention to input and information gathered through the employee survey process is important. It is especially important to close the loop on this communication by reporting back to the employees what was learned and what actions management will be taking as a result.

Social media—today's society of social media has fostered a convergence of business and personal information at our finger tips. Much can be learned about businesses and people with communication through the various mediums of social media.

Organizational grapevine—a vital form of communication that is sometimes overlooked by leaders is the organizational grapevine. Being close to the scuttlebutt through the grapevine helps leaders keep their fingers on the pulse of the organization.

THE SOUNDS OF SILENCE—BEYOND THE WORDS BEING SAID

According to Seth S. Horowitz, auditory neuroscientist at Brown University and author of The Universal Sense: How Hearing Shapes the Mind, **"The richness of life doesn't lie in the loudness and the beat, but in the timbres and the variations that you can discern if you simply pay attention."** Many times, the true communication message lies beyond the actual words being said. The true meaning of the communication message is typically found in body language, gestures and facial expression, voice tone and inflection, and the underlying emotions that accompany the communication message from the sender.

> **Leaders must pay attention to what is not being said, probe a bit deeper, and be active and empathetic listeners and observers in order to clearly grasp and accurately interpret the true meaning of the communication message.**

Moreover, many times the true communication message and its meaning lie in what isn't being said in the message. Therefore, leaders must pay attention to what is not being said, probe a bit deeper, and be active and empathetic listeners and observers in order to clearly grasp and accurately interpret the true meaning of the communication message being sent in the various communication mediums and environments where communication takes place.

In the article *Why Leadership Means Listening*, Carmine Gallo states that "***great leaders are great listeners.***" In today's environment, employees want to be asked for their input and opinions and to be listened to by leadership. What problems and challenges do employees face in their work? How do employees view key policies and procedures? What is the level of teamwork and collaboration that exists, and how can it be improved? Where are the opportunities to reduce waste and improve service at the point of care delivery?

It seems the old axiom just may be true for leaders: being born with two ears and one mouth just might mean we should listen twice as much as we speak.

FEEDBACK

Sam Odle states, ***"I think there has to be regular feedback. When I talk about feedback, there has to be communication both ways: where the leader is giving feedback on the performance of the organization, but the leader is also listening to the employees about their observations as well. And then making sure we're asking the basic questions about 'what can we do for you to help you be more successful?' Because when people feel like the organization has their best interest at heart it is going to be more easy for them to sustain having the organization's best interest at heart. If they feel like they're just being used, then they aren't going to be engaged, they aren't going to be loyal, and they aren't going to be looking for improvements. But [if] they feel like that organization cares about them, they are going to do a good job when they are there. I think a lot of feedback, both ways, and then making sure we're asking not just what the organization needs but the employees what their needs are and how we can help them do a better job, and how we can do a better job of letting them actualize their aspirations."***

Judy Monroe, MD, states, ***"Feedback is the breakfast of champions. I love that quote because I learned long ago when I was the [family practice] residency program director [at St. Vincent's Hospital in Indianapolis, Indiana] I went to a conference where they made the distinction between feedback and evaluation. They said the annual evaluation that's really long-term, looking back to see if they met their goals and objectives. Feedback is where the gold is. So if feedback is the breakfast of champions, and you want a champion team, feedback has to be timely—on the spot—because otherwise it becomes an evaluation and you've lost the moment. I am a big believer in the value of feedback. If it's done correctly, then it is a very powerful tool for employee engagement."***

A LEADER'S INNER CONVERSATION

A leader's inner voice—the one in his or her head that never leaves his or her mouth—is very powerful. An argument can be made that the most powerful conversation that any leader will have is the one inside that never gets verbalized. That inner voice or conversation that never leaves a leader's head structures everything he does and feels. It can be positive and affirming, or it can be negative and destructive. Being aware of one's inner voice is step number one. Managing it and reprogramming it as necessary is step number two.

Judy Monroe, MD, says to ***"Listen to that little voice. Even in practicing medicine I remember hearing others articulate this. If you are going to bed at night and you're thinking about a patient and you are a bit worried, get up and go check it out. Call the nurse if the patient is hospitalized. When that little voice inside is trying to rear its head, you'd better listen. That is [a lesson] that I've carried with me."***

Leaders' inner voices are very powerful, as they provides them with the information that structures everything: what they think, how they think, feedback to themselves and whether it is affirming and encouraging or negative, what they like, what they don't like, etc. A leader's inner voice is where his or her intuition, or "gut" feeling, lies—a very powerful tool but only if it is recognized and utilized.

UNDERSTANDING INFORMAL COMMUNICATION

Informal channels of communication, sometimes referred to as the "grapevine," are very important channels of communication in a health service organization. Leaders need to be in touch with the important communication messages that are transmitted over informal communication channels. By understanding the informal channels and communication messages that are occurring within the organization, a leader can then effectively understand the perceptions of employees; internal issues or problems that need to be addressed; and opportunities for improvement.

DISCUSSION QUESTIONS

1. What are some of the important considerations that should be made when crafting communication?
2. Describe the important and powerful role that listening plays for effective leadership.
3. What does it mean to listen beyond the actual words that are said?
4. What role does feedback play in effective leadership?
5. What are the major differences between formal and informal channels of communication in a health service organization?
6. What do you believe are a few of the most important communication mediums and environments in a health service organization?
7. What role does a leader's inner communication play in his or her effectiveness as a leader?
8. What does it mean for a leader to be an empathetic listener?
9. How important is a leader's body language in his/her communication, and why?
10. What does Judy Monroe, MD mean when she says "You can never listen too much. You can never go wrong with listening"?

FIGURE CREDIT

14

Creating Vision and Strategy

Creating vision and strategy is a fundamental function and responsibility of senior leadership in a health service organization. Creating vision and strategy is paramount for any health service organization to have an overall direction and path to improve its internal operations and external position in the market in order to fulfill its mission, compete, and remain a sustainable healthcare asset. What does a strategic plan represent to the health service organization's stakeholders, such as the employees? How about to the physicians? To the leadership? To patients and families? To the community at large? When an organization doesn't have a clearly defined overall direction and path to improve its internal operations and external position in the market to best serve its customers, it risks being blown off track from a variety of internal and external factors and forces. There is an old Sioux proverb that supports this axiom: "***If you don't know where you're going, any path will get you there***" and another similar saying: "***If you always do what you've always done, you'll always get what you've always got***"(source unknown). Country music artist Toby Keith, from his CD *Bullet in the Gun*, says "***If you don't know where you're going, you might end-up someplace else.***" And, here is one more saying that is apropos: "***A goal without a plan is simply a wish***" (source unknown). Goal setting is bringing the future into the present, so the organization can do something about it now and help to create its own future state.

OBJECTIVES

1. Understand and appreciate the importance of the strategic planning function and process for a health service organization.
2. Learn about a common process and structure for strategic planning and strategic plan document development and implementation.
3. Learn and apply key components of the strategic thinking and strategic momentum processes.

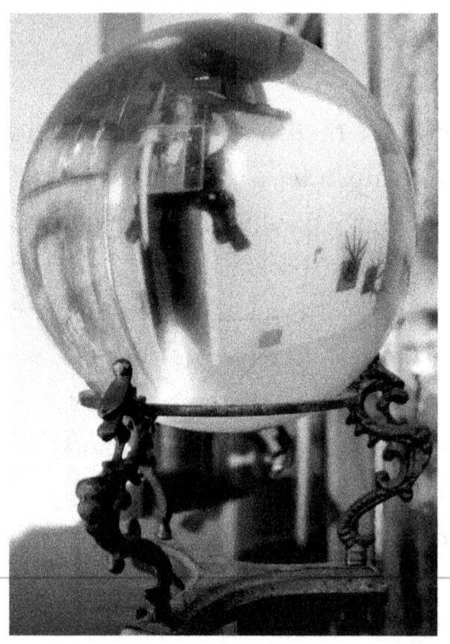

FIGURE 14.1 Crystal Ball

PLANNING AND STRATEGY

Planning is one of the four basic functions of management. Planning is determining organizational goals and a means to achieve them (*Effective Management*, Chuck Williams). According to Chuck Williams, there are five benefits of planning:

1. Planning ***facilitates intensified effort***–managers and employees put forth greater effort when following a plan
2. Planning ***provides direction***—encouraging managers and employees to direct their efforts toward activities that help accomplish their goals
3. Planning ***leads to persistence***—working hard for long periods of time
4. Planning encourages the ***development of task strategies***
5. Planning is ***proven to work*** for both companies and individuals

Strategy is the means an organization chooses to move from where it is today to a desired state sometime in the future, pursuant to achieving its vision, mission, goals, and objectives (*Effective Management*, Chuck Williams). Strategic planning is the process used for assessing a changing environment to create a vision of the future; determining how the organization fits into the anticipated environment based on its institutional mission, strengths, and weaknesses; and then setting in motion a plan of action to position the organization accordingly (Strategic Management of Health Care Organizations, Sixth Edition, Linda A. Swayne, W. Jack Duncan, and Peter M. Ginter).

THE PLANNING HORIZON

The planning horizon is the period of time in the future being targeted by the organization in its strategic planning. The planning horizon can be 1, 3, 5, or 10 years or longer. However, in today's rapidly changing environment the conventional wisdom is that a one- to three-year planning horizon is probably as far into the future that health service organizations should strategically plan. Clearly, there are exceptions to this rule, particularly as it relates to planning for a major construction project, like a new or replacement hospital facility. Moreover, a health service organization's existing strategic plan may be considered current, and the organization may only want to go through a modified or abbreviated strategic planning process in order to update those components believed to be appropriate for and in need of updating. Peter Drucker, considered by many to be the founder of modern-day management, stated that **"We greatly overestimate what we can do in one year. But we greatly underestimate what is possible for us in 5 years."**

THE STRATEGIC PLANNING PROCESS

How a health service organization goes about developing its strategic plan matters. Many consider the strategic planning process as important as the strategic plan document itself. Why? Because as Sam Odle states "***if you have a vision, and no one else shares it, then it might as well be a nightmare because you*** **[the leader]** ***are going to try and get there but these other people*** **[employees]** ***don't share your vision, and they're not marching or following you.***" Therefore, one of the most important aspects of the strategic planning process is creating a shared vision among key stakeholders about the type of future state the organization should create. The strategic planning process should be designed to accomplish that important task: gain consensus towards a shared vision. Getting key decision makers and stakeholders involved in the process is important to accomplish this objective.

One of the most important aspects of the strategic planning process is creating a shared vision among key stakeholders about the type of future sate the organization should create.

Many health service organizations create a strategic planning committee that is a board-level committee consisting of the board of directors, physician leadership, and senior management. In addition, the CEO, COO, or Vice President for Planning or Development are typically the type of positions that take the lead to facilitate and coordinate the process. Sometimes, the organization will hire an outside consultant to help spearhead the process and perform some or all of the legwork in developing the strategic plan document for the organization. Many times the strategic planning process is initiated with a strategic planning retreat.

THE STRATEGIC PLANNING RETREAT

The strategic planning retreat is a common venue for starting a strategic planning process, and it is many times held outside the organization in another location. The objectives typically include education, review and update on the status of implementation of the previous strategic plan, and review and discussion regarding one or more components that have been updated or newly created for the new strategic plan in a working draft format. Many times, there has been a survey, a questionnaire, or individual stakeholder interviews conducted with members of the strategic planning committee before the retreat to gather input, feedback, and perceptions from that group about the process, what is being done effectively, what can be improved and other questions and points relevant to the new process.

BUILDING A WORKING DRAFT DOCUMENT

In addition to the strategic planning retreat, holding several additional meetings with the strategic planning committee during the process in order to share an updated working draft document of the strategic plan as it is being developed is a good way to get input and feedback from key decision makers and stakeholders during the strategic planning process. A typical strategic planning process can take three to six months to complete; therefore, allowing ample time for gaining the input and feedback needed from others. Moreover, involvement from others is important to create the needed support and buy-in for a shared vision of the organization's future.

THE STRATEGIC PLAN DOCUMENT

The structure/organization of a strategic plan document for a hospital or health service organization can vary greatly; however, a typical strategic plan document structure can include the following major components or sections.

- Executive Summary
- Directional Strategies
- Environment Assessment
- Service Area Analysis
- Market Share Analysis
- Competitive Analysis
- Internal Analysis
- Strengths, Weaknesses, Threats, and Opportunities (SWOT) Analysis
- Strategic Initiatives
- Strategic Implementation Plan

EXECUTIVE SUMMARY

This section provides a brief overview of the organization, along with any key points, characteristics, or factors that are appropriate about the organization. This section can also highlight the key objectives for both the strategic planning process and the plan document. Outlining clear and specific objectives can help stakeholders more clearly understand the desired objectives to be achieved, why elements of the process or the plan document are the way they are, and even their role in the strategic planning process.

DIRECTIONAL STRATEGIES

The directional strategies include the mission, vision, and values statements of the organization.

Mission statement—a summary statement or statements that describe the organization's enduring purpose or reason for being.

Vision statement—a summary statement or statements that describe the organization's desired future state, ideally with clarity and specificity. The vision is what the organization will look like or what it will be doing when it is meeting its mission in the future.

Values statement—statements of guiding principles that direct desired actions and behaviors and represent the values of the organization to be lived out.

ENVIRONMENTAL ASSESSMENT

This section identifies key strategic factors in the external environment—both in the general and specific environments—that may have implications for the organization's strategy. The process used to complete an environmental assessment is referred to as environmental scanning, or searching the environment for important events or issues that might affect an organization. The general environment is the economic, technological, sociocultural, and political factors and trends that indirectly affect all organizations. The specific environment is the customers, competitors, suppliers, industry regulations, and advocacy groups that are unique to an industry and directly affect how a company does business. These strategic factors are typically summarized into key findings, changes, and trends that have the greatest possible relevance to the organization and implications for its possible strategy.

SERVICE AREA ANALYSIS

This section identifies the health service organization's primary and secondary geographic service areas and describes the demographics and health status of the service area population. Strategic factors identified in this section can be summarized into key findings, changes, and trends that have the greatest possible relevance to the organization and implications for its possible strategy.

MARKET SHARE ANALYSIS

This section identifies the market share of the health service organization along with its primary competitors and will break down the market share by major service lines if the data is available. Market share is the proportion of total sales of a product or service (or patients, visits, or procedures) secured by one organization. Strategic factors identified in this section can be summarized into key findings, changes, and trends that have the greatest possible relevance to the organization and implications for its possible strategy.

COMPETITIVE ANALYSIS

This section identifies the health service organization's primary competitors and describes key factors, characteristics, actions, strengths, weaknesses, or possible future actions. Strategic factors with the competition identified in this section can be summarized into key findings, changes, and trends that have the greatest possible relevance to the organization and implications for its possible strategy.

INTERNAL ANALYSIS

This section identifies clinical and operating outcome data, statistics, ratios, and/or benchmarking that compares its internal operations, results, and performance typically over the prior two fiscal or calendar years and the most current year. Strategic factors identified in this section can be summarized into key findings, changes, and trends that have the greatest possible relevance to the organization and implications for its possible strategy.

STRENGTHS, WEAKNESSES, THREATS, AND OPPORTUNITIES (SWOT) ANALYSIS

This section summarizes the health service organization's major strengths and weaknesses, along with the key opportunities and threats in the local service area or general or specific environments. An organization may identify a competitive advantage it possesses, whereby it provides greater value for customers than competitors can. A competitive advantage is something an organization will want to take advantage of and build into its strategy whenever possible. It is recommended the SWOT analysis be completed towards the latter part of the process as most of the major, key elements to be summarized in the SWOT analysis should have already been identified in the other areas or components of the strategic plan. Strategic factors identified in this section can be summarized into key findings and changes and trends that have the greatest possible relevance to the organization and implications for its possible strategy.

STRATEGIC INITIATIVES

This section identifies the health service organization's strategic goals or initiatives that it proposes to pursue and attain. These strategic initiatives should be major goals and priorities for the organization; have high impact when achieved; are typically not easily achieved; typically take time, resources, and considerable effort to achieve; and should be no more than 5 to 10 in number. In most cases, each strategic initiative is driven by one or more strategic factors, as identified in the SWOT analysis or in the strategic factors having implications for strategy key findings, changes, and trends section of one of the other major components in the plan. In other words, the answer to the question "What are the strategic initiatives based on?" are the key findings, changes, and trends identified in the major components of the strategic plan completed heretofore in the process.

STRATEGIC IMPLEMENTATION PLAN

This section outlines a plan of action to implement the strategic goals or initiatives. A suggested format includes breaking down the strategic initiatives into specific actions steps; identifying the administrator responsible for coordinating the completion of each action step; a target date for completion of each step; and a section for recording the progress, status, or other appropriate comments on each step. This strategic implementation plan—also called an action plan—can be used as a reporting and communication tool for the ongoing implementation of the strategic plan at various levels in the organization.

CREATING A SHARED VISION

Sam Odle talks about the importance of vision as it relates to leadership being able to create positive change in a hospital or health service organization. Mr. Odle states that "***You have to be able to define a future state that is better than where you currently are. The status quo is very powerful: this is the way we do things around here, so people are very comfortable [(with the status quo)]. So if you want them to move to another level of performance, you [(the leader)] have to define a vision—a future state—that is compelling and better than what they [(employees)] have today. Then people will start to move forward with that. But if you have a vision, and no one else shares it, then it might as well be a nightmare because***

you [(the leader)] are going to try and get there but these other people [(employees)] don't share your vision and they're not marching or following you. So you have to have vision, and to define it, and you have to be able to build shared vision. That's where you [(the leader)] explain the "why" and allow people to ask questions and help to improve upon that vision if they have suggestions. It's about creating vision, and then building shared vision."

Vince Caponi states that ***"It takes clarity around what it is you are trying to accomplish, along with a well thought-out strategy that is well understood. This isn't done alone. This is a strategy where you've taken a hard look at the analytics; you've connected with others and you've gotten their input. And now you are going to recommend to someone who is going to decide and you are going to have to check with different people who are going to have to agree. Eventually you're going to have to perform. The leader has to make sure all those bases get covered. You have (to create) that sense of clarity; that sense of honesty; that sense of a clear picture."***

Dennis Dawes states that ***"Having the ability to put together a plan and to convince the Board of Trustees and the county government that this hospital needed to move in these directions–all those different times that I would [refer to as] building times, expansion of the building expansion of services, all of those through the years were defining moments. I don't know what would've happened if I was not able to convince the powers to be that I had to convince."***

STRATEGY AND CAPITAL EXPENDITURES

Dennis Dawes talks about a joint venture project with the YMCA to create the Hendricks County YMCA and Hendricks Regional Health outpatient center in Avon, Indiana. That project took a significant capital investment, as well as a number of years in the decision-making and planning process. ***"This project—on the hospital side of it—was about $25 million dollars: not small change. The bigger risk before this project was a $70 million expansion of the hospital campus in Danville. This building in Avon houses what is called the Hendricks Regional Health YMCA, but the same building also houses Hendricks Regional Health Medical Services. We are in the same building under the same roof providing services [including] physical therapy, cardiac rehab, doctors office space, etc., along with YMCA programs serving lots of people: all kinds of activities that are going on. Probably five years before the board said 'Yes' to the idea of doing this [project], we were talking about doing something in Hendricks County. Five years before this [project was approved by the hospital board], we were talking to the board about the fact that Hendricks regional health needs to not just be an illness care providing facility, we need to be in the business of providing wellness care to the people in this community as well. We need to do something that really speaks to that in a major way. We need to develop a major fitness facility or something like that to provide that aspect of healthcare. The board said 'No,' that's not our mission that's not our role. We are to provide inpatient care, outpatient care and these types of hospital services and we're not thinking outside of that. It took a long time to convince them that is a good concept, the right concept, and we need to pursue that. It really jelled when we brought to them***

the joint venture between Hendricks regional health and the YMCA. But it took many years to let that seed soak in with them and we would keep bringing it up. I was told 'No' by the board I don't know how many times. At one point I was even told 'No,' and let's don't talk about it again. Yet it wouldn't get out of my mind. That was probably a defining moment. I just thought of it as this is important and I've got to keep doing this."

BUSINESS PLANS

Mr. Dawes states that ***"We really did put together solid business plans for things, as well. It wasn't just an idea and a half-page of written notes and concepts, and by the way will you approve this $20 million expenditure? We developed solid business plans with adequate financial information, even to the point of showing the board and others this may not be the best financial decision to make, but it's the right decision to make for providing a service that doesn't have the best financial reward. But it is something that needs to be done. Being in a big business requires good business planning."***

Developing a business plan is an important step when a major new service line, expansion project or other major capital investment is being proposed or considered. A business plan is a written document that outlines and specifies important details regarding the proposed creation of a new business, service, or program or the expansion of one that already exists. Development of a business plan is an important step in the process of analyzing and evaluating the feasibility of the new or expanded service. There are many important purposes and uses for a business plan, including a document or tool that: 1) contains both the qualitative and quantitative data and analysis for the proposed service; 2) provides analysis regarding the business case, feasibility, and projected financial impact; 3) facilitates the presentation of a concept or definitive proposal; 4) facilitates date-driven decision-making regarding a proposal or investment; 5) assists in the process of securing funding, whether the funding source is internal or external; 6) provides budgeting and resource allocation planning and evaluation metrics; and 7) helps to facilitate consensus towards embarking on a new venture.

TAKING RISK

Dennis Dawes talks about risk as ***"Part of an executive level management position involves risk, no-matter what. That's just a part of it. There aren't any classes that I'm aware of on risk and what risk, and how you deal with that in a work career: it's just there. I always encourage my staff do not be afraid of taking risk. I'm not going to fire you: you need to be willing to take risks at your job as well. I always tried to keep reminding myself to give credit to people when they developed something and it was their project, and to not take all the credit for that. If something failed, to make sure that I took the blame for that." As CEO, "I am at the head of the organization, I allowed it to happen, and I am going to stand up and take that hit. To a certain extent I could be a buffer to people and buffer the risk they were taking.***

If I felt like the board might come down somebody, I always felt I wanted them to come down on me. To me is just proper management."

PLANTING SEEDS

Dennis Dawes says he would ***"plant a lot of seeds in different places and see if something would grow from those seeds or not. It could be a seed planted with a medical staff leader that I could see (whether he) accepted my idea or not, or convince me not to go there. Planting seeds was always an approach I used at different levels, especially with the board as well."*** Mr. Dawes goes on to say ***"it might take a few years to convince everybody, and occasionally it did. We would plan something out, and we couldn't get there, and I would say to myself 'find another way to get this done.'"***

Planting seeds is a leadership philosophy and style that can help a healthcare leader to: 1) test a new idea or concept with others and get their reaction; 2) help the leader to think through the idea or concept further by soliciting other thoughts, ideas, insights and considerations; 3) identify other action steps that may need to be taken in order to rework the idea or concept before taking it any further; 4) evaluate and assess the level of support and enthusiasm overall for the idea or concept and where pockets of support, as well as opposition, may rest; and 5) determine how others perceive the idea or concept in relationship to other goals and priorities of the organization.

MISSION DRIVES VISION

Mr. Dawes states, ***"I can't say there was a time when I felt like it might be a decision this way might be a career-ending decision or [conversely] have a positive impact on me or another person. I never thought of it that way. I always thought of it as we need to make this decision for the sake of providing healthcare in this community to people who need it. And if we don't do this, someone else is going to do it, and the mission of the hospital is to provide this and we need to do it. Figure out a way to get it done."***

PUSHBACK ON VISION

Mr. Dawes states that ***"Some tough defining moments? I guess I would say were steps to increasing the services of Hendricks Regional Health in the community that we serve. There were times when I would have major pushback from the board, maybe physicians, maybe the county government since the county owned the hospital. But I never felt like it would be such a moment in time that I would have to leave. I just felt like this was the right thing to do and I need to press ahead to get it done."***

COMMITMENT TO A STRATEGIC PLANNING PROCESS IS CRITICAL

Mr. Stella states, ***"And the hospital association just popped-up. I followed a legend (Mr. Elton Tekolskie). I told the board during my interview—I told Mr. Strausheim, Hicks, and Gent—if you want to hire me we've got to do a strategic plan. And I will tell you during my interview, right now, if you're not committed to change that a strategic plan is going to call for—and we don't know what it will say—then don't give it [(the job)] to me, because I will fail. They gave that position to me. And the two consultants and I drove from the Ohio River to Lake Michigan, and we talked to everybody in this state. Jerry McMannnis and a lady by the name of Jerry Stewart and myself. We were everywhere developing that plan. So when that plan came out—it had us organized, and the issues articulated, and it had the emphasis which was going to be regulatory and public policy."*** In addition to securing the commitment needed for a strategic planning process, Mr. Stella utilized a participatory leadership process in his approach to the strategic planning process. Soliciting input from key hospital process owners and stakeholders was a vital element in his success to develop a strategic plan for the entire hospital association with the support of its member hospitals.

IMPLEMENTING A STRATEGIC PLAN

Mr. Stella reflects upon an experience when he was the CEO at Morgan County Hospital in Martinsville, Indiana, and was spearheading a strategic planning process. ***"My achievements in Martinsville were the Martinsville community and the hospital community coming together and implementing a plan, and getting that done. I really can't say that I made that plan. That [strategic planning] committee made that plan: the community made that plan. My job was to implement it. The first part of that [plan] was physician recruiting. And I look back on the physicians we recruited together and used the community to help us as well. But to look back on those physicians that came in: they trusted us; they trusted the plan; they trusted if they came they would get the [new] facilities. That was accomplished in a four year window of planning, then getting it implemented. It was some of the most exciting times to be honest. In many ways I felt like a football coach because every time a physician would commit they were coming—it was like winning the Super Bowl. I still remember one evening when the front page [of the local paper] had pictures of four new physicians who were coming to town along with their specialties and bios. It was exciting. Then going on and seeing the [new] facilities constructed."***

FIVE INTANGIBLE BENEFITS OF HOSPITAL STRATEGIC PLANNING

The U.S. healthcare system is complex and confusing, according to a majority of respondents to the 2012 Deloitte Consumer Survey. Many consumers don't understand what factors cause limited access or uncoordinated care; requirements and limitations involved with both public and private health insurance coverage; conflicting interests amongst healthcare providers; or even high charges that leave many dumbfounded, disillusioned, or even financially broke. Those working in healthcare frequently see the industry as overly complex and confusing, as well, with rapid changes in the external environment producing a sense of turmoil and chaos within the organization. The complexity and confusion—both outside and within the industry—are sure to increase as a result of the Patient Protection and Affordable Care Act of 2010 and related reforms to health policy, regulation, and reimbursement.

Most hospital boards of directors, leadership teams, medical staffs, and employees are feeling a sense of uncertainty in this turbulent healthcare operating environment—and for good reason. Healthcare reform and other numerous forces at play are creating a disruptive state in the healthcare operating environment, including significant cuts in governmental reimbursement; consolidation of the market and systemization; growing consumerism; increasing competitive pressures; physician practice variability and integration issues; the growing impact of social media; and our instant, in-a-hurry society. What does all this mean? For one, the critical and multifaceted role hospital strategic planning plays today is increasingly vital to a hospital's ability to proactively plan for and respond to dynamic changes and trends occurring in the external environment.

Hospital organizations—and their employees—want to know what the future of healthcare has in store, where the organization is going, and how it will get there. Moreover, employees want to be reminded their work is important and understand how it contributes to the hospital's mission and vision for the future. Understanding how the work they do connects with and supports the organization's vision is critical for employees to appreciate the valuable role they play on the healthcare team. Helping employees make this powerful connection takes effective leadership.

While effective leadership requires many essential elements, creating and executing a shared organizational vision may be more imperative today than in any other era in the history of healthcare. Given all of these external changes, a strategic planning horizon of three years is probably optimal for most hospital enterprises with an annual process for updating. Strategic plans are most effective when they become dynamic, working documents that provide organization, structure, and reporting for organizational planning and business implementation processes.

Strategic plans are most effective when they become dynamic, working documents that provide organization, structure, and reporting for organizational planning and business implementation processes.

In addition to spotting key changes and trends in the external environment, there are multiple internal benefits a hospital can realize from a strategic planning process and plan development and strategic implementation:

- Clarity amongst chaos
- Operating in vision, not circumstances
- Employee motivation and engagement
- Transformational leadership and accountability
- Organizational collaboration

CLARITY AMONGST CHAOS

During periods of dynamic environmental change like we are experiencing today, it is easy for an organization and its people to become bewildered and confused. Employees, physicians, and other stakeholders want to know the organization has a bright future and what that will look like once the vision is achieved. In other words, they want to know where the organization is going and how it will get there.

An effectively developed and executed strategic plan can provide needed clarity amongst the chaos. A strategic plan should articulate key strategic issues and provide a roadmap to the organization's vision for the future, as well as a game plan to get there. This helps give employees and stakeholders the confidence they need to make a financial, emotional, and psychological commitments to the organization. In the case of employees, that commitment extends to their overall career, as well as their daily work, and can result in increased productivity and a higher level of employee engagement in the workplace. In the case of patients, that commitment is about trusting the hospital with their health or even their very lives.

OPERATING IN VISION, NOT CIRCUMSTANCES

Developing and sharing a vision through a participatory process can have a powerful impact on all levels of the organization. Employees are inspired by a well-crafted and clear vision that vividly describes a compelling future state. There will be challenges, however, to bringing the organization's vision into fruition.

Just as individuals must confront challenges, every organization must deal with forces and circumstances of all kinds. An organizational culture that operates or lives in circumstances—only to constantly react to negative changes with no planning or vision—won't ever see what's possible. Consequently, leaders who live in circumstances and not vision will prevent the organization from believing in an achievable future state or vision. A strategic plan and well-articulated vision that is properly developed, communicated, and executed can elevate an organization above its circumstances and connect it and its people with a future of possibility that is both inspiring and achievable. It is only when individuals and organizations live and operate in vision that they will ultimately realize a better future—one that is much more compelling and powerful than their current state.

EMPLOYEE MOTIVATION AND ENGAGEMENT

An aspect of organizational behavior getting more attention today—and increasingly being recognized as a critical success factor for organizational performance—is employee engagement. Employee engagement impacts everything from patient safety, quality, and service delivery to innovation, problem-solving, and financial performance. The level of employee engagement in the organization is an expression of employee beliefs and attitudes that is made manifest by the degree of effort teams and individuals give—otherwise known as discretionary effort.

Every employee makes a decision as to the amount of discretionary effort they give at work—every shift. Discretionary effort refers to the extra effort an employee has to give. Tapping into this employee discretionary effort inspires them to give over and above the "minimum acceptable standards" as outlined in a job description or performance evaluation form. Tapping into employee discretionary effort takes leadership; however, leadership alone isn't enough. Employees won't be inclined to give their discretionary effort for an organization that doesn't have an inspiring vision or a game plan that is well communicated and understood as to how the organization will get there. For many employees, it boils down to this thought: Why give extra effort for an organization going nowhere? This is a matter that moves beyond transactional leadership into the realm of transformational leadership.

TRANSFORMATIONAL LEADERSHIP AND ACCOUNTABILITY

Transformational leadership is about a leadership style that transforms an organizational culture and inspires its people to perform better. Transformational leaders use techniques well documented in today's organizational behavior literature. Moreover, transformational leaders are skilled at communicating the organization's vision, the steps to get there, and each employee's key role for its realization. Transformational leaders are effective in getting followers to understand and believe in their own individual and collective abilities to achieve higher levels of performance.

Sam Odle states that ***"I still reflect back on Dr. Goldberg and his telling me what a good leader I was, but the way I was doing it made me look bad. I could do better. That made me reflect upon how I treat people; how I got results—not just getting the result—but how I got the results was really important. That's where I changed my leadership style to one of followership. You get people to follow you; then they will be more productive and do things even better than what you thought they could. I always tell people good ideas don't come from my office—they come from people out there doing the work. But I have to create an atmosphere where they think I want to hear their ideas versus I'm just barking orders and they are to just follow the next order."***

Mr. Odle also says, ***"Going back to the difference between management and leadership, I look at it as being all leadership, management is more focused on the transactional leadership. If you're a unit leader–if you're managing a section—you're managing the buyers, or the x-ray technicians, etc. There are incremental transactions that have to be done, no matter if they are patient care, business, or whatever. Hopefully what happens [through a healthcare manager's career is the healthcare leader] masters the transactional skills and then makes it up to the vision and strategy. That's right where transformational leadership comes in. You don't lose your transactional skills, but you develop transformational leadership skills."***

Sam Odle says, ***"It's all one big family: it's all interconnected. If you use that philosophy of making the decisions that have the most positive impact on the most people, you'll make different decisions."***

Dave Handel says that ***"I was involved in a lot of things over my career. Everything I was involved in, the accomplishments were done by a team: not by me or any one individual. It's clear to me the key is 'can you be an effective part of the team?' In a [healthcare] leadership role it is creating effective teams. And it is also making sure you attract and retain really talented people who are going to populate those teams as well."***

Helping employees understand the important role they play in achieving the organization's mission and vision is crucial. Moreover, using a management by objectives, or MBO, process is needed to help everyone in the organization work together and create a common understanding. In this approach, individual employee objectives and plans are created in alignment with overall organizational goals and objectives. In addition, an effective MBO process includes regular reports on progress toward goals, along with holding individuals and teams accountable for effort and results. Therefore, transformational leadership takes both vision and accountability.

ORGANIZATIONAL COLLABORATION

Cooperation, collaboration, and team unity are essential to deliver high quality patient care, great service and organizational performance. Employees must work from the same "playbook" and pull in the same direction. Teamwork is essential for hospitals to improve their performance in critical areas of operation. An effective strategic plan implemented using an MBO approach for organizational alignment can be a powerful tool that fosters organizational collaboration.

An effective strategic plan implemented using an MBO approach for organizational alignment can be a powerful tool that fosters organizational collaboration.

A word of caution here. Many times the strategic planning process breaks down during implementation. A strategic plan's execution involves clear communication and understanding at all levels of the organization; an organized, decentralized approach to push implementation and execution throughout the organization; responsibility, accountability, and authority for implementation; evaluation metrics and reporting; and a supportive and collaborative spirit of cooperation and support.

The execution of a strategic plan takes organization, performance accountability, and teamwork, just as quality care and service takes interdisciplinary professionals at all levels working together in a spirit of cooperation, collaboration, and team unity—with a single-mindedness of purpose.

A well-crafted, properly executed strategic plan can provide numerous intangible internal benefits for an organization's culture, working environment, and employees. In the dynamic healthcare operating environment of today, with expectations of hospital operating performance growing, the benefits create a compelling case for hospital strategic planning.

REASSESSING THE DIRECTIONAL STRATEGIES

Historically, the mission and vision for most health service providers and organizations haven't materially changed; however, today these directional statements/strategies are in a state of change—just like the healthcare industry at large. As new incentives, structures, and expectations in healthcare dramatically shift, providers are reassessing and reevaluating exactly what their organization's mission and vision really mean, if they still remain appropriate, and what they should be; how to go about obtaining the mission and vision in a new era of healthcare reform; and what true organizational success looks like, along with the path to get there. Now more than ever, boards, CEOs, and senior leadership of health service organizations should be spending ample time contemplating and having dialogue about their mission and vision. If changes seem to be in order to these directional statements/strategies, well, change appears to be moving rapidly in healthcare wherever one may look. How will health service organizations respond to this rapidly changing environment?

The U.S. healthcare industry is transitioning from a fee-for-service environment to one based on value, performance, and accountability. Bundled payments for episodes of care; value-based purchasing and pay for performance; capitated or modified capitated reimbursement; and reimbursement withheld when the care rendered doesn't meet the prevailing standard of care are increasingly the way healthcare services are being reimbursed. At the same time, payors are getting into the provider business, and providers are getting into the health insurance business. The health insurance marketplace is making more health insurance plans available with the click of a mouse. Retail and worksite clinics are proliferating, and mid-level and alternative providers alike are increasingly being accepted by consumers and employers. Mergers and acquisitions are creating large, integrated delivery systems, providing a complete continuum throughout each level of care. The majority of physicians in the U.S. are now employed, including many specialists and sub-specialists. Proprietary delivery systems continue to flourish. And, the roles of various health service organizations, as well as the service offerings they are providing and ventures they are involved in, are no longer neatly marked by clear lines of demarcation. In other words, the metamorphosis of traditional healthcare organizations is being spurred by healthcare reform, and much more is yet to come. What are the implications for health service organizations?

To be sure, the implications of this new healthcare environment are varied, complex, and far-reaching. It is clearly no longer business as usual. And health service organizations shouldn't approach their annual or three-year review of their mission and vision statements (along with the organizational values referred to as the "directional strategies") as business as usual, either.

Historically, boards, CEOs, and senior leadership teams of some health service organizations have approached the review of the organization's mission and vision as nothing more than a perfunctory exercise to just get through as quickly as possible. But those days—like the "good old days of healthcare"—are over. The mission and vision should truly be used as strategies to provide direction for the organization and should be carefully reassessed for pertinence, applicability, and appropriateness. Change to a health service organization's directional strategies may well be needed in light of the evolving delivery models and payment structures for care; shifting roles and ventures of various health service providers and organizations; new incentives and structures in today's healthcare environment; and health service organizations' need to evolve in an industry for which the landscape is dramatically shifting. More than ever, health service organizations need clear direction for their future, and that direction begins with a clear understanding and articulation of the organization's purpose and reason for being (mission) and the state it desires to attain in the future when it is achieving its mission to the community and people it serves (vision).

DEFINITIONS

The Mission Statement—1) defines the reason for the organization's existence; 2) provides overall direction for organizational priorities, strategies, and decision-making; 3) declares what the organization does and who it serves.

The Vision Statement—1) defines the desired future state of the organization; 2) describes what the organization will look like in the future when it is meeting is mission; 3) provides direction for strategies, goals, and tactics for the organization's future course of action.

Along with the organizational values—or guiding principles—the mission and vision comprise the directional strategies that provide needed guidance and direction for everything the organization does or implements, including its strategic plan; community health needs assessment implementation strategy;

capital and operating budgets; corporate scorecard; corporate goals, policies, and priorities; service offerings; marketing plan, strategies, and tactics, and much more.

Given new operating paradigms in healthcare, like population health management or accountable care, how does a health service organization go about making important decisions, such as: Should the health service organization become involved in an accountable care organization, bundled payment program, or health insurance product? What role should physician integration and clinical co-management play? What about involvement in risk-bearing reimbursement models or vertical integration into other health care ventures? What services does the organization consider its "core?" How involved should it really be in expensive, long-term community initiatives? While the mission and vision statements alone won't answer these or similar questions, these directional strategies can provide much-needed guidance and direction for decision making at all levels of the organization. Three key points for decision making by boards, CEOs, and senior leadership teams that warrant mentioning here are: 1) staying true to the mission throughout all endeavors; 2) truly using the directional strategies in setting organization direction, strategy, policy, and action; and 3) fostering and promoting alignment from the directional strategies throughout every level of the organization, including the individual work performed by each and every caregiver and employee of the organization.

SPECIFICITY IS KEY TO FOSTER REAL, CLEAR DIRECTION

Now is the time for health service leadership to reassess their mission and vision for the specificity and clarity needed to articulate real direction and guidance to the organization and communicate its strategies, priorities, tactics, and actions. When re-assessing the mission and vision statements, the following questions might be helpful to determine what changes may be warranted:

1. Does the mission and vision articulate enough specificity and clarity for the board, leadership, and employees to truly understand what the organization's purpose, role and direction should be in the new era of healthcare reform?
2. Does the vision create a clear picture or mental construct for what the organization should be doing in the future when it is meeting its mission to patients and the community?
3. Does the mission and vision articulate select key service lines the organization should offer, markets it should serve, and corporate relationships or structures it should embrace?
4. Does the mission and vision provide clear guidance and direction for organizational decision making at all levels?
5. Does the vision provide ample clarity and specificity for assessing organizational success within a specific period of time?

USING THE MISSION AND VISION FOR REAL GUIDANCE

In an environment where regulation, incentives, and priorities are changing rapidly, it has never been more imperative for health service organizations to know who they are and what they want to be in their service provision to patients and the communities served. Using the mission and vision to help set and guide strategic direction and decision making has never been more important. The winds of change can blow any health service organization—large or small—off course without notice. The mission and vision serve as the rudder and steering wheel for the organization to steer its way through the choppy waters and storms it is confronting in a sea of change in the healthcare industry.

The mission and vision serve as the rudder and steering wheel for the organization to steer its way through the choppy waters and storms it is confronting in a sea of change in the healthcare industry.

Using the mission and vision for real guidance requires boards and leadership teams to actively use the mission and vision—once it articulates the clarity and specificity needed—in corporate-level, departmental, and service-level decision-making. This requires referring to the mission and vision statements regularly and prospectively when decisions are being discussed and contemplated. Moreover, it requires referring to the mission and vision regularly and retrospectively after decisions are made to assess for alignment and congruency. This includes when discussing and contemplating strategies and policies, as well as tactics and actions for implementation at the lowest levels in the organization.

ONGOING ORGANIZATIONAL COMMUNICATION

Regular, ongoing communication of the mission and vision is important, including using specific examples of how these statements are being used to help set strategic direction; drive and support policy formulation and decision making; and structure operations, including work processes, priorities, standards, and performance expectations. The board and senior leadership should model the way and provide examples and illustrations of how corporate strategies, policies, and decisions are being made with the support and direction of the mission and vision. This type of leadership by example is a powerful method for instilling the importance of using these statements in real practice and reinforcing the culture for doing so.

The mission and vision can be powerful statements that provide much needed guidance and strategic direction to a health service organization, especially given the dramatically changing landscape and operating paradigm health service organizations are operating within today. Moreover, rapidly changing regulations, incentives, and opportunities are driving many health service organizations to re-examine and rethink their purpose, role, corporate relationships and structures, target markets, policies, and service offerings. Given this new healthcare environment, the mission and vision statements should truly be used to provide the needed guidance and direction for organizational strategy, policy, decision-making, tactics, and actions. Does your health service organization's mission and vision provide the clarity and specificity needed to effectively provide guidance and direction in the midst of the dynamic and chaotic healthcare environment? If not, it might be time for reassessment.

THE COMPELLING CASE FOR AN INSPIRING VISION

What will the organization look like in 10 years? What future state is the organization striving to create? An old nautical saying succinctly summarizes the compelling case for an inspiring vision: ***"No wind favors the ship that has no chartered course."*** Or the old Sioux proverb which also summarized the need for an inspiring vision: ***"If you don't know where you are going, any path will get you there,".*** These old adages underscore the need every organization has for a clear, inspiring, achievable vision. A vision is the starting point for the organization's destination. Strategic positioning of the organization to meet its mission, achieve its strategic initiatives, and prosper in the future begins with a clear vision of what the future state could be if the organization was achieving its potential.

An organization's vision statement provides direction for the development of strategic initiatives and key strategic decision making. The operating environment for hospitals will increasingly become more dynamic as the major provisions of the Patient Protection and Affordable Care Act and the Healthcare and Education Reconciliation Act of 2010, commonly known as "Healthcare Reform," become effective. It is this increasingly dynamic and complex operating environment that makes a compelling case for clarity, direction, and purpose for the organization more critical than ever.

With an increasingly dynamic healthcare environment comes anxiety, confusion, and uncertainty—all requiring organizational clarity among the chaos. This significant type of external change creates a compelling case for the important role of a clear and inspiring organizational vision statement to provide needed direction and clarity to where the organization is going and how it wants to be strategically positioned. However, the organizational vision statement must not only motivate and inspire, but also be perceived as achievable and realistic. Leaders and employees alike will not be as motivated or inspired by an organizational vision statement they perceive as a "pipe dream" or unrealistic.

According to Alan M. Zuckerman, ***"A shared vision is the target, whereas strategic planning is the arrow."*** Creating a shared vision involves engaging key stakeholders in the process. This process calls for utilizing the classic management approach of participatory leadership to effectively create support, commitment, and "emotional ownership" for the vision. The process of creating the vision statement follows a similar path to that of creating the mission statement; however, mission statements typically aren't time-specific while a vision statement is. Vision statements are usually of a longer-term duration, with a 10-year horizon pretty standard. Although most organizations will reaffirm their existing mission statement, the vision statement will probably require some modification to adequately represent the future state desired in a dynamic environment. Effective vision statements should be somewhat idealistic, unique, future-oriented, realistic, somewhat of a stretch to attain, and descriptive of what is truly possible.

A proven approach to effective strategic planning—at any level—is to visualize the end state or the future conditions, achievements, or performance, then work backward to identify the milestones and steps necessary to create the desired future state. To be effective, therefore, the vision statement must articulate the desired future state and describes the (general) conditions to portray a clear and vivid picture of the organization's future. A vision statement isn't the roadmap, but rather the destination, and should clearly answer the question all employees have: "Where is the organization going in the future?" Or, "Does this organization have a future, and what does it look like?"

Another critical role for the vision statement is to provide direction for the development of organizational strategic initiatives. Every organization is challenged with the task of developing strategic initiatives that create alignment with the mission and facilitate the creation of the future state or vision desired. Once the strategic initiatives have been developed, an implementation plan (or action plan) can be created in order to break the larger strategic initiatives down into action steps that can be pursued and accomplished.

Given the amount of external change occurring in healthcare today, alignment of daily operational decision making with the vision and other directional strategies may be more challenging, as well as more important, than ever. Staying the course toward mission and vision attainment takes clarity, determination, commitment, persistence, and leadership. It also takes an organization of stakeholders knowing and understanding exactly where the organization is heading, why, and how their individual and departmental contributions contribute to the attainment of all the directional strategies. Without a high level of stakeholder understanding and connection with the vision, a gap in expectations and performance may occur. It is leadership's job to engage, educate and inform stakeholders of key changes and trends in the external environment that are impacting the organization and its future. Moreover, it is leadership's job to help employee's clearly understand how their important work supports the organization's mission and vision.

PUSHING THE BOUNDARIES OF STRATEGIC THINKING

Strategic management is both a philosophy and a process for optimally positioning the healthcare organization in the market. One of the three components—and the foundation of strategic management—is strategic thinking. What is strategic thinking? It is an intellectual and conceptual process for considering how to renew or reinvent the organization due to dramatic change in the environment. Strategic thinking involves questioning, analyzing, and projecting current assumptions and trends that are occurring or emerging and contemplating the company's strategy, actions, offerings, and image to transform the organization and optimally position it within its changing environment and service area. In this regard, there is much for strategic thinkers to consider with the changing environment.

Changes to consider include the needs, wants and preferences of consumers; advancements in technology and clinical know-how; changes in the organization's service area demographics; competitive threats; changes in the economic, political, or regulatory environments; or even national or local manpower or resource shortages. All of these, as well as other changes and trends, must be carefully considered regarding their current and future impact on the organization. These considerations then lead to the overarching strategic question: "How should the organization respond?"

Strategic thinking is a process that can help stretch the thinking about the organization; its mission, vision, and goals; and the future position it can hold in the market. How can the board and executive leadership push the organization beyond the boundaries of its current market offerings, organizational culture, and practices and create a future above that which it has experienced? Strategic thinking is the first step in breaking the boundaries of the complacency of ordinary, operational thinking. That's not to say that operational thinking isn't a good thing. To the contrary, solving problems, addressing challenges, and making everyday decisions is critical for effective daily operations. However, strategic thinking elevates us above the ongoing problems and demands of daily operations to help us see the big picture and consider what is really possible for the organization and its future.

In his book *Thinking for a Change*, author John C. Maxwell provides the business case for the critical role a change in thinking plays in changing your situation at a personal or organizational level. Furthermore, Maxwell reinforces the need to continue a change in thinking in order to see the vision and steps for achieving that vision. In other words, strategic thinking is an ongoing process, and persistence is required. Strategic thinking should, therefore, not be a singular, episodic event, but a process that is given the focus and attention that it needs to become the creative, strategic, insightful, and conceptual process foundational to strategic management. Given its rightful due diligence, strategic thinking can be highly effective in producing understanding, insight, and vision for where the organization should go and how it should get there. Below are 10 steps for effectively engaging a strategic thinking process.

1. **Permission to Think Big**—Many people in the organization—including leaders—need permission to think big, to dream, to consider possibilities. Without permission, many people won't stretch their thinking beyond the ordinary and commonplace.
2. **Start with the Endpoint in Mind**—The organization's vision represents the endpoint: a point in time in the future and what the organization can be and what it can look like. Start with the vision or the endpoint in mind and work backwards to today, outlining the initiatives and specific steps needed to create the desired future reality. The focus of strategic thinking is about that vision or endpoint.
3. **Search for Ideas that Inspire**—Great ideas can inspire others. Many times, we can develop great ideas for our organization derived from ideas used by others. Look around and see what other organizations are doing. It has been said that, in order to be great, one needs to study greatness. What can you learn? What are other organizations doing that can be modified to work well for your organization?

4. **Connect with Your Own Creativity**—Strategic thinking may well be more of a right brain process. Tapping into your own creativity, intuition, and innovative skills is necessary to create a vision or picture of what is possible for the organization and its future.
5. **Use the Brainstorming Technique**—A proven process that is effective in generating new ideas and ways of thinking, brainstorming can be useful in developing possibilities for the future. The use of the brainstorming technique can be particularly effective in a retreat or other similar meeting setting. Be sure to follow the procedure of not judging or critiquing ideas before getting possibilities out and on the table for exploration and analysis.
6. **Make the Process Inclusive/Seek Multiple Perspectives**—Nobody has a monopoly on good ideas. Seeking input from a variety of disciplines and perspectives is important so that critical elements can be seen or viewed differently while, many times, shedding new light on the situation or sparking new ideas. Moreover, making the process inclusive reduces the possibility for overlooking or minimizing key strategic factors.
7. **Consider the Opportunity Costs for Not Changing**—The natural tendency is to analyze possibilities from the perspective of what the cost might be if considered; however, many times the cost of not giving proper consideration to an idea (and subsequently not changing) can be greater. Be sure to examine costs from both an opportunity cost standpoint, as well as a resource allocation standpoint.
8. **Tolerate the Unstructured and Disorganized Nature of Creativity**—The creative process is not a logical, structured, linear process. Moreover, the creative process is a disorganized, unstructured, and potentially sloppy process. Be sure to acknowledge, accept, and tolerate this fact as you move through the process.
9. **Find The Right Emotional Space**—It is difficult to be creative and think about the "Big picture" when one is in the emotional space that comes with the normal routine of daily operations. For effective creative, strategic thinking to occur, participants must be in both a conducive physical space and emotional space to be at their height of creativity. Setting the right tone, attitude, framework, or mood for participants is critical to maximize their ability to think creatively.
10. **Use Outside Facilitation**—Our familiarity, routine, and close relationships with our organizational team is vital for fostering teamwork and productive working relationships. However, familiarity can breed more familiarity. Therefore, utilizing an outside facilitator should be considered to help provide the necessary "Ground rules," emotional space, and experiences and perspective that can help spur creative, strategic thinking.

STRATEGIC MOMENTUM

Strategic momentum is an essential ingredient for effective strategic plan execution. Momentum is one of the most powerful forces there is in business today. So much can be accomplished when positive momentum propells individual and team effort for organizational performance; however, without big motivation, not as much seems to get accomplished. When a leader attempts to implement the directional strategies and strategic initiatives, the same is true. How can senior leadership use strategic momentum to make an organization's vision come alive? What are the forces at play, and what are the implications for senior leadership?

Implicit with organizational momentum is executive management providing organizational leadership: the inspiration and motivation for others to be engaged, achieve organizational goals, and give their best. Managing a healthcare organization and its people includes leading others toward achieving important organizational goals and objectives, attainment of the organization's mission, and achieving a shared vision of the future. Creating a shared vision, along with the strategic momentum to attain that vision, is at the core of leadership performance and organizational effectiveness. In his book *The Functions of an Executive*, Chester Bernard states that ***"Belief in the real existence of a common purpose is the essential executive function."***

Strategic momentum concerns the management of day to day activities to achieve the strategic goals of the organization. Active management and implementation of the strategic action plan developed to achieve the organization's strategies is essential. Therefore, strategic momentum includes more of the basic functions of management: planning, organizing, leading, and controlling. Activating, organizing, and directing managerial action toward the achievement of goals and objectives is fundamental to pursuing and attaining organizational directional strategies. These managerial actions are either supported or deterred by the organizational culture, structure, systems, and financial and human resources.

So, what elements or ingredients are essential for creating, driving, and sustaining strategic momentum in a health services organization?

STRATEGIC MOMENTUM'S 10 KEY WORK INGREDIENTS

A carefully crafted strategic plan can be instrumental in positioning the organization to respond to external changes and opportunities—but only if effectively executed with strategic momentum. Strategic momentum concerns the daily activities of managing the organization's strategy to achieve the strategic goals of the organization. The remainder of this chapter features 10 key elements essential for creating, driving, and sustaining strategic momentum in any health services organization. These 10 key elements are functions of effective leadership and take the effort and support of the governing board, CEO, and executive leadership team for implementation.

Only through understanding will acceptance occur.

Educate and Inform—Only through understanding will acceptance occur. A key role of executive leadership is to inform and educate the board, management team, employees, and physicians about changes and trends in the external environment, as well as key strengths and weaknesses of the organization. Key stakeholders need to know and understand how changes, trends, and issues impact the hospital, and how future strategic action being contemplated will help position the hospital effectively for the future. A variety of communication mediums can be used for this purpose.

Realistic and Inspiring Vision—Every health service organization should have a realistic and inspiring vision statement that describes the desired future state of the organization fulfilling its purpose. What could the organization achieve if it was reaching its performing potential and fulfilling its purpose? A vision should help inspire and motivate leaders and employees to achieve organizational goals. However, leaders need to help all employees clearly see and understand how their work fits into this vision.

Strategic Initiatives Supporting the Vision and Mission—Ongoing, effective communication by executive leadership is needed to help the management team, employees, and physicians understand how the major initiatives of the strategic plan support the vision and mission of the organization. How do the strategic initiatives drive the organization toward achieving its vision and fulfilling its mission? Again, leaders need to help all employees clearly see and understand how their work supports the directional strategies.

Consistency of Message—Research supports the important role repetition plays for any message to be heard, understood, and retained by its intended audience. Key talking points about the organization's mission, vision and strategic initiatives (collectively called the directional strategies) must be consistently communicated internally using various communication mediums.

Supportive Culture of Participatory Leadership—The organization's culture affects its performance at all levels. A culture of shared decision making is participatory leadership at its fullest, allowing employees input into decisions about things that affect them, the work they do, and their future. Making a concerted effort to solicit input from employees when developing the strategic initiatives sends a strong message of teamwork and respect, creating a sense of ownership for the strategic plan.

Management by Wandering Around—As CEO, would you like to know how effective the information and message about vision, mission, and strategic initiatives is getting out, and what people know and understand? There is really no more effective way to find out than making rounds and talking to employees and physicians. Moreover, personal interaction at the "grass-roots" level can facilitate inter-organizational dialogue, provide a forum for words of encouragement that motivate and inspire, and promote greater understanding and appreciation for the strategic plan.

Board and Key Physician Leadership—The "three-legged stool" of power in a hospital includes the board, medical staff, and administration. The working relationship and business partnership that exists in this triad is critical to effective organizational leadership and performance. Meaningful involvement of the board and physician leadership in the development and implementation of the strategic plan is critical. Moreover, keeping these two groups informed of progress being made and problems encountered during strategic plan implementation is vital for accountability. Written progress reports and verbal presentations should be consistently provided throughout the organization.

CEO or COO as Designated Strategic Plan "Champion"—Top management—and one identified executive as champion—must take the responsibility to drive the strategic planning process internally. Using an outside consultant to do the "leg work" to develop the strategic planning document and facilitate the planning process can be instrumental in the plan's overall development. However, the CEO or COO needs to be the plans "owner" and take ultimate responsibility and accountability for the process and plan, as well as its implementation and overall success.

Implementation Planning and Execution—Development of action plans for the implementation process of the strategic plan is every bit as important as the strategic plan itself. Strategic implementation takes leadership initiative, guidance, and direction; activation of people and resources; collaboration and discipline; and accountability. Senior leadership must hold itself and others accountable for implementation progress and take corrective action to drive results.

Department Specific Objectives and MBO—Asking departments to create specific objectives in alignment with and support of the broader strategic initiatives and organizational goals provides the important connection between strategy and the worksite. Moreover, MBO can help facilitate employee engagement, support, and emotional ownership for the vision, mission, strategic initiatives, organizational goals, and department objectives.

Strategic momentum can be a significant ally to a healthcare executive who uses its powerful force to help make the organization's vision come alive. If carefully planned and executed, these daily activities will provide executive leadership with the force—the momentum—to move the organization forward toward achieving its vision and fulfilling its mission. Strategic momentum is about creating leadership that will transform the organization into a much more efficient, effective, and well-positioned health service organization in its operating environment and the community it serves.

Ken Stella talks about taking a planning course one summer at Indiana University, Bloomington, from Professor John Meade when he was working on his graduate degree. Mr. Stella states that ***"I just remember learning so much from him and yet things that were very simple. He walked into class the very first day and wrote 'PIE' on the blackboard. He said That is all we are going to talk about this summer. We'll start with 'P'; we're going to end with 'E'. We're going to start in June and we're going to end in August. The month of June will be 'Plan', July will be 'Implement' and the month of August will be 'Evaluate'. So you plan, you implement and then you evaluate. And then you start all over again."***

A word of advice may be in order from Michael Angelo, the great artist, who said "***The greater danger lies not in setting our aim too high and falling short, but in setting our aim too low and achieving our mark.***" It seems appropriate that Michael Angelo's advice may be apropos for health service leaders as they embark on a strategic planning process.

DISCUSSION QUESTIONS

1. Describe why the strategic planning process is so important to health service organizations?
2. List two or three of the major components of the strategic plan document, and explain what they are about.
3. What is strategic thinking and how is it different from operational thinking?
4. What is strategic momentum, and why is it important?
5. Identify two or three functions or steps for effective strategic momentum to be carried out in a health service organization.
6. What are a few of the purposes or uses for a business plan when considering a new or expanded program or service?
7. What does Dennis Dawes say about "planting seeds," and what are a few of the reasons to do so?
8. What does it mean to start with the end in mind when doing strategic planning?
9. What is meant by the planning horizon?
10. How can a leader apply the concept of participatory leadership by creating a strategic plan working draft document?

FIGURE CREDIT

15

Results-Driven Change

Results-driven change is driving individual, team, and organizational performance by focusing on the measurement and improvement of the desired results to be achieved. Results-driven change is foundational to Goal-Setting Theory. Goal-Setting Theory states that people will be motivated to the extent to which they accept specific, challenging goals and receive feedback that indicates their progress toward goal achievement. Whether the healthcare leader wants to foster and drive individual, team, or organizational performance, the use of goals to help structure motivation and effort towards desired performance is essential.

OBJECTIVES

1. Understand the important role that goal setting plays in results-driven change.
2. Understand and appreciate the power of management by objectives (MBO) in a health service organization.
3. Learn why clearly defining success and establishing clear goals in the beginning of a process are essential to drive performance and results.

PLANNING

Planning is determining organizational, departmental, or individual goals and a means for achieving them. Planning is essential to providing focus for work and energy. Planning is fundamental to driving performance by focusing on the desired results to be achieved. There are a myriad of different types of plans that are typically developed and used in a health service organization, including strategic plans, operational plans, financial plans (i.e., a budget), performance improvement plans, marketing plans, patient care plans, treatment plans, risk management plans, emergency preparedness plans, departmental plans, recurring plans (i.e., written policies and procedures), action plans, and work plans. Again, plans are important, as they provide focus for work and energy and help drive performance by focusing on the desired results to be achieved. Another way in which plans can be helpful is in the process of being developed and approved, particularly when a participatory leadership process is utilized. Participatory leadership is a leadership style in which the leader consults employees for their suggestions and input before making decisions.

Two plans to mention here briefly are an action plan which outlines the specific steps, people, timeframes, and resources needed to accomplish a goal. An action plan can be used for breaking down a strategic plan into a form that can be implemented. An action plan can be used to outline the work and steps needed to complete a multi-step task or project. Action plans can be used to help organize the work into manageable, structured, organized sections or parts and allow leaders to monitor and track progress being made toward goal achievement. A second plan to mention briefly here is the contingency plan, which outlines alternative means, options, or scenarios for achieving an organizational goal or pre-established objective, task, or project. The use of contingency planning is sometimes overlooked as leaders don't plan or account for the possibilities and "what ifs" as they should. An example of a contingency plan is an emergency preparedness plan that outlines policies, procedures, processes, and other details relating to how the organization will respond to unpredictable natural or man-made emergencies that may occur. Here is a short list of common plans and their definitions:

Action plan—the specific steps, people, resources, and timeframe needed to accomplish a task or goal.

Business plan—a plan that outlines and projects the important elements and considerations for starting a new business or service line.

Capital budget—a plan that outlines a company's future expected expenditures on new assets, such as for land, physical plant or facility, and equipment.

Operating budget—a financial plan that indicates financial projections and targets and administration for a set period of time, typically monthly and annually.

Operating plan—a daily plan, developed and implemented to produce or deliver the organization's products or services over a 30-day to 12-month period.

Policy—a standing plan that indicates a company's official position or the general course of action that should be taken in response to a particular issue, event, or situation.

Procedure—a standing plan that indicates the specific steps that should be taken in response to a re-occurring activity, action or process, or event or situation.

Pro forma income statement—a financial plan or forecast of projected revenue, expenses, profitability, and related assumptions for a new service, program, or future state being considered.

Rolling budget—a statement that indicates financial projections and targets that is reviewed in a specified timeframe (monthly or quarterly) and updated.

Strategic plan—an overall company plan that clarifies how the company will serve customers and position itself in the market against competitors over the next one to three years or more.
Tactical Plan—Plan created and implemented that specifies how the company will use resources, budgets, and people over a set time period, such as 6 months to 2 years, to accomplish specific goals within its mission.

Work Plan—the specific steps, people, resources, and timeframe needed to accomplish a specific project or multi-task activity.

Planning occurs at all levels in a health service organization. However, senior-level administrators, as well as the board of Directors of the organization, are typically involved in the development and/or approval of major policies and procedures, budgets, strategic plans, and other more organization-wide plans. Middle managers such as department heads or service line managers are involved in implementing plans developed and approved at the senior level, as well as development and approval of plans more specific to their areas of responsibility, such as tactical plans for the department, policies, and procedures specific to the service or function, or related plans. Front line managers are usually involved in implementation and enforcement of plans and polices with input into those specific to their area of responsibility.

MANAGEMENT BY OBJECTIVES (MBO)

MBO is a practical application of goal setting theory that has been proven to drive results and performance, typically at the individual employee level. MBO uses the participatory leadership process, which is a leadership style in which the leader consults employees for their suggestions and input before making decisions. MBO's participatory process makes it a powerful technique to gain individual employee support, buy-in, and emotional ownership. MBO works. It is fairly simple and straightforward process to use. Sam Odle talks about using MBO as a central aspect of his healthcare leadership during his career, using several different versions and models, but all based on MBO's four-step process. The four-step MBO process is as follows:

1. Supervisor and subordinate meet to discuss possible objectives for the employee;
2. Supervisor and subordinate agree upon objectives the employee will work to achieve;
3. Supervisor and subordinate share information and discuss strategies and tactics that could lead to achievement of objectives;
4. Supervisor and subordinate meet regularly to review and discuss employee progress made towards goal achievement and take corrective action as needed. It is important for the supervisor to help the subordinate, as needed, with support, advice, suggestions, coaching, providing additional resources, or other appropriate means to assist the employee in meeting his objectives, as needed. This doesn't mean the leader does the work, but provides the conditions necessary for the employee to succeed in achieving the objectives.

Sam Odle states that ***"Management by Objectives is a fundamental tool that we [(leaders)] use to define what it is we are going to try and accomplish, along with tactics that go with that, so we don't just accidently get through the year but there clearly are some things we are going to try and accomplish. Especially in complicated organizations where there is a lot of autonomy, leaders need to make sure those MBOs are aligned. That means senior leadership has to cascade them from the top. You have to decide on what are the priority areas. Sometimes organizations call these pillars, or areas of emphasis: the 5 or 6 important areas of emphasis that leadership wants everyone to focus on. These get cascaded down [to the department level] and departments have to decide how to accomplish each objective or pillar [at the department level]. Eventually it has to cascade down to the individual employee level. So [senior leadership] has to start and make certain that they align those [(corporate)] objectives and areas of emphasis as they cascade them down throughout the organization so that everyone is rowing the boat in the same direction."***

DEFINING SUCCESS

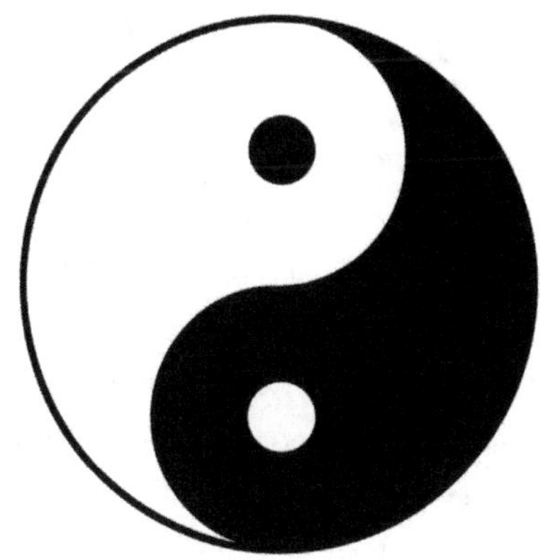

FIGURE 15.1 Yin and Yang

Many times the process of defining specifically what desired future success looks like—in terms of results, performance, and goal attainment—is overlooked or given cursory or minimal emphasis, time, and effort in some organizations. When this occurs, many times there isn't the clarity and consensus needed to generate or produce the understanding or motivation and organizational alignment at all levels needed for Results-driven change to be optimally effective. Therefore, the process used to identify and foster commitment to the goals and objectives that define success—the results and performance desired—is critical and should be given careful thought and attention by the healthcare leader. The following old cliché is apropos here: "***You can't hit a target you can't see.***" And, if you can't define the future success that is desired, or what that success should look like in terms of results and performance, then clarity needed to drive effort and performance in the same direction is lacking.

Sam Odle says that ***"One of the traits of a really great organization is that leaders hold themselves accountable and leaders hold others accountable for their performance as well. That comes from making sure the metrics of success around those objectives are real clear. If the objectives are real clear, people want to be successful. But the organizations that struggle are those [in which] the metrics aren't clear. [For example,] we all are going to do better this year. Well what's better? You have to make it real clear. Because if its not, then people will be out there doing things they think are the right things to make it better, but you don't have a common understanding of the objectives and the metrics."***

> Being clear and specific about what success looks like and what goals and objectives for results and performance should be one of the first tasks of any newly formed group.

Many times the process of defining success is skipped or given cursory attention when a new committee or task force is formed to tackle a problem, improve a process, or pursue an opportunity. Being clear and specific about what success looks like and what goals and objectives for results and performance should be one of the first tasks of any newly formed group. These goals and objectives for results and performance are also called Key Performance Indicators, or KPIs. Healthcare organizations can establish KPIs for any respective department, function, or service, as well as overall for the organization. KPIs established for the organization as a whole can also be referred to as critical success factors, a corporate scorecard, or a balanced scorecard.

CORPORATE SCORECARD AND TRANSPARENCY

The terms Corporate Scorecard or Balanced Scorecard or synonymous. The concept of a balanced scorecard was first conceived and promulgated in 1992 in an article written by Robert S. Kaplan and David P. Norton. The idea is to create a "dashboard" of KPIs for the organization as a whole that establish priorities for operating results and performance, and drive effort and work processes at all levels of the organization. This point is key: driving effort and work processes at all levels of the organization is critical to creating alignment of effort at all levels. A metaphor for this is to visualize a crew of eight rowers in a rowboat—four rowers rowing on each side—rowing to propel the boat forward in a straight line. If there isn't synchronicity of effort, timing, and rhythm, the boat won't go as fast or as straight. Why? Without the synchronicity of timing, effort, and rhythm, there will be forces contradicting or working against others, and the results and performance won't be optimal. The same applies for the operations of different departments, functions, services, and staff in a healthcare organization. Pulling together in the same direction towards the same goals and objectives is hypercritical.

Sam Odle states that ***"One of the best examples is the corporate scorecard and transparency. You make the metrics [of success] understood, and then you make the measurements really transparent so that everybody can see it. If my objectives are in the red, then I should have a plan of how I am getting from red to yellow and then to green. It's all around that transparency, and being willing to let people see how you [(the leader)] are doing and that you are holding yourself accountable for getting [the objective] from red to green. Sometimes that can be done in a very short period of time, and sometimes it may take a long time. Patient satisfaction is an example where we made it very transparent, not only to the employees but to the patients, the visitors, everyone. We posted those scores and we had a goal to get to green. It took two years just to get [the objective] to yellow. But you could see the metrics were moving a little bit all the time towards the positive. We were holding ourselves accountable saying we were going to get there. We were willing to hold that out there and let everybody see it."***

GOAL CLARITY AND ALIGNMENT

Sam Odle states that ***"Leaders need to make sure they are really clear on whatever the problem or opportunities are they are working on. We do a lot of things in groups, and we may go after one issue and we are not in agreement as to what the issue is; so we are working at odds with each other. When you are talking about cost controls, which is a big part of leadership is to make sure the budget is met and that you are being as effective with the resources you have as you can. An example would be looking at your operating costs. A lot of times you are trying to tighten-up all the [different] department's operations so you can have a better bottom line and invest more in the operations. Are you trying to get everyone to run faster, or are you trying to figure out that we don't have to run as many races as we are trying to run. So we have to make sure we are working on the right problem. The model for improvement is a standard way of thinking: what are we trying to solve? How would we measure success? And then***

trying some small scale changes—running PDSA cycles—to test your theories about how you can make improvements. It is one tool to keep the team from getting off track and working on the wrong things."

As Sam Odle stated, alignment of goals and objectives at all levels in the organization is important. Alignment is important for synchronicity of work and effort. Without alignment in synchronicity of work and effort, there will be suboptimization occurring in different departments, functions, and services. Suboptimization is when performance improvement efforts in one part of the organization result in decreased results, effort, or performance in another part. Many times, suboptimization results from the creation and implementation of policies, procedures, workflow processes, and practices that may assist an individual area achieve its goals and objectives but at the expense of others. It is taking a myopic approach towards policies, procedures, workflow processes, and practices in a different department, function or service without consideration to the impact elsewhere. Most of the time when suboptimization occurs, there is no malice or negative intent involved: rather it's the result of a lack of conceptual skills being used or applied.

Conceptual skills are the ability to see the organization as a whole, understand how the different parts affect each other, and recognize how the organization fits into and is affected by its environment. It is vital that a healthcare leader have good conceptual skills, as there are so many different departments, functions, services, and work processes that are connected and interrelated. Knowing and understanding how a change in one area (with a policy, procedure, practice, process, or workflow change) will impact others is vital for effective leadership decision-making. Without good conceptual skills, a healthcare leader will make decisions that will lead to suboptimization. Conceptual skills also apply to understanding how a health service organization fits into its community and its environment.

Sam Odle talks about goal clarity and alignment when he was an x-ray technician and radiology department supervisor. ***"When I was an x-ray technician and working in that small, microcosm of the x-ray department I realized that in order to get the work done in the timeframe that was desired, you really had to have everybody working as a team. Somebody had to work in the dark room; somebody had to do the barium enemas; somebody had to do the GI work; somebody had to do the IVPs. Everybody had a role to play. A lot of times those roles might change from day-to-day. But each member of the team had to be enthusiastic that day about the role they had—even if it wasn't the most desirable role—they had to say 'I'm going to do it the best I can do because it will make a difference for the whole team.' Seeing that at that small level was influential, and I took that philosophy with me as I moved up in the organization."***

DISCUSSION QUESTIONS

1. What is Results-driven change, and why is it important?
2. What recognized motivational theory is Results-driven change part of?
3. What are conceptual skills, and why are they particularly important in healthcare leadership?
4. What are the four steps in the MBO process?
5. Describe the role that clearly defining success plays in Results-driven change.
6. What example does Sam Odle use for leadership teams to hold themselves accountable?
7. What is meant by goal alignment, and why is it important?
8. What is a corporate scorecard and what is it purpose?
9. What is the definition of a policy?
10. What is the difference between a capital and a operating budget?

16

Thinking For Change

What do you do in your life that doesn't first start with a conversation? Anything? The answer is not too much. Other than things that occur automatically, such as the beating of your heart or the blinking of your eyes, everything you do starts with a conversation. Really—is that right? For many people, the first conversation of the day starts when the alarm clock goes off in the morning. The first conversation might go something like this: "*Is it time to get up already? I'd better shut the alarm off—it is so annoying. How do I feel? Did I sleep well? Should I get right up or lay here in bed for just a minute or so*?" That is how a lot of people start their morning—with a conversation similar to this. It's a conversation that isn't spoken verbally. It's that inner voice in your head, conversation that each of us have throughout our day. And, those thoughts and inner conversation structure everything we do. Sometimes our inner thoughts can be categorized as blaming and complaining or ones that are of intention and responsibility. These thoughts can be demotivating or affirming and encouraging. These thoughts can make us be passive and complacent or drive us to take action. This also applies to healthcare leaders and how they approach their jobs and think about themselves and their leadership—everyday.

OBJECTIVES

1. Understand and appreciate the role a healthcare leader's inner voice or conversation plays in his every day leadership.
2. Realize how a leader must first change his thinking in order to change his leadership style.
3. Understand that, for a leader to learn and grow through his experience, he must be reflective.

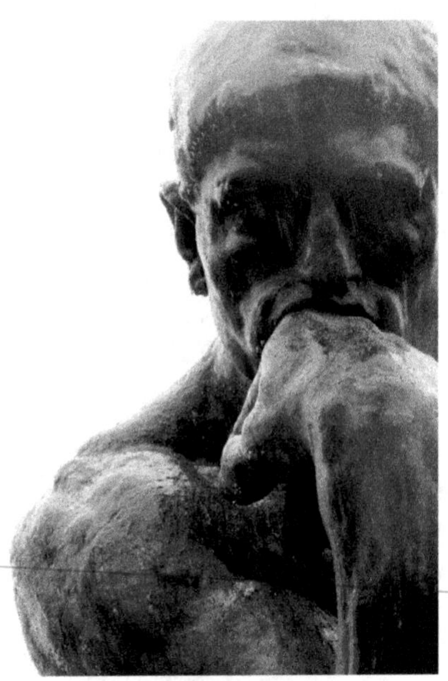

FIGURE 16.1 Close up of Thinker
Copyright © innoxiuss (CC BY-SA 2.0) at http://commons.wikimedia.org/wiki/File:The_Thinker_Musee_Rodin.jpg.

THE POWER OF THOUGHT

If you want to change your situation, position, or circumstances in life—and in leadership—you must first change your way of thinking. Everything you do starts with a thought, sometimes at the sub-conscious level and sometimes after considerable conscious thought, deliberation, and evaluation. Just like the old saying "form follows function;" action follows thought. Want to change your leadership actions, behavior, or style? Change your thinking.

The decisions that you've made, the processes you've followed, and the leadership style you've employed have resulted in the accomplishments, results, performance, and legacy you've created to date in your career. These have also resulted in the mistakes and failures you've experienced as well. If you want to be more effective and successful as a leader in the future than you have in the past, you will have to change something: maybe the decisions, processes, or leadership style you've employed. Why? Because if you always do what you've always done, you'll always get what you've always got. And changing your leadership style begins with a change in thinking.

Albert Einstein, considered one of the brightest and most intelligent persons to have ever lived, said "***We cannot solve our problems with the same thinking we used when we created them.***" www.brainyquotes.com. As a scientist, Einstein was also very conversant with the scientific method (see graphic below). Simply put, a healthcare leader should reflect on what aspects of his leadership style have been effective and which ones haven't. Those aspects that haven't been effective should be identified, and an action plan should be developed and implemented that features changes—use of a different leadership style, methods, techniques—and then reassessed. Did the changes result in improved effectiveness?

But the power of thought goes far beyond structuring your actions and behaviors. The power of thought plays a central role in your feelings and emotions, as well as your attitudes, beliefs, and values. Consequently, the power of thought cannot be underestimated nor undervalued in its critical role of structuring your life and how you distinguish the world around you and everything in it. Moreover, whether you are happy and satisfied with your work and your career or not; whether you hear or feel the affirmation from others that you help, support, and assist, or not; or whether you see the difference your work and efforts are making for the organization and community you serve or not; it's all about how you distinguish and think about the world you interact with every day.

THE STORY OF AN INSIDE JOB

A story is told of an elderly patient who became increasingly unable to care for herself. Consequently, she was being sent to a nursing home where she would be properly cared for and live the rest of her life. The elderly lady's family didn't live close by and wasn't able to take care of her: there really was no choice. So, on the day she was being admitted to the nursing home she was sitting in the lobby waiting for one of the staff members to escort her to see her room where she would be living. When the staff member approached the elderly woman, she inquired "***Would you like to see your room now***?" To which the new patient said with a big smile "***Oh, it's beautiful***!" The staff person replied, with a bit of a perplexed look on her face, "***But you haven't even seen the room yet.***" The new patient then replied "***Yes, I have—I've seen it in my mind, and I know it's beautiful and that I am going to be very happy here.***"

In leadership, just like in life, happiness and satisfaction with your job and your career is an inside job.

Here's the key point: in leadership, just like in life, happiness and satisfaction with your job and your career is an inside job. If you don't yet follow this belief, then change your thinking and your distinctions: it could change your life and your world.

THINKING ABOUT LEADERSHIP STYLE

Leaders will never change their leadership style—they won't make improvements; incorporate learning; apply new or different methods or techniques; reflect upon what they are observing or hearing; or even reflect on their own experiences and what they may do differently in the future to be a more effective leader—until they first think about it. As talked about in an earlier chapter, leadership is a journey, a journey that involves learning, growing, and developing as a leader through both formal and informal processes. But, a requirement for learning and development to occur is thinking about your leadership effectiveness and what has or is working effectively and where you could or should make changes and improvement with your leadership style. Thinking for change in your leadership style begins with reflection and asking yourself questions, such as:

- Are you being reflective around your leadership style and experiences? Are you spending ample time in reflection?
- What area or areas do you need additional knowledge and what opportunities, settings, or methods would be the most effective and appropriate to consider?
- What feedback have you received from others regarding your leadership style? What should you consider the most important, relevant, or informative, and what action should you be taking as a result?
- What changes have you incorporated into your leadership style, and what have your experiences been so far with those changes?
- What do you need to start thinking about doing that you have not been doing to be more effective as a leader?
- What do you need to stop doing to be more effective as a leader?
- What do you need to think about continuing to do to be more effective as a leader?
- What are you observing from other leaders that you might consider incorporating into your leadership style that might help you be more effective?
- What have you observed from other leaders that you might consider incorporating into your leadership style but in a different way to help you be a more effective leader?
- What have you observed from other leaders that you don't want to incorporate into your leadership style that would prevent you from being as effective as possible?

ORGANIZATIONAL CHANGE

At the heart of leadership lies the goal and responsibility of the leader to help make things better: the organization and its performance; the working environment and working relationship with employees; the quality of care and service delivery; the organization's competitive position in the market; compliance with laws and regulations; and reducing operating costs and improving financial performance. It's about improving everything that can and should be improved. This doesn't mean to change something working well. This means that a fundamental role of a healthcare leader's job is to be aware and look for opportunities to make different aspects of the organization better and take the appropriate action needed to do so.

Judy Monroe, MD, states ***"We are in some tough economic times and government is feeling the squeeze. Here at CDC we are trying to decrease the amount of cost for offices, so we are going to hoteling and tele-work. We have opened the doors to engage employees in problem solving around this. How do***

we decrease the amount of space we need and still produce what we have to?" Engaging employees to help improve the organization through change that will affect them—including how and where their work gets done—is most effectively done using a participatory leadership process. Participatory leadership is a leadership style in which the leader consults employees for their suggestions and input before making decisions. But sometimes the organizational culture can be an obstacle or impediment to organizational change. Judy goes on to say ***"When there is an organizational culture that is unproductive—either not a healthy culture or not productive—that is the job of the leader to change that culture."*** Driving organizational change requires the leader to understand and be completely in tune with the organizational culture and the organization's readiness for change or its receptivity and motivation to change. A leader must first give careful thought and contemplate the organization's readiness for change.

Driving organizational change requires the leader to understand and be completely in tune with the organizational culture and the organization's readiness for change or its receptivity and motivation to change.

In order for a healthcare leader to positively affect needed change in the organization, they must first be in-tune with the informal channels of communication; understand employees, physicians, trustees, and other internal stakeholders and how they will react to change; understand the organization's readiness for change or its receptivity and motivation to change, along with any resistance forces that support the existing state of conditions in the organization. Many times, change should be introduced as incremental change or change that is implemented in a planned or methodical process with small, intermittent amounts of change over a period of time. It is critical for a healthcare leader to think about and plan for change and how it should best be introduced and implemented. It can be a major mistake for a leader to attempt to drive too much change when resistance forces are high and readiness for change is low. Many times, the use of informal and/or formal change agents can be highly effective in driving change within the organization. An informal change agent is someone who helps to drive change but is not in a management position of authority. Informal change agents rely on their informal influence and relationships in the organization to gain support to help drive change. A formal change agent is the person formally in charge of guiding a change effort and typically occupies a management position of authority. A healthcare leader needs to think about whether to use formal and/or informal change agents to drive a needed change within the organization and determine how best to facilitate this.

It can be a major mistake for a leader to attempt to drive too much change when resistance forces are high and organizational readiness for change is low.

Creating change first starts with having vision about what that change should accomplish. Sam Odle talks about the importance of having vision as it relates to leadership being able to create positive change in a hospital or health service organization. Mr. Odle states that "***You have to be able to define a future state that is better than where you currently are. The status quo is very powerful: this is the way we do things around here, so people are very comfortable [with the status quo]. So if you want them to move to another level of performance, you [(the leader)] have to define a vision—a future state—that is compelling and better than what they [(employees)] have today. Then people will start to move forward with that. But if you have a vision, and no one else shares it, then it might as well be a nightmare because you [(the leader)] are going to try and get there but these other people [(employees)] don't share your vision and they're not marching or following you. So you have to have vision, and to define it, and you have to be able to build shared vision. That's where you [(the leader)] explain the 'why' and allow people to ask questions and help to improve upon that vision if they have suggestions. [It's about] creating vision, and then building shared vision.***"

> **So if you want them to move to another level of performance, you [(the leader)] have to define a vision—a future state—that is compelling and better than what they [(employees)] have today.**

Given the changing operating environment that health service organizations are operating in today—a dynamic external environment, changes with healthcare reform initiatives, increasing regulation, and reductions in reimbursement to name a few—the amount of change most health services organizations are experiencing is unprecedented. It is leadership's role and responsibility to facilitate the change needed within the organization and this first starts with the healthcare leader thinking for change.

DISCUSSION QUESTIONS

1. What do you do in your life that doesn't start with a conversation?
2. What does a leader have to do first in order to change his leadership-style? Please explain.
3. Describe the role your inner voice plays in your life.
4. How does the power of thought impact your feelings and emotions?
5. List two or three questions a leader should ask him or herself when reflecting on his or her leadership style and effectiveness.
6. What is participatory leadership, and how can it be used by a leader when facilitating change?
7. What does the term readiness for change mean? Please describe
8. Describe why healthcare leaders today must be effective change agents.
9. What role does the organizational culture play in the process of organizational change?
10. What is your reaction to Einstein's famous quote: "We cannot solve our problems with the same thinking we used when we created them."

17

Business Planning and Development

As the U.S. healthcare system's operating environment becomes more demanding, multifaceted, and complex—even confusing—many healthcare organization's clinical and program services offerings are changing. Health service organizations are reassessing their mission and vision, what services they should be offering, and how they are positioned in the market to compete. A health service organization must respond to its ever-changing environment in order to best meet the needs of its customers and stakeholders, comply with evolving regulations, and compete for business, including patients. Moreover, when the external environment—including both the general environment and the specific environment—are changing rapidly, it can create a sense of instability, turmoil, and uncertainty for a health service organization and its employees. The general environment includes the economic, technological, sociocultural, and political trends that indirectly affect all organizations. The specific environment includes customers, competitors, suppliers, industry regulations, and advocacy groups that are unique to an industry and directly affect how a company does business. This type of dynamic environment calls for good business planning in order to address changes occurring in the environment and how the health service organization should respond and optimally be positioned in a dynamic healthcare environment. Therefore, good business planning includes a process for reassessing the directional strategies, as well as the organization's business development function and processes.

OBJECTIVES

1. Understand and appreciate the important role business planning and development has in health service organizations today.
2. Examine how the organizational culture and leadership philosophy of senior leadership determines how the business planning and development function is structured and organized.
3. Learn about and apply a business development framework that can be used to develop new or expand an existing service or program.

ORGANIZATIONAL CULTURE AND STRUCTURE

The organizational culture greatly influences how the business planning and development function is handled in a health service organization. In most small hospitals or health service organizations, the CEO or CFO takes the lead and is responsible for new business planning and development. In large hospitals or health service organizations, there may be a senior-level manager, or even a department, devoted to and responsible for new business planning and development. How the function is organized, structured, and performs is typically a matter of the CEO or COO's philosophy and approach. What's the organization's appetite for risk? How supportive of innovation is the leadership team? Does the organization operate in a highly competitive market? Is the organization financially sound with ready access to capital? Many variables are at play that impact how an organization approaches business planning and development.

The business planning and development function, in many health service organizations, is administered by the same leader or department responsible for managing the strategic planning function. Why? Business planning and development is a similar function to strategic planning with similarity in terms of its process and some components. Moreover, the marketing function can also be part of the same leader or department's responsibilities as business planning and development. Again, the organizational structure is highly variable from one health service organization to another.

The decision-making process for a new venture also varies greatly by organization; however, the final decision-making authority typically rests with the board or CEO, depending upon the approval authority granted to the CEO by the board of directors. Moreover, depending upon the nature of the new venture, the CEO may want board approval, or at least board support, even if he has the authority to approve the request for capital expenditures needed to fund the new venture.

BUSINESS PLANS

A business plan is a written document that outlines and specifies important details regarding the proposed creation of a new business, service, or program or the expansion of one that already exists. Development of a business plan can be an important step in the process of analyzing and evaluating the feasibility of the new or expanded service. There are many important purposes and uses for a business plan, including a document or tool that: 1) contains both the qualitative and quantitative data and analysis for the proposed service; 2) provides analysis regarding the business case, feasibility, and projected financial impact; 3) facilitates the presentation of a concept or definitive proposal; 4) facilitates decision-making regarding a proposal or investment; 5) assists in the process of securing funding, whether the funding source is internal or external; 6) provides budgeting and resource allocation planning and evaluation metrics; and 7) helps to facilitate consensus towards embarking on a new venture.

WABASH COUNTY HOSPITAL
Statement of Revenues and Expenses
(UNAUDITED)

	Current Month Ending		30-Apr-09		30-Apr-08
	Actual	Budget	Variance	Variance %	Actual
PATIENT REVENUE					
Inpatient Services	$1,054,532	$1,067,742	(13,210)	-1.2%	$1,176,634
Outpatient Services	3,789,205	3,665,098	124,107	3.4%	3,727,005
Swing Beds	0	0	0	0.0%	0
Skilled Nursing Care Unit	264,391	224,500	39,891	17.8%	203,531
Home Health Agency Care	251,263	257,153	(5,890)	-2.3%	248,809
Total Patient Revenue	5,359,391	5,214,493	144,897	2.8%	5,355,979
DEDUCTIONS FROM REVENUE					
Charity	80,420	78,773	1,647	2.1%	189,311
Medicare Contractuals	1,575,083	1,490,433	84,650	5.7%	1,697,471
Medicaid Contractuals	295,832	283,240	12,592	4.4%	274,112
SNF Deductions	107,196	91,585	15,611	17.0%	79,202
Swing Beds	0	(48)	48	-100.0%	0
HHA Deductions	13,098	36,557	(23,459)	-64.2%	16,801
Other Deductions	428,324	418,088	10,236	2.4%	461,086
Total Deductions	2,499,952	2,398,628	101,324	4.2%	2,717,983
Deductions as a % of patient revenue	47%	46%			51%
Net Patient Revenue	2,859,438	2,815,865	43,573	1.5%	2,637,997
Other Operating Revenue	55,105	54,222	883	1.6%	160,739
Net Operating Revenue	2,914,543	2,870,087	44,455	1.5%	2,798,736

FIGURE 17.1a Wabash County Hospital

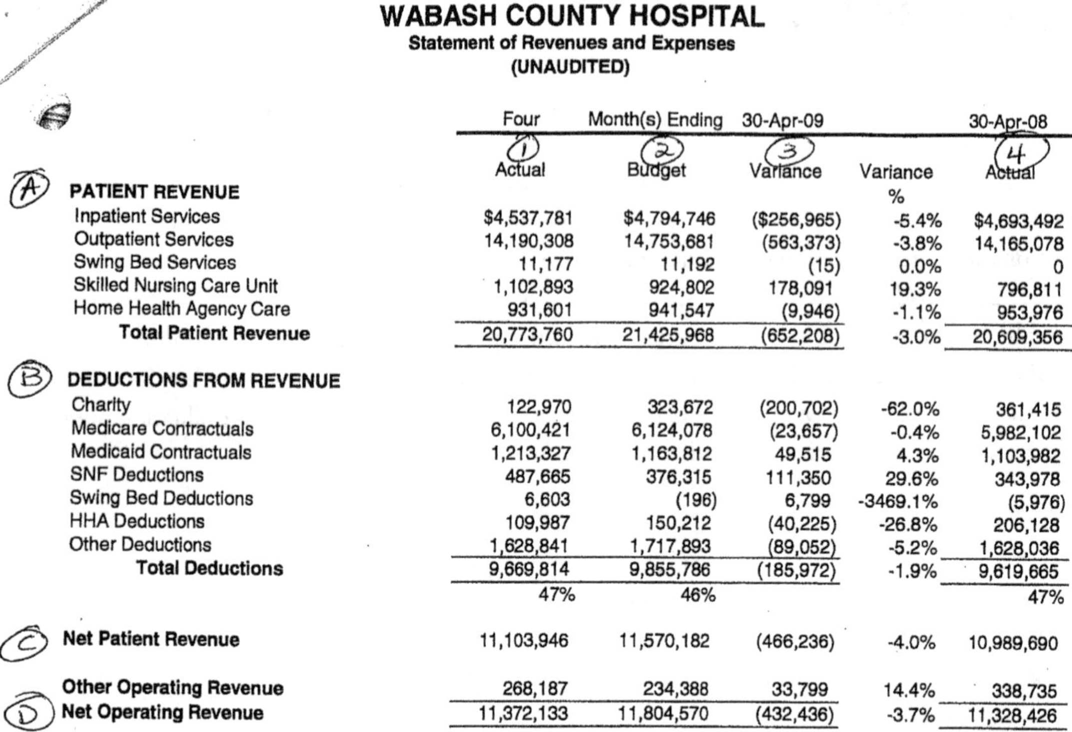

WABASH COUNTY HOSPITAL
Statement of Revenues and Expenses
(UNAUDITED)

	Four Month(s) Ending 30-Apr-09				30-Apr-08
	Actual	Budget	Variance	Variance %	Actual
PATIENT REVENUE					
Inpatient Services	$4,537,781	$4,794,746	($256,965)	-5.4%	$4,693,492
Outpatient Services	14,190,308	14,753,681	(563,373)	-3.8%	14,165,078
Swing Bed Services	11,177	11,192	(15)	0.0%	0
Skilled Nursing Care Unit	1,102,893	924,802	178,091	19.3%	796,811
Home Health Agency Care	931,601	941,547	(9,946)	-1.1%	953,976
Total Patient Revenue	20,773,760	21,425,968	(652,208)	-3.0%	20,609,356
DEDUCTIONS FROM REVENUE					
Charity	122,970	323,672	(200,702)	-62.0%	361,415
Medicare Contractuals	6,100,421	6,124,078	(23,657)	-0.4%	5,982,102
Medicaid Contractuals	1,213,327	1,163,812	49,515	4.3%	1,103,982
SNF Deductions	487,665	376,315	111,350	29.6%	343,978
Swing Bed Deductions	6,603	(196)	6,799	-3469.1%	(5,976)
HHA Deductions	109,987	150,212	(40,225)	-26.8%	206,128
Other Deductions	1,628,841	1,717,893	(89,052)	-5.2%	1,628,036
Total Deductions	9,669,814	9,855,786	(185,972)	-1.9%	9,619,665
	47%	46%			47%
Net Patient Revenue	11,103,946	11,570,182	(466,236)	-4.0%	10,989,690
Other Operating Revenue	268,187	234,388	33,799	14.4%	338,735
Net Operating Revenue	11,372,133	11,804,570	(432,436)	-3.7%	11,328,426

FIGURE 17.1b Wabash County Hospital

Mr. Dennis Dawes states that ***"We really did put together solid business plans for things as well. It wasn't just an idea and a half-page of written notes and concepts, and by the way will you approve this $20 million expenditure? We developed solid business plans with adequate financial information, even to the point of showing the board and others this may not be the best financial decision to make, but it's the right decision to make for providing a service that doesn't have the best financial reward. But it is something that needs to be done. Being in a big business requires good business planning."***

FRAMEWORK FOR A BUSINESS PLAN

The following is an outline and brief description of each section that can be used in developing a business plan. Typically the greater investment or risk associated with a venture, the more detail required in the business plan. For a smaller venture, such as increasing the hours of an immediate care center, a minimal amount of information may be required, such as the financial impact. For a much larger venture and financial investment such as initiating an open heart surgery program, a more comprehensive and complete business plan would be appropriate.

OVERVIEW/EXECUTIVE SUMMARY

This section provides an overview or summary description of the proposed new program or service. This section should consist of a brief overview or summary providing a high-level description of the new program or service, including the vision, its purpose, or any key business trends or opportunities it is intended to take advantage of or unmet clinical needs it will address.

GOALS AND OBJECTIVES

This section summarizes the overarching goal for this new program or service and enumerates the corresponding objectives that are to be achieved. Objectives should be written as SMART objectives—specific, measurable, achievable, realistic, and timely or time-specific.

PROGRAM/SERVICE DESCRIPTION

This section provides a brief description of the new program or service and any key points or corresponding factors for its start-up, operation, or marketing.

ORGANIZATIONAL STRUCTURE AND PERSONNEL

This section defines how the new program or service fits into the organizational chart, including management responsibility and chain of command and how it supports the organization's mission and vision; additional personnel that will be needed by skill, discipline, or position; initial training required; and any other key points or factors relating to organization or personnel.

START-UP MARKETING PLAN

This section outlines the start-up marketing plan needed for pre-startup marketing and for the first 90 to 120 days of operation. Include any factors impacting visibility or access; referral sources and referral development; physician support and outreach; internal marketing; and promotion, advertising, or sales.

PRICING AND REIMBURSEMENT

This section outlines the suggested pricing for the new program or services; projected payer mix; and projected reimbursement method(s), including projected contractual allowance, discounts, or other elements impacting net reimbursement.

COMPETITIVE ANALYSIS

This section outlines the competition's strengths and weaknesses and competitive dynamics in the market that will impact the new program or service. Any particular strategies relative to creating or maximizing an existing competitive advantage should be outlined here.

INITIAL INVESTMENT

This section defines any start-up capital or investment required and how the project will be funded or financed, including any implications for a future capital budget.

ASSUMPTIONS DRIVING THE *PRO FORMA* INCOME STATEMENT

List all the key assumptions being made and used in the pro forma income statement regarding volume, reimbursement, costs, etc. These can be listed separately or with the pro forma income statement.

PRO FORMA INCOME STATEMENT

Develop the pro forma income statement outlining the projected financial performance for the first year or first three years of operation. The pro forma income statement can serve as the initial operating budget for the new or expanded service. A pro forma income statement is a projection of revenue, expenses, and net income for a new or expanded program or service based on known and projected volume and financial data and assumptions.

KEY ACTIVITIES AND ACTION STEPS FOR DEVELOPMENT AND IMPLEMENTATION

This section outlines the various key activities and action steps for the development and effective implementation of the new program or service.

IMPLEMENTATION TIMELINE

A timeline or Gantt chart can be used to depict the major steps and milestones involved in development, implementation, and start-up.

Other Factors to Consider in Developing a Business Plan:

- Who's your audience for the business plan?
- Is there a story that will help your audience of decision makers gain a clearer understanding or make a stronger connection to this plan and how it supports the organization's mission, vision, and strategies?
- What's the purpose of the business plan?
  - Planting a seed to see if it grows?
  - Board or Executive Leadership decision making or formal approval?
  - Soliciting investor support or funding?
  - Forecasting/budgeting/resource allocation?
- What are the possible or anticipated obstacles or roadblocks?
- What type of internal or external stakeholder support is needed? Who are/will be some of the biggest existing supporters for this plan?

DISCUSSION QUESTIONS

1. What is a pro forma income statement and what is its purpose?
2. How does the leadership philosophy and organizational culture impact an organization's approach to business planning?
3. What are a few examples of different decision criteria that might be used when evaluating the feasibility of a new service?
4. How is the business planning and development function typically organized in a health service organization?
5. Describe the role that business planning and development have in a health service organization.
6. What is a business plan?
7. Describe two or three purposes of a business plan.
8. What are some of the components typically found in a business plan?
9. What administrative position is typically responsible for administering the business planning and development function in a small hospital or health service organization?
10. Identify one or two other administrative functions or processes that are similar and comparable with the business planning and development function.

BUSINESS PLAN PRO FORMA TEMPLATE

BUSINESS PLAN PRO FORMA TEMPLATE

	YEAR 1	YEAR 2	YEAR 3
Volume / Units of Service			
Gross Revenue			
Contractuals & Discounts			
Net Revenue			
Operating Expenses:			
Salaries & Wages			
Benefits			
Rent & Utilities			
Supplies			
Marketing			
Other			
Total Operating Expenses			
Net Income			

Assumptions:

- Pricing
- Payor Mix
- Contractual Allowance Percentage
- Managed Care Discounts
- Volume / Clients
- Units of Service Rendered by Service Type
- Staffing
- Hourly Rates of Pay
- Benefits as a Percentage of Salary / Wages
- Supply Expense as a Percentage of Revenue or Expenses
- Market Share

FIGURE CREDIT

18

Marketing Health Services

Over the past several decades, marketing has become increasingly recognized as a legitimate business function that is important for a community hospital or other health service organization. The marketing function can be defined as: (1) actions undertaken to elicit desired responses from a target audience, including identifying and meeting human and social needs profitably; (2) the process of planning and executing the conception, pricing, promotion, and distribution of ideas, goods, and services to create exchanges that satisfy individual and organizational objectives; (3) an organizational function and a set of processes for creating, communicating, and delivering value to customers and managing customer relationships in ways that benefit the organization and its stakeholders (American Marketing Association, 2004). (Kotler, Philip & Keller, Kevin Lane, 2007. *A Framework for Marketing Management,* Third Edition. Pearson Prentice Hall. ISBN: 0-13-145-259-2)

In its simplest form, marketing is about maximizing exchanges between the organization and its customers.

OBJECTIVES

1. Learn about the marketing function and how its effective application can add real business value for a hospital or health service organization.
2. Understand the important roles internal marketing and public relations play in communicating about a health service organization and services offered.
3. Learn about strategies and techniques used in advertising and promoting a community hospital to its consumers and potential consumers.

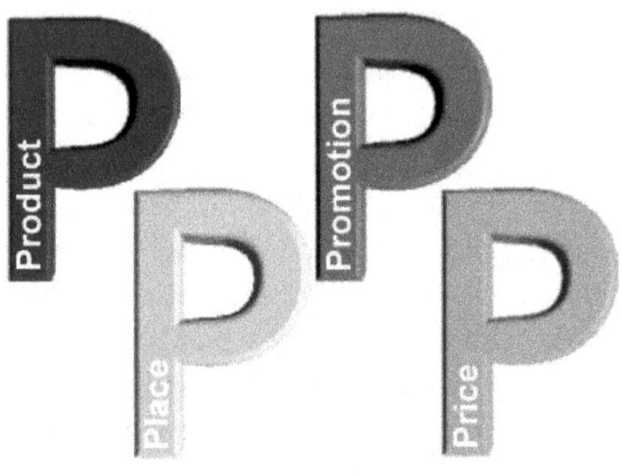

FIGURE 18.1 Four Ps

Davin7, "Four P's," http://commons.wikimedia.org/wiki/File:4P%27s-nl.png. Copyright in the Public Domain.

The basis of the marketing function is the marketing mix, also referred to as the four P's of marketing: product, price, place, and promotion. The product represents the goods and services—both tangible and intangible—the organization provides in its service offering. Product positioning involves how a product is perceived in the minds of consumers relative to defined attributes and competing products. Product differentiation is a strategy of altering one or more marketing mix elements to respond to the various wants and needs of different groups. Product life cycle refers to the stages a product goes through as it exists in the market from its first introduction to its final withdrawal. Product advertising is used to promote a particular product or service. There are three types of product advertisements: 1) informational, which explain the service, how it can be accessed, or its objectives; 2) competitive, which are persuasive ads comparing the company's services over that of the competition; and 3) reminder, which is follow-up communication with the consumer.

Price represents the amount charged for the goods, services, and related policies, practices, and strategic positioning associated with pricing. This also includes contracting for services with different third-party payors and directly with employers, in addition to the use of sliding-fee scales with patients for their out-of-pocket obligations. A hospital or health service organization's policies and practices toward the collection of the patient's out-of-pocket portion of the bill is increasingly important with the push for price transparency and the proliferation of high-deductible health plans placing greater financial responsibility on the patient for payment of health services received. In addition, pricing includes the different methodologies used in charging for services, such as *per diem* rates, case rates, and bundled rates and their reimbursement.

Place represents the location and points of access where healthcare products and services are made available to consumers. New developments in this area include retail health clinics, worksite health clinics, retail pharmacy service line expansion into immunization and related services, and resurgence toward providing care and service in the least restrictive environment, including the patient's home. Advancements in smart phone and digital technologies will continue driving this trend. Furthermore, as greater emphasis and value is placed on the delivery of primary care services, hospitals and other health service organizations have increasingly focused on strategies that create greater patient access to primary care.

Promotion represents the area for which marketing is most widely known and thought of and involves communication with various audiences through the promotional mix of advertising, public relations, personal selling, and sales promotion. Although there can be many forms and types of advertising, the two primary forms of advertising in healthcare are institutional advertising and product or service advertising. Institutional advertising has as its goal to strengthen the organization's visibility and image in the community. Service advertising focuses on a particular product or service offered by the organization. A separate, but somewhat related, function to the marketing mix is corporate communication, which is communication that represents the official position of the organization.

PRODUCT

- Organization's service offering
- Service line branding
- Quality outcomes
- Patient service outcomes/patient experience/patient satisfaction
- Points of parity
- Points of differentiation
- Service or product guarantee
- Service recovery
- Patient scheduling, registration, and admitting
- Patient gowns, socks, etc.
- Televisions and programming
- Food service: food service on request
- Housekeeping—cleanliness and appearance
- Facilities and the environment of care
- Physician recruitment
- Physician credentialing
- Athletic-trainer coverage at football games
- JCAHO accreditation

PRICE

- Managed-care contracting
- Rate negotiations
- Pricing strategy
- Chargemaster review
- Financial-assistance policy
- Collection policies and procedures
- Collection-agency usage
- Monitoring insurance payment remittance advices and payment per contract
- Discount practices for prompt payment on out-of-pocket balances
- Payment plans for out-of-pocket balances

PLACE

- Hospital campus and location
- Physician offices and location
- Urgent care centers
- Parking
- Valet parking
- Transportation services
- Off-site outpatient clinics
- Ambulatory surgery centers
- Freestanding diagnostic centers
- Worksite clinics
- Retail pharmacies
- Hospital-based or off-campus MOBs
- Signage
- Ambulance service
- Emergency helicopter service

PROMOTION

- Referral development, outreach, and sales
- Billboard advertising
- Television advertising
- Radio advertising

- Newspaper advertising
- Newsletters
- Brochures, flyers, and postcards
- Websites
- Healthcare topic educational sessions for the public
- Fee-screening clinics
- Saturday football clinics
- Ball field signage
- Sports program advertisement
- Physician relations and recruitment
- News releases
- Clinical education and training with high school and college students
- Service club participation and program presentations
- Concierge services

It is common for hospitals and other health service organizations—particularly larger organization's—to have personnel in personal selling positions. Many times, these positions have titles like Physician Liaison or Outreach Coordinator, and these roles typically emphasize education and need satisfaction or consultative selling. Need-satisfaction selling is where the focus is on developing, identifying, and fulfilling the physician or other referral source's needs. Consultative selling is where the representative serves more as a consultant using his or her expertise to support and assist the physician or referral source.

FACTORS AND VARIABLES IMPACTING THE HEALTH SERVICE MARKETING FUNCTION

The organization, structure, and strategies of the marketing function can vary immensely from one hospital or health service organization to another, depending on a number of different factors and variables, including the following:

- Position the organization holds in the market and in the hearts and minds of the service area population
- Number and type of competitors in the service area, their respective positions in the market, and how aggressive they may be with marketing
- Service offerings in the market and extent there is duplication
- Supply of physicians, as well as physician satisfaction, referral patterns, practices, and preferences
- Image and reputation of the organization
- Payor mix of the organization

- Service area demographics, psychographics, and growth trends
- Patient experience and satisfaction
- Employee satisfaction and morale and the internal culture of communication
- Local price competition in service area
- Local market health plan restrictions and steerage
- Leadership philosophies and practices
- Number and type of media outlets and associated advertising costs
- Past marketing activities and practices and their effectiveness
- Budget and available resources

PUBLIC RELATIONS

The public relations function is typically an active and vibrant function in most hospitals and health service organizations today. Public relations is any indirectly paid presentation of goods, ideas, or services designed to promote or protect a hospital or health service organization's image or its individual products. Public relations, or PR, when done effectively, can be viewed more as a source of objective or non-biased and credible information than other forms of organizational promotion.

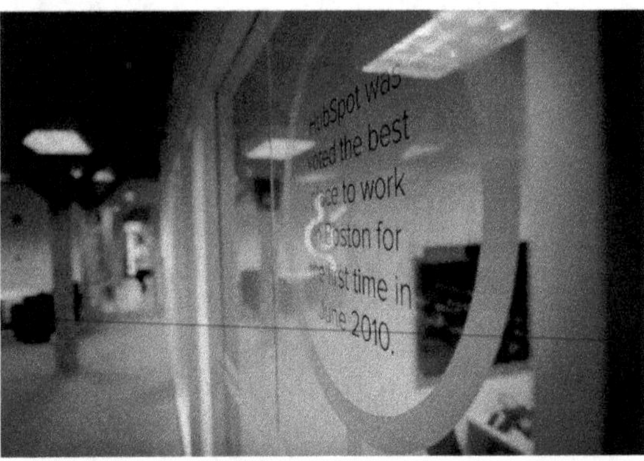

FIGURE 18.2 HubSpot Glass Wall

A FEW RULES OF THUMB FOR THE PUBLIC RELATIONS FUNCTION

Invite local media in routinely. Give them good stories about your hospital or health service organization. Build a relationship with the local media before you really need it. Conduct ongoing internal scanning for good stories (about new technologies, new procedures, human interest stories, local impact of national stories, etc.). Provide local media with press releases and summaries that are newsworthy. Identify leaders and physicians who are good with media and in front of the camera for public relation stories that might be of interest to the media. Provide media training to key internal clinical and administrative staff who can act as spokespersons on public relations stories. Establish clear and specific goals, objectives, and a plan for public relations. Review the media relations policy and procedure periodically and modify it as needed. Present and discuss the policy with leadership and the board before it is needed. As a rule of thumb, develop "talking points" for important internal or "corporate" public relations communication and external media communication.

DEVELOPING MEDIA RELEASES

The primary goal is to develop media releases that provide a consistent, coordinated, and organized approach/process to generating positive public relations. Objectives for developing media releases includes: 1) to increase attention, visibility, and a positive image for the health service organization in the community; 2) to increase connections with customers/potential customers; 3) to utilize public relations as a vehicle for increasing believable, credible stories that promote the services and capabilities of the hospital or health service organization and top-of-the-mind awareness in the community.

DETERMINING IF THE PUBLIC RELATIONS STORY IS NEWSWORTHY

Below are five important criteria for determining if a prospective news story from the organization is newsworthy of a media release.

Timing—Current topics are good news. If it happened today, it's news. If the same thing happened last week, it may not be interesting or newsworthy any longer. This criterion includes trying to find a local angle or story for a national news story or trend.

Unique—Is it something that is the first of its kind in the city, community, or state? Is it a first for the hospital or health service organization? Is it a new or novel approach to an old way of doing something? Is it innovative and revolutionary?

Human Interest—Human interest stories appeal to emotion. Putting a human face on a story shows how a particular treatment, program, or device actually benefits real people. (Tell the story of the war through the eyes of a soldier). Human interest stories also show how a field of work or an opportunity made a difference in someone's life.

Significance—The number of people affected by the story is important. It's also important to address the readers'/viewers' questions: "So what? What does this mean to me?" Furthermore, it is important to show how the event or potential story impacts the health of the organization's patients and/or local community.

Prominence—Famous people get media coverage, because they are famous. If a famous person suffers or dies from a particular disease, the public interest and desire to understand the disease increases.

TALKING POINTS

Talking points refers to creating an outline of the key communication message points that you want to convey in an important communication message, along with a few points of explanation or examples that illustrate each key talking point. Use of talking points can help to manage internal communication from department managers and frontline supervisors to department employees and provide for consistency of message. Talking points can be used for external communication, including presentations or interviews with media. It is usually a good idea to outline your key talking points and supporting points of rationale into "sound bites" or short statements that are clear and specific in communicating or explaining the desired message.

Use of talking points can help to manage internal communication from department managers and frontline supervisors to department employees and provide for consistency of message.

EXAMPLE OF TALKING POINTS

For example, if the organization is a hospital undergoing a reduction in force (RIF) the Single Overriding Communication Objective (SOCO) for this action step might be: A reduction in force is necessary in order to remain financially viable in the long run and remain the vibrant healthcare asset our community depends on given the cuts in reimbursement we, like all hospitals, are experiencing.

EMPLOYEE LAYOFFS	TALKING POINTS
• Laid-off 20 employees; 15 full-time equivalents • How was the RIF determined? • What RIF process or policy was followed? • Why is this action being taken now?	• Followed board-approved reduction-in force policy and procedure • Policy based upon seniority by job classification • Impacts six different departments • Areas affected in lower quartile on productivity as benchmarked against peer group • Patient Protection and Affordable Care Act—significant cuts in reimbursement to hospitals • Employer pressure to reduce costs: can't keep cost-shifting in future as hospital have done historically

In developing talking points, identify key target audiences. Who will be listening to the communication message: board, leadership, employees, patients, employers, regulators, the public, etc. What key messages should you send to each target audience? How do they feel? What do you want to tell them? What do they need to hear from you? How will people react? What are your biggest critics thinking? Talking points can assist in providing consistent communication at all levels of the organization and to manage internal messages to help prevent distortion of the facts or rumors. Remember: If no word is forthcoming, then staff (and everyone else) creates their own story! Employees want to hear from both executive leadership and their direct supervisor. Don't overlook the need to communicate to the board and medical staff. Use multiple channels to communicate the message. On important communication, repetition of the communication message is mandatory to be sure it has reached its intended audience and that clear understanding of the message has occurred.

> **If no word is forthcoming then staff (and everyone else) creates their own story!**

MARKETING RESEARCH

Many times, a situation will call for marketing research to be conducted in order to answer a key question about the market and to learn about and understand consumer wants, needs, and preferences. Clearly defining what needs to be learned or understood is critical in order to establish a marketing research plan that will provide the information needed. Marketing research is performed using primary and/or secondary data. Primary data is information acquired or collected to address the specific purpose of the research. Secondary data is information that already exists and is acquired or collected from some other intended purpose. The basic steps in the marketing research process are 1) define the problem or better understand something; 2) establish research objectives, 3) create the design for the research, 4) gather and organize data, and 5) analyze and evaluate results. Techniques commonly used in healthcare to acquire and collect primary data include observational, experimental, and survey research. Observational research can include direct observation or mystery shopper methods. Experimental research can include test marketing or pilot programs designed to provide a trial run or experience that can be evaluated and assessed for effectiveness. Survey research can include conducting focus groups, telephone interviews, personal interviews, or mail or internet-based electronic surveys.

HEALTHCARE CONSUMER BEHAVIOR

Healthcare consumer behavior is changing in our electronic world of advancing technology. According to the Deloitte Consulting Group 2012 Healthcare Consumer Survey, healthcare consumers are more interested in interacting with their physician via email; more reliant on the internet for gathering information about healthcare services and comparing providers; and looking to academic health centers as providing the most credible sources of information on diseases, clinical healthcare, and related information.

It's critical that a health service organization and its leadership truly understand the healthcare consumer in order to best design programs and services and the optimal marketing mix to provide exactly what the consumer desires. Marketing research can be useful in helping to determine the needs and preferences of healthcare consumers. Consumers typically go through a decision-making process when facing a healthcare-purchasing decision that includes 1) recognizing the problem; 2) searching for information; 3) evaluating alternatives 4) making the purchase; and 5) evaluating the purchase after the fact. Clearly understanding the evaluation criteria healthcare consumers' use in making different purchasing decisions is paramount. Post-purchase decisions are evaluated critically by the consumer as to whether the purchase decision met their needs and if they are satisfied overall. Cognitive dissonance is a mental state of anxiety brought on because the consumer is unsure of the chosen alternative or purchase made. The question asked by a typical healthcare consumer post-purchase is "Did I make the right choice or decision?" Post-purchase information, support, consultation, and follow-up are important for a health service organization to reinforce the consumer's belief about his or her purchase decision.

INTERNAL MARKETING

The employees and physicians of any hospital or health service organization are the marketing ambassadors for the organization in the community. The employees and physicians interact and communicate with patients and prospective patients in the community and are frequently asked about what is happening where they work and what they think about issues and happenings in healthcare in general. How employees and physicians interact and respond to people in their community about the organization and related issues impacts the image and reputation of the hospital or health service organization. Therefore, internal marketing to employees and physicians can help to better prepare and equip them to speak about the organization. Keeping the organization's internal audiences aware and informed is a key marketing function on an ongoing basis. Moreover, employees and physicians are typically interested in knowing about what is happening in their organization and sensitive about hearing or reading information for the first time about their own organization through various outside forums, including the media. Communicating with internal audiences first is almost always the rule of thumb to follow, as it impacts employee morale, satisfaction, and engagement.

MARKETING TOUCH POINTS AND PATIENT SATISFACTION

Marketing "touch points" are those experiences or situations where the patient or prospective consumer interacts with the hospital or health service organization in some way. Examples of "touch points" include seeing or hearing an educational advertisement or promotional message about the organization; scheduling a visit or test; or receiving services, a bill, a follow-up telephone call regarding services rendered, or a patient survey. The concept of the value chain categorizes these touch points into pre-service, service, and after service. How is the organization interacting with its patients and prospective patients from the vantage point of these three categories? What impressions are being created? How can improvements be made that will enhance the image and brand of the organization in the minds of consumers?

Delivering a great service experience to patients—either in the pre-service, service, or after-service phases—is increasingly becoming important from not only a quality of care standpoint, but also from a business standpoint. Developing extremely satisfied, loyal customers is an important goal of marketing. Customer loyalty represents repeat business for the organization, and a potential greater share of the patient's future overall healthcare purchases. Having loyal patients reduces the cost of acquiring new patients; increases repeat business and overall revenue per patient over time; improves the organization's profitability; may result in the loyal patient being willing to pay a premium for services; are typically more forgiving if a mistake is made; and improves word-of-mouth marketing. Relationship marketing is the effort to develop a long-term relationship with patients and consumers and to develop long-term loyalty. "Hardwiring" an organization to deliver the very best in customer service involves creating the type of organization, structure, and processes within the fabric of the organization and its culture to focus its priorities, processes, and systems on customer service. This can include processes and systems such as routine meeting agendas that include customer service goals, plans, and performance outcomes reporting, so they are regularly discussed; orientation and training programs to include customer service training; performance expectations and appraisals that account for customer service behaviors; merit-based compensation practices that include customer service delivery and performance; and the establishment of goals at all levels of the organization, including part of the corporate or balanced scorecard.

BRANDING

Branding is creating mental structures and helping customers organize their knowledge about products and services in a way that clarifies their decision making and, in the process, provides value to the organization.

Brand equity is the added value endowed to products and services, reflected in how consumers think feel, and act with respect to the brand, as well as the prices, market share, and profitability that the brand commands for the firm. This is an intangible asset that has psychological and financial value to the firm. Brand loyalty is a situation in which the consumer regularly chooses the same product or service to fill a recognized need. Brand promise is the marketer's vision of what the brand must be and do for consumers. Brand knowledge consists of all the thoughts, feelings, images, experiences, and beliefs that become associated with a brand.

Ken Stella says that ***"All the large hospital systems have their marketing people and they are doing focus groups, telephone surveys, and it's almost become like political campaigns. These systems are spending millions of dollars as far as major advertisements. I compare it a little bit to Miller High Life and Budweiser. You heard Miller and you heard Budweiser commercials. And they were fighting for market share, and they were trying to brand. And I think that is what we have going in healthcare today. We are trying to do this branding, and I think it is going to continue. We now see it filter down in the smaller communities as we see more affiliations. And that will continue."***

SOCIAL MEDIA

The use of social media as a marketing strategy has been slow to be adopted in healthcare, probably for a variety of reasons, including the fact that healthcare services are not purchased in the same way as many other goods and services. However, the adoption of social media by hospitals and health service organization as a marketing strategy has, and will probably continue to, increase. As the functionality and overall use of social media evolves, organizations are developing strategies to provide relevant and useful information to consumers to help them solve problems and add value to their lives. Organizational website design and operation, along with the use of different social media vehicles, should be part of most hospital or health service organizations' marketing strategy. As social media promotes the convergence of business and personal information at the fingertips of consumers, hospitals and health service organizations need to clearly articulate their goals and strategy for communicating using these newer social mediums.

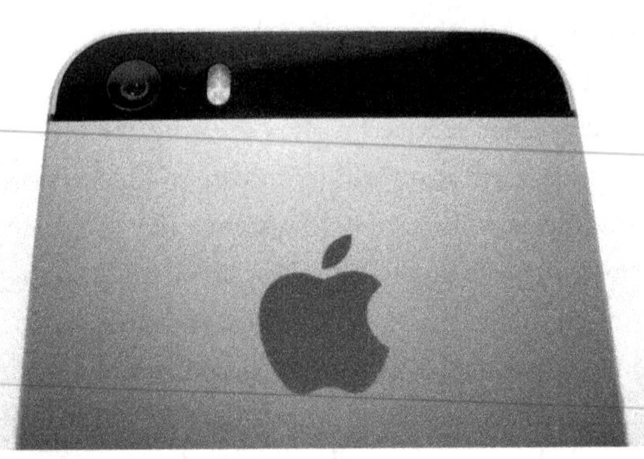

FIGURE 18.3 iPhone 5

MARKETING STRATEGY

The marketing strategy for many small hospitals is really about the various communication messages the hospital wants to communicate out to various customers or markets. Increasingly, more of the communication messages from hospitals are focused on health education, prevention and wellness. Most of this type of health education is disease specific; however, sometimes hospitals get involved in health fairs and other preventive or screening services that can also help to heighten awareness within the community about preventive care and services. If a concern shows up through a screening test, the hospital and its physician are then available to provide the medical care needed or refer the person someone that can.

The marketing function for a community hospital typically places significant emphasis on marketing communication using various mediums targeted at various audiences. Creating visibility and awareness about the different programs and services a hospital or health service organization offers is paramount. Connecting with the organization's target audiences is critical to creating the awareness, understanding, and motivation for various consumers to seek access to the programs and services the organization offers. While the referral preferences of the patient's physician is still a primary determinant of where a patient may seek care or treatment, the drivers of referral and preference are multi-faceted and varied in every situation.

What are effective strategies and techniques in crafting different communication messages, and what mediums are effective in reaching and connecting with the target audience? The local newspaper in many small towns and communities today is still a viable medium for local news and information. The same is true about the local radio station as well. Direct mail can also be used to target certain geographic areas with a specific communication message. Magnets that can go on a refrigerator; pens with the hospital's name and logo on it; or other similar materials can be used as well. Health fairs, community outreach programs, and participation and support of important community initiatives is also a great way for the organization to connect with and be engaged with the community.

Nationally, approximately 54 percent of all hospital admissions come through the emergency department (ED or ER). The emergency department is, therefore, considered the "front door" to the hospital. "However, the emergency department can be a challenging department to manage given the episodic nature of the care that is provided. Moreover, the growing expectations on the part of healthcare consumers is also a factor as well. Creating a patient experience in the emergency room that is satisfying and meets the patient and families expectations is challenging but imperative, particularly for small hospitals in small communities where one bad experience can spread quickly over the communication grapevine. Still today the word-of-mouth marketing plays a big role."

Mr. Ken Stella says that ***"I maintain the best [hospital] marketing starts at the ER. When I used to go around the state and talk to small rural hospitals, I used to tell them you have limited dollars. The real marketing for you is when a farmer rolls his tractor putting in the spring crop, and he comes in crushed, that you are able to stabilize him, keep him alive, and transfer him to the trauma center. And that's going to say more about your ER. Or when somebody comes in at night with their child. So I used to say spend your limited resources on making your ER as good as it can be because your ER is your front door. If I was leading a small rural hospital today, I would probably be marketing my ER to the local community."***

Mr. Stella goes on to say, ***"Something I learned from Allen Hicks is what I call 'Barbers and beauticians marketing'. When somebody goes in to get a haircut, or somebody goes into the beauty shop, they are there for about 30 minutes and the conversation usually goes like 'What's new? What do you know?' And they are either talking local sports or politics, or somebody got hurt or they are sick. I advocate that hospitals entertain barbers and beauticians a couple times a year and make sure they know about the programs and services the hospital offers because you will instantly have about a hundred people out there talking about the hospital. The other marketing is the hospital volunteers or guild. They need to know your plan, no different than your employees, and what it is you are trying to accomplish. That to me is rural marketing. You don't need to be doing a bunch of television. In Martinsville, back before HIPPA, we had a five day a week radio show. It was admissions, discharges, births and deaths. It just so happened that the lady I had doing that show was the local high school football coaches' wife. Martinsville had a pretty good football team. The subject on Friday after the announcements was 'Marilyn, how's the coach think the team's going to do tonight?' Marilyn would not only talk about the football team, but she would also throw something out about the hospital. We started talking about things we had going on at the hospital. Those were some of the little techniques we used. Marketing on a broader base today has become a profession."***

Should a small hospital constantly be doing something in the area of advertising and promotion to stay in front of the local community and be visible to create awareness? How do you decide what to promote from a service line perspective? There are many variables at play that impact the decision about marketing; however, when the hospital acquires a new piece of medical or surgical technology; recruits a new physician; starts a new service or program; or reaches some important milestone, these are all occasions to advertise and/or promote the hospital and its services. In addition, if the hospital offers a program or service that is perceived as being better than the competition; is somewhat unique in the area; or generates a strong financial margin, it is probably a candidate for advertising and promotion.

MARKETING TO BE USEFUL

A marketing strategy that is gaining more momentum in today's world is marketing that will be useful to current or prospective customers. How can the organization be useful and helpful to current or prospective customers? What can the organization do to promote education and provide information that will be useful? If you sell a service, you will have made a customer for a day. If you help someone in a useful way, you might have earned their loyalty as a customer for life. Earning of trust and reliability is something that should be nurtured over time by an organization in its quest to develop loyal customers, as well as prospective customers who will look to the organization in their time of need. If a health service organization doesn't generate and foster a high level of trust and reliability, it is in trouble. Consumers have options, and they are not interested in going to a physician or hospital they don't have high regard for or don't trust. A health service organization needs to be viewed as putting the health of patients ahead of profits. Making the health service organization useful in ways that may not generate immediate revenue for the organization is a long-term marketing strategy. This strategy is about putting the needs of patients and prospective patients as a top marketing priority and, in doing so, believing there will be a handsome payoff for the organization that executes this strategy effectively and stays the course over time.

> **If you sell a service, you will have made a customer for a day. If you help someone in a useful way, you might have earned their loyalty as a customer for life.**

MARKETING PLAN

A marketing plan typically outlines and describes the strategies, goals, objectives, and action steps for the marketing function of the organization. A marketing plan can include an analysis of the service area, the competition, and statistics regarding performance of internal operations that help form the basis for which strategies, goals, and objectives can be planned and developed. Planning for the marketing function should ideally be done in concert with other organizational business planning processes in order to reduce duplication of effort and increase efficiency, effectiveness, integration and alignment. Other business planning functions to coordinate with the development of a marketing plan include strategic planning, budgeting, and community health needs assessment processes. See the example of a marketing plan outline at the end of this chapter.

TEN CRITICAL SUCCESS FACTORS FOR A MARKETING PLAN

The following are ten critical success factors for the development, implementation and execution, and communication and evaluation of a marketing plan.

1. Consider putting together a "plan-to-plan" executive summary for the marketing-planning process. Include a few summary highlights and key trends of the market, organization and/or previous marketing strategy and tactics, along with the proposed timeline, milestones, and process for the marketing-planning process and plan development.
2. Conduct a marketing-education and strategy-setting retreat with the objectives to help educate the board, executive leadership, and physician leadership about the marketing function and past marketing strategies, tactics, and action steps along with successes, failures, and key points of learning. Incorporate learning into the new process and plan.

   a. Provide an update on the organization's current state and trends in key areas such as admissions, surgeries, market share, patient satisfaction, etc.

3. Solicit insight, market intelligence, understanding, and perspectives from key stakeholders by developing a structured questionnaire; interviewing a number of key stakeholders, including a few external to the organization; and recording important information obtained and a few key quotes made during those interviews that highlight key findings or perspectives. Summarize and share the results.
4. Involve key leaders in the development of a preliminary working draft of the marketing plan, soliciting and incorporating their input and feedback on information and data gathered, analyzed, and displayed, along with proposed marketing strategy and tactics.
5. Be sure to include the organization's mission, vision, values, and strategic priorities and initiatives, and reference same to be sure proposed marketing strategies and tactics are in total alignment with directional strategies.
6. Present a preliminary working draft of the marketing plan to key internal stakeholders, including the board, for their input and feedback prior to finalizing.
7. Incorporate the input and feedback from key internal stakeholders into the final marketing plan document.
8. Provide updates and status reports to the board and executive leadership during the marketing plan development process at pertinent milestones.
9. Develop a communication plan for internal education and marketing of the marketing plan, and use these communications to educate, inform, and inspire internal stakeholders.
10. Establish evaluation metrics along with the marketing strategies and tactics, and use these to evaluate effectiveness, performance, and success.

DISCUSSION QUESTIONS

1. What are the four P's of marketing?
2. What is the difference between primary data and secondary data?
3. What are one or two criteria to use in determining if a public relations story is newsworthy?
4. Describe the marketing function and its important role in healthcare delivery.
5. Describe the marketing mix.
6. Describe the PR function and a few key elements of PR for a health service organization.
7. What are talking points, and how might they be used?
8. What are the five steps of the marketing research process?
9. Identify two or three touch points for patients with a hospital.
10. Describe one or two strategies discussed by Ken Stella for marketing a community hospital.

MARKETING PLAN OUTLINE

I. **Name, address, and brief description/overview of the health service organization.**
A brief description should be one or two paragraphs and probably no more than one-half page in length. This is an overview of the health services organization (type, tax-paying status, ownership, size, general description of services, general description of the market, etc.) and any relevant key characteristics or aspects worth noting. The mission and vision can also be included to provide overall direction and guidance.

II. **Situational Analysis**

A. **Environmental Assessment**
Provide an overview of the organization's key products and services offered; key general environmental changes and trends; position in marketplace; key competencies or competitive advantage; summary of competitive environment, including major threats and opportunities; overall image and reputation; key strategic factors, changes or trends in the general environment or with consumer trends or preferences; and key strategic factors that have implications for its marketing strategy, goals, and recommendations. The use of narrative and bullet points is appropriate. This section should be approximately one to five pages in length.

B. **Service Area Analysis**
This section analyzes the demographic and related data, key findings, and changes and trends of the population in the organization's service area. This can include an analysis of the health status of the service area's population and any key aspects noted.

C. **Competitive Analysis**
Describe the competitive environment in which the health service organization operates. Identify the top competitors, along with their images and competitive positions in the market; each competitor's points of differentiation, core competencies/strengths and weaknesses, and any competitive advantage they may enjoy; and marketing strategies and their key tactics. Identify any opportunities or threats that may exist in the market.

D. **Market Share Analysis**
Complete a market share analysis by major service line (if the data is available) to determine the current market share, as compared to competition, and any changes and trends worth noting.

III. **Internal Analysis**

Describe the competencies/strengths and weaknesses of the health service organization that identifies strengths and weaknesses of key programs and services offered and key financial, operational, quality, and service outcomes and trends. Identify the organization's position in the market, points of differentiation, core competencies, and any competitive advantage it may enjoy.

IV. **Strengths, Weaknesses, Opportunities, and Threats (SWOT) Analysis**

Complete a SWOT analysis that summarizes the key strengths and weaknesses of the health service organization, along with the opportunities and threats that exist in the market. The SWOT analysis should be a summary and approximately one page in length.

V. **Marketing Audit**

Complete a marketing audit on the health service organization's existing marketing strategies and action steps. Identify current strategies and actions and your assessment of their effectiveness. Identify strengths and weaknesses of the current strategies and action steps, including elements, such as its mission, vision, website, brochures, logo, slogan, newsletters, corporate communications, advertising campaigns, public relations efforts, pricing, access, service offerings and brand image. What is the current state of the organization's marketing function and its overall performance and effectiveness? This section should be one to two pages in length.

VI. **Top Target Market Segments**

Identify the top one to three target market segment(s) for your health service organization (overall) and provide a brief explanation of each along with the rationale/business case. This section can be up to one page in length.

VII. **Marketing Research Plan**

What information is needed from the primary market segment(s) being targeted in order to gain greater understanding that will assist in the development of a more effective marketing plan and strategy than what currently exists? If warranted, outline a marketing research plan following the five-step marketing research process: 1) problem identification or understanding needed, 2) establish research objectives, 3) create the design for the research, 4) gather and organize data, and 5) analyze and evaluate results. Identify the sources of secondary market research data (if any) that are available and can be used to better understand the needs, wants, preferences, and perceptions of the identified target market segment(s). This section should be one to three pages in length.

VIII. **Goals and Objectives**
Articulate the key goals and objectives for the new marketing plan. These goals and objectives should clearly identify what programs, services, strengths, weaknesses, opportunities, or threats are being targeted for strategy and why. Be as clear and specific as possible.

IX. **Marketing Strategies and Major Action Steps**
Identify 5 to 10 marketing strategies recommended for the health service organization. Identify these marketing strategies in reference to: 1) the value chain, 2) the marketing mix, 3) the promotional mix, and 4) the budget. Identify the key action steps that will need to be taken to implement each marketing strategy. These marketing strategies and action steps should connect to the key findings, changes, and trends identified in the Situational Analysis, Competitive Analysis, Internal Analysis, SWOT Analysis, Marketing Audit, and Marketing Research Plan sections in some fashion.

X. **Evaluation Process and Metrics**
Outline the process, timeframe, and metrics recommended to evaluate the effectiveness of this plan and the attainment of the goals, objectives, evaluation metrics, marketing strategies and action steps.

FIGURE CREDITS

Figure 18.1: Davin7, "Four P's," http://commons.wikimedia.org/wiki/File:4P%27s-nl.png. Copyright in the Public Domain.

Figure 18.2: Copyright © RebeccaChurt (CC BY-SA 3.0) at http://commons.wikimedia.org/wiki/File:HubSpot_voted_best_place_to_work.jpg.

Figure 18.3: Copyright © aconcagua (CC BY-SA 3.0) at http://commons.wikimedia.org/wiki/File:IPhone_5s_true_tone_flash.jpg.

19

Making a Business Presentation

As COO of a two-hospital group—a 350-bed, not-for-profit, community hospital and a 25-bed critical access hospital—I attended all Board of Director monthly meetings, and routinely presented the request for privileges coming from the Medical Executive Committee to the board. However, an upcoming Board of Directors meeting had me scheduled to make a business presentation on a proposed initiative to start a hospitalist program. I would be requesting the board's formal approval. Clearly the numbers needed to speak to the financial viability of the new program. Should the presentation have been all about the numbers, and should I have just let the numbers speak to the rationale and justification to start the hospitalist program? In any presentation, it is important to connect with the audience in order to effectively convey the communication message and for that message to be effectively received and understood. There are two primary ways a presenter connects with his audience: cognitively and emotionally. Providing the numbers and making the business case will help connect on a cognitive level, but how could I connect emotionally? After some reflection, I realized I had an appropriate personal story that could help me connect emotionally in presenting the hospitalist proposal. Moreover, my personal story would be the way I would open the presentation. Here is how I opened my presentation on the hospitalist program to the Board of Director's that day.

> "Having the right physician, in the right place, at the right time, makes all the difference."
>
> It was Monday, Memorial Day, 2005, and I was attempting to remove a broken piece of cracked ceramic tile from my bathroom floor. All of a sudden, a piece of tile broke loose and cut my middle finger on my right hand at the middle joint before I knew what happened. In a moment I knew my cut was more than what a band aid would handle. I grabbed a rag, wrapped my hand, and jumped in the car, driving myself to the hospital's emergency department. On my drive to the ED, I was thinking about three things: 1) I hoped I didn't cut my finger too badly (I didn't want to look; just kept it wrapped), 2) I hoped the ED wasn't crowded when I arrived, and 3) I hoped my friend, hospital Medical Director and ED physician Dr. Leach, would be working. I checked in at the registration desk and didn't get a chance to sit down as I was quickly escorted back to an ED treatment room. On my way to the treatment room, I saw Dr. Leach—and he saw me—down the hallway. He immediately came walking towards me and asked ***"What's going on? Are you alright?"*** The first words out of my mouth were ***"Boy, am I glad to see you!"*** Dr. Leach fixed me up that day, which included suturing the tendon in my finger back together—which had been partially cut. I would soon, thereafter, be as good as new. The funny part of this story was arriving back home with a splint on the middle finger of my right hand sticking out and my youngest son, after taking one look at me, exclaiming ***"You'd better be careful dad, that's your middle finger!"***
>
> "Having the right physician, in the right place, at the right time, makes all the difference."

It felt like my personal story connected emotionally with my audience, which included the board and senior leadership team in attendance that day. I'm pleased to say the board unanimously approved implementing the hospitalist program. The financial break-even point for the program was an average daily census (ADC) of 16 patients, which was quickly exceeded after only a few months.

A FEW POINTS ABOUT MY PRESENTATION THAT DAY

1. I knew that most every trustee in that room had experienced some type of injury or illness before; sought medical care for it at the hospital emergency department, and could relate to my story experiences.
2. I knew that most every trustee in that room respected Dr. Leach and would probably feel the same way I did about hoping Dr. Leach would be working that day.

3. I wanted to make the key point, through my story, that providing care and treatment to hospital patients is about more than just numbers: it's about providing the type of care and medical resources that each of us would want for our family and ourselves.

OBJECTIVES

1. Appreciate how becoming a more effective presenter of business presentations can help augment your performance and career as a healthcare leader.
2. Learn how a presentation is about connecting with your audience on two primary levels.
3. Learn methods and techniques to help deliver an effective business presentation.

Healthcare leaders frequently make business presentations to various internal and external audiences. As a result of these presentations, healthcare leaders are judged—whether it is fair or not—as to their level of knowledge and competency, motivation to lead and leadership ability, caring and passion, empathy and understanding, and overall effectiveness. Healthcare leaders must be skilled and adept at making business presentations to be effective. Like any other communication technique, giving effective presentations is a skill that can be learned and developed through practice and experience.

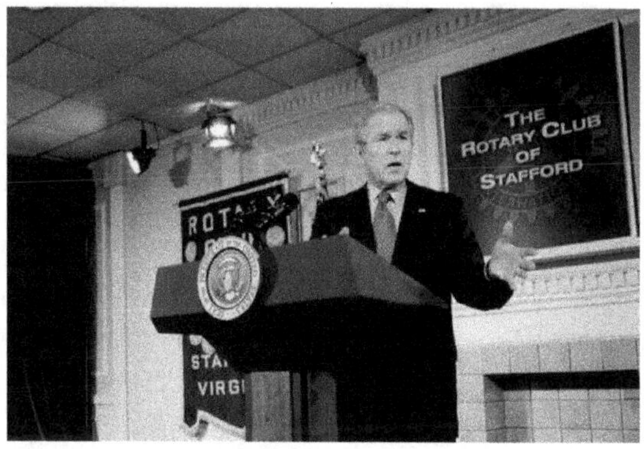

FIGURE 19.1 President Bush
Chris Greenberg, "President George Bush at Podium," http://commons.wikimedia.org/wiki/File:Bush_Dec_17,_2007.jpg. Copyright in the Public Domain.

Business presentations vary greatly by subject matter, type, and size of the audience, whether the purpose is to inform or persuade, or whether it is a formal or informal presentation. Regardless of the type of presentation, most of the fundamental presentation methods and techniques discussed here are applicable. The remainder of this chapter will highlight a number of important guidelines, methods, and techniques for making an effective business presentation.

GENERAL GUIDELINES FOR PRESENTATIONS

When delivering a presentation or planning your remarks for a speech, spend ample time developing how you will deliver the presentation, not just the words you want to use. Communication is a combination of words, voice, and body, with more based on voice and body than the actual words used.

1. Communication is:

    1) 7% - Words
    2) 38% - Voice, tone, and inflection. Remember that sameness is the enemy of the speaker.
    3) 55% - Face and body: Be cognizant of your stance, posture, movement, and body language. (Therefore, don't spend all your time preparing for just the 7%).

Most presentations should have transitions—mainly natural transitions —just like transitions in a song or movie. Alfred Hitchcock said ***"A movie is like life with all the dull parts left out."*** Think about having a conversation with your audience. Good presentations are delivered conversationally; the only difference is the conversation can be planned, edited, tightened-up, and structured as a logical conversation ahead of time. That is what a presentation should be: a conversation with all the dull parts left out.

It is OK to use notes; however, don't read from a script! Deliver your presentation, don't read it.

Presentations are about being personable—not perfect.

Presentations are about being personable—not perfect. Hands should stay out of your pockets, and don't clasp them together in front of you in what is referred to as the "fig leaf" position. Use your hands naturally in speaking or to gesture to make key points. Display energy and interest in your topic/subject. If you aren't, and don't, act interested, why should the audience be interested? Everything you do during a presentation either adds to or distracts from your message. Practicing giving business presentations is important to develop and perfect both the skill and art that are involved. Are you practicing to improve, or just reinforcing bad habits? What are you doing naturally that is effective? What are you doing that is distracting from your delivery and message?

Don't be afraid of silence—use it to make a point or allow your audience to think about and process a key point you've made. Think about the past, present, and future. How does the past relate to the present or the future on this topic? Where is this topic going in the future, and what is your prediction? Regarding humor, don't use it unless both the setting and subject matter are conducive to humor. If humor would be appropriate, is there a "lighter" note or something humorous or ironic the audience might find funny? Remember, the truth can be the most humorous. If you lose your place during the presentation remember: the answer is always right in front of you, but sometimes you have to pause to find it. Specificity builds credibility. If you are making a claim, taking a position, or offering a compelling case you need to back it up with a statistic or example. Use case examples, personal examples, illustrations, stories, logic and metaphors to make key points. And, try to have a balance of the main key points or "takeaways" you want to leave with the audience versus detail.

Three goals for any business presentation are: 1) simplify and demystify (complexity confuses people), 2) speak to be remembered and repeated, and 3) speak to inform, persuade, convince, and/or sell. When practicing your presentations skills, learn to do the following effectively: speak in shorter sentences than you might do in normal conversation; use visual words that help to describe the situation and provide greater clarity and context; emphasize key words, phrases, or points; repeat key words and messages; and tell stories.

STORY TELLING

In everyday conversations, we tell stories. Stories can help make a key point very simple and understandable and help you connect with your audience. Presentations connect on two primary levels: cognitive/intellectual and emotional. Emotion is the internal drive of life. Great speakers connect effectively on both levels. People don't remember so much what you say, but rather what they see or visualize in their minds when you say it.

Telling a short but pertinent story that delivers a relevant point that helps to provide an explanation or meaning in a way the audience will clearly understand can be powerful. An audience would rather hear a simple story well told than a long story told badly. In healthcare, there are lots of stories that can be told about great care, service, and people. Stories can be told from the perspective of the patient, the family member, the doctor, the nurse, or even from a personal perspective. Telling a story that conveys some key point of meaning that will create an emotional impression or impact with the audience can help them personally relate to your message. Don't explain a story, let the story explain the key points of meaning it conveys or reveals. Practice your stories and deliver them using the appropriate dialogue of the characters, emotion, and drama for full effect. And, provide eye contact with your audience when you are telling a story to help connect with your audience.

THE I/YOU RATIO

Be cognizant of the "I/You" ratio. Focus on "You"—the audience. Speak as an audience advocate. Structure the presentation to be as much about the audience as possible. How does your topic impact or relate to your audience? Why should they be interested? What do you and the audience have in common? Think of a simple, common experience that you have had that the audience probably has experienced too that will articulate a key point of wisdom. Find a connection with the audience that you can present. What is your audience thinking? What is your biggest critic thinking? Anticipate and address your biggest critic's point/counterpoint during your presentation.

USING POWER POINT IN A PRESENTATION

General guidelines for using power point slides include using very short, summary points. Remember that less is more. Don't use long narrative, as it requires your audience to read it, which means they won't not be paying as much attention to what you are saying. Don't put too much detail on one slide. You don't want to inundate your audience with details so they lose sight of key points or the big picture. Make your slides visual, where possible. Remember the old saying: A picture is worth a thousand words. Charts and graphs that highlight key points can be very helpful. Direct your audience's attention to key points you highlight on each slide. Everything you say should not be on a slide. Alternatively, you don't have to say everything that is contained on your slides. Power point slides help to augment the presentation; however, they are not the presentation.

DEVELOPING THE PRESENTATION

A good way to start developing the presentation is by designing the message first, using visual words; then, design the structure/organization and power point slides to help deliver the message. It is typically a good rule-of-thumb to develop your Single Overriding Communication Objective (SOCO) in the initial phase of developing your presentation. What is the SOCO? It is the one single overriding message that you want to convey and what you want your audience to think, do, or act as a result of your presentation. Is this presentation to educate and inform; influence and persuade; sell a concept, idea, or new initiative; or receive formal support and approval for a financial investment? Determine in the very beginning of developing the presentation what your SOCO is, and then, build the structure that supports your SOCO. Moreover, the SOCO may be something that should be featured in the opening and closing of the presentation in an interesting or engaging way in order to connect with your audience. In the opening of this chapter, you read about the story of the presentation I gave to the hospital board requesting approval for the hospitalist program. The SOCO for that presentation was: *Having the right physician, in the right place, at the right time makes all the difference.*

When developing the structure of your presentation, keep this in mind; this point process is more like taking a field trip than working in a laboratory. It can be a bit messy to start out, and it is clearly not a linear process. In many ways, this is a creative process that relies on the brainstorming and thinking of ideas and different possibilities as to what key points, stories, examples, illustrations, data, quotes, or other methods are germane and pertinent for use. As ideas and key points develop, jot them down, and then, go back and edit. Many times just getting ideas on paper helps the creative development process start to flow, other ideas to evolve, and direction to start developing.

Another helpful practice is to use three main points of wisdom overall for your presentation. Using three main points of wisdom is a technique that can help provide a flow or rhythm to your presentation. This technique can also help provide structure and organization, so your audience can identify, follow, understand and remember what the key points of the presentation are, along with the SOCO.

Once you have your presentation outlined, and the opening and closing scripted, go back and edit. Focus your editing on four key elements: clarity, specificity, visual words, and emotional connection. Think about your presentation outline and material as either adding to and enhancing your presentation or distracting from it. Delete anything that doesn't support your SOCO of educating, persuading, influencing, selling, or convincing. Remove content that isn't essential and doesn't really connect with your audience to achieve your SOCO. Think critically when editing.

LEVEL OF ABSTRACTION

It is important to know your audience in terms of their role and knowledge of the subject matter. For example, say you are giving a business presentation on healthcare to the local Rotary Club, which consists of a diverse group of managers and non-managers, from different industries. In this case, you'll need to use a combination of broad, general words, phrases, and descriptions without a lot of industry-specific terminology; however, you may want to provide some detailed, specific information that does contain some limited industry-specific language. The idea is to match the level of abstraction to your audience. Another way to think about this concept is to balance the "big picture" with supporting details. If the Chief Medical Officer was addressing a group of physicians about new clinical protocols being adopted, this presentation would feature much more detailed, specific, even technical clinical language. However, in the case of a hospital leader speaking to the local Rotary Club on the topic of healthcare reform, the level of abstraction would need to be bigger picture with some supporting detail and data. Being overly detailed using industry jargon would not work well with the Rotary Club audience, as many wouldn't have the background or familiarity with industry-specific terminology and dealings in healthcare to understand all the terminology or detail.

MOVEMENT

Something that many presenters overlook is movement. Don't distract from your own message with unnecessary movement. At the beginning of a presentation, it's best to stand still. Standing still can visually indicate the stability of your ideas and your authority of the subject while also making you feel comfortable. When telling a story or emphasizing a key point, it is also advised to stand still. Movement during a presentation should be on purpose, during a transition between thoughts or points, or to emphasize a specific phrase. When the speaker is moving during a presentation it is very obvious to the audience, including nervous movements that can be distracting. Again, are your movements adding to or distracting from your presentation?

ASK KEY QUESTIONS

Asking your audience key questions at appropriate times throughout the presentation can be engaging. You can also build credibility by stating a question you've heard from someone in the audience prior, and make a point or comment to demonstrate your insight and understanding of the audience's challenges, perspectives, or other point from the audience's view. A big question with no real answer, or with multiple possible answers, is also a good way to connect and engage and get the audience thinking about their own perspectives. A technique to consider using is to comment on a provocative question you've posed that will make your audience think to themselves "Yeah, that's right."

THE OPENING AND CLOSING

The two most important parts of any presentation, in this order, are:

a. The closing—remember that *last words linger and are remembered.* One can use a rhetorical question that ties to your premise; use a call for action; or circle-back to your opening. What do you want your audience to do as a result of your presentation?
b. The opening—the second thing that will be remembered. The opening is the "flavor" scene, as it sets the tone for the entire presentation. Work on scripting your opening and closing. It is a good rule of thumb to only try to script the opening and closing, along with a few other key points or quotes. Everything else presented should flow conversationally.

DISCUSSION QUESTIONS

1. What is important when it comes to the presenter's movement during a business presentation?
2. How can becoming more effective at making business presentations help augment a leader's career?
3. What are the two primary levels for the presenter to connect with the audience during a business presentation?
4. What role do voice, tone, inflection, and body language play in a presentation?
5. Describe what is meant by the "I/You" ratio.
6. What can a short story, told well, help the speaker do?
7. What are the two most important parts of any presentations?
8. What is the SOCO, and why is it important when developing a presentation?
9. Describe two or three guidelines to follow when using power point slides in a presentation.
10. Describe what is meant by the statement "Developing a presentation is more like a field trip than working in a laboratory."

Most of the content for this chapter comes from several training sessions I have personally attended, along with email newsletters provided by my friend Patricia Fripp.

Patricia Fripp, CSP, CPAE
Sales Presentation Trainer, Keynote Speaker, Executive Speech Coach
527 Hugo Street, San Francisco, CA 94122
(800)634–3035, (415)753–6556, Fax (415)753–0914
PFripp@fripp.com, www.fripp.com

FIGURE CREDIT

Figure 19.1: Chris Greenberg, "President George Bush at Podium," http://commons.wikimedia.org/wiki/File:Bush_Dec_17,_2007.jpg. Copyright in the Public Domain.

20

Dealing With the Media

Healthcare is under the microscope. A hospital or health service organization's business practices are under public and regulatory scrutiny like never before. With the ongoing implementation of the Affordable Care Act of 2010; continued increases in costs; advancements in care, treatment, and related technologies; increasing expectations of all stakeholders; and numerous healthcare reform initiatives, the ongoing debate about what changes are needed to improve the U.S. healthcare system is likely to continue for the foreseeable future. Healthcare is increasingly being scrutinized at all levels, and that includes the media. In general, people are interested in the developments occurring in the healthcare system on a national level, as well as with their local hospital and other health service providers. The healthcare operating environment is ripe for media coverage and scrutiny like never before. Attention hospitals and health service organizations! Get your media relations and crisis communication media plan ready now—you're going to need it.

OBJECTIVES

1. Understand and appreciate how the new healthcare landscape is drawing greater scrutiny for hospitals and other health service organizations and their business practices.
2. Understand the technique of developing and applying talking points, when needed, to manage and be consistent with internal or external communication.
3. Learn what to say/not say and how to prepare for an interview with the media or conduct a press conference.

MEDIA RELATIONS

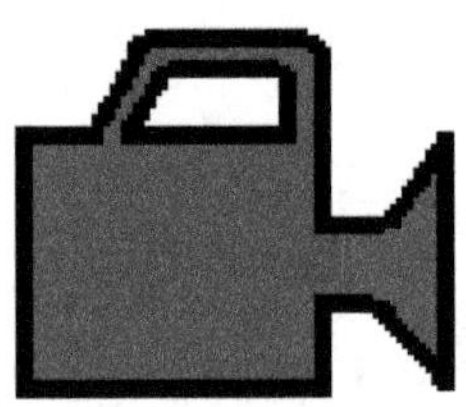

FIGURE 20.1 Blue Video Camera

A good rule of thumb is for a hospital or health service organization's Marketing Director and/or hospital CEO to build a strong, positive relationship with local media well in advance of ever needing it. Make no mistake; at some point, that relationship will be vital.

PUBLIC RELATIONS: A FEW GENERAL GUIDELINES

- Invite local media in routinely. Give them good stories about your hospital or health service organization.
- Do ongoing internal scanning for good stories (new technologies, new procedures, human interest, local impact of national stories, etc.).
- Inquire about what types of healthcare stories various local media are most interested in.
- Provide local media with press releases and summaries.
- Identify leaders, physicians, and other clinicians who are good with media and in front of the camera.
- Provide media training to key internal spokespersons.
- Establish goals, objectives, and a plan for public relations.
- Review the media relations policy and procedure periodically and modify, as needed. Present and discuss the policy with leadership and the board periodically.

- Don't overlook the important role of internal marketing. Employees are ambassadors for your health service organization in the community. Communicate with employees about what's going on in the organization, and provide them with good information about the organization to share in the community. Why not equip them to speak about topics and stories that can help with positive public relations in the community? Moreover, employees want to know and hear about happenings in the organization before they read or hear about them in the media.
- Talking points are an effective way to organize key points of communication. Consider developing talking points for important internal "corporate" (official) communication, as well as external media communication.

DEVELOPING MEDIA RELEASES

A key goal is to develop a consistent, coordinated, and organized approach/process to generate positive public relations, including media releases.

Here are a few primary objectives for public relations and media releases:

- To increase exposure and visibility for the health service organization in the community.
- To increase the sense of personal connection customers/potential customers have with the organization.
- To serve as a vehicle for increasing believable, credible stories that will promote the services and capabilities of the hospital.

When considering whether a story might be newsworthy for preparing as a news release, consider the following five criteria.

- **Timing**—Current topics are newsworthy. If it happened today, it's news. If the same happening occurred last week, it probably won't be interesting or newsworthy any longer. This includes attempting to find a local angle or story for a national news story, happening, or trend.
- **Uniqueness**—Is it something that is the first of its kind in the city, community, or state? Is it a first for the hospital? Is it unique? Is it a novel approach to an old way of doing something? Is it innovative and revolutionary?
- **Human Interest**—Human interest stories appeal to human emotion. Putting a human face on a story shows how a particular treatment, program, technology, or device actually benefits real people. (Tell the story of the war through the eyes of a soldier). Human interest stories also show how a field of work, innovation, or technology has made a difference in someone's life.
- **Significance/Impact** -The number of people affected by a story is important. It's also important to address the readers'/viewers' questions: "*So what? What does this mean to me*?" How significant is the story? Furthermore, it is important to show how the event or potential story impacts the health of patients and the local community.

- **Prominence**—Famous people get media coverage, because they are famous. If a famous person suffers or dies from a particular disease or is treated with a new procedure or medical technology, the public interest and desire to understand the disease or new procedure increases. This can be on a national, regional, or even local level.

TALKING POINTS

The use of talking points is always a good idea when attempting to manage internal or external communication and foster consistency of key communication messages, including to department heads and supervisors and from them to their staffs. The use of talking points is also a good idea for external communication when preparing to meet with the media. Outline the agenda and key talking points, with rationale, into "sound bites."

An example of this might be for a hospital that is experiencing a reduction in force (RIF). Here is a simple layoff for how this might look.

EMPLOYEE LAYOFFS QUESTIONS	TALKING POINTS
• Laid-off 20 employees; 15 full-time equivalents • How was the RIF determined? • What RIF process or policy was followed? • Why is this action being taken now?	• Followed board-approved RIF Policy and Procedure • Policy based on seniority by job classification • Impacted six different departments • Areas affected in lower quartile on productivity as benchmarked against peer group • Affordable Care Act of 2010—cutting reimbursement to hospitals • Employer pressure to reduce costs: can't keep cost-shifting in future, as hospital have done historically • Will continue to provide the highest quality care and service to patients.

When developing talking points, be sure to develop and articulate your Single Overriding Communication Objective (SOCO). An example of this is building a replacement hospital. The SOCO might be "*A new hospital is necessary in order to become the hospital of choice and meet the needs and expectations of all our stakeholders, including our patients—and what they are seeking—even demanding.*"

It is also important to identify key target audiences. What key messages should you send to each target audience? (Who will be listening to the communication message: the board, leadership, employees, patients, employers, patients, regulators, etc.?) What do you want to tell them? What should you tell them? How do they feel? What do they need to hear from you? How does your proposed communication message feel? How will people react? What are our biggest critics thinking?

When communicating key messages internally, these must be communicated repeatedly through various mediums (verbally in staff meetings, in written communications, etc.). Here are some key points regarding internal communication.

a. Control internal messages to manage distortion/rumors. If no official word is forthcoming, then staff (and everyone else) will create their own story.
b. Employees want to hear from both executive leadership and their direct supervisor.
c. Don't overlook the need to communicate with the board and medical staff.
d. Use multiple channels to communicate the message.
e. Repetition of the communication message is important for it to be heard and understand.

INTERVIEWING WITH THE MEDIA

Interviewing with the media is something that should be practiced and prepared for. As previously mentioned, the preparation and use of talking points to convey key messages in the form of short sound bites is advisable. Below is a list of key points to consider when preparing for an interview with the media:

- Ask, in advance, what the interview is about and what questions will be asked. You can specify what you will and won't talk about; however, this still has to be managed (i.e., be prepared for anything).
- You are always "on the record." There is no such thing as "off the record." This includes when the camera is being set up or taken down after an interview. Always assume the camera or tape recorder is rolling.
- The biggest questions your audience has: 1) are you being honest (are you believable?) 2) are you likeable?
- Control the interview agenda. Prepare your key talking points in advance. Transition to your key talking points, as appropriate, throughout the interview. Remember: you are the subject matter expert!
- Keep your composure.
- Always be honest with your responses and never distort the truth.
- Control the location of the interview, when possible.
- If you don't know the answer, then say you don't know (but also say something like "We are trying to make that determination," "We are still investigating that," "We haven't concluded our analysis of the situation," or "I don't know the answer to that, but I will find out and get back with you," and then, follow through and get back with the answer as soon as possible.
- Don't speculate—only provide facts that are known.
- During a hostile interview when the interviewer interrupts you, say something like "May I finish my response first please." Be more likeable than your interviewer!

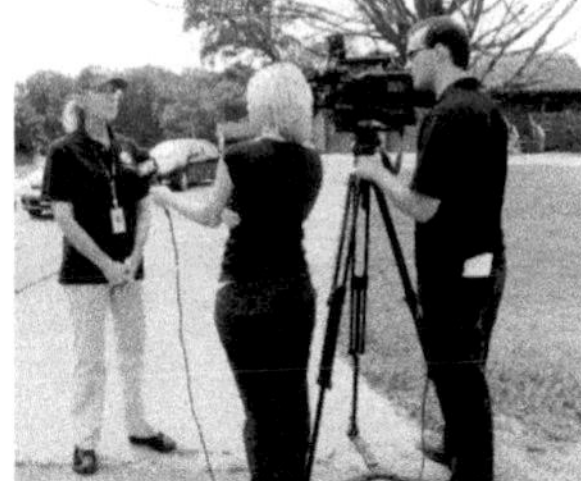

FIGURE 20.2 Woman Being Interviewed
Patsy Lynch / FEMA, "Woman Being Interviewed," http://commons.wikimedia.org/wiki/File:FEMA_-_44946_-_FEMA_public_affairs_offcer_giving_interview_with_media_in_IL.jpg. Copyright in the Public Domain.

- Posture and body language matter: be aware!
  - Remember that communication is 7 percent words used; 38 percent voice, tone, and inflection; and 55 percent face and body.
- Know who you are really speaking to regarding your interview. Who's listening? What do you need to tell them?
- Dress for your role. Avoid stripes and plaids for TV interviews (stripes and plaids will looked washed out on TV).
- Be forthright and honest; however, manage your messages.
- Talk in shorter sentences than normal—think about sound bites:
  - Sound bites are more likely to be used.
- Avoiding long sentences can help prevent interview "splicing," as well as getting off-track and wandering "into the weeds" or talking about something you don't want to.
- Practice interviewing/role playing with a colleague. There is no substitute for practice and being prepared for questions and anticipating what to expect.
- You can always ask to see the typewritten interview copy, audio track, or TV interview tape before it is aired.

PATIENT SAFETY ISSUES AND CRISIS EVENTS

Patient safety issues and crisis events are matters that must receive critical focus, attention, and preparation in order to handle them appropriately. Here are a few additional key points to keep in mind:

- Outline steps the organization is taking to address the situation (and, in the event of a sentinel/never event, making sure it doesn't ever happen again to another patient).
- If appropriate, extend sympathy and condolences to those affected by a patient safety incident.
- Answer the question, but immediately bridge to your key talking points.
- Don't repeat negative words, phrases, statements, or questions.
- Avoid humor.
- Remember: there is no such thing as "off the record."
- When can the media expect your next update? Let them know and stick with this schedule, even if you don't have any new information.
- Keep the media in a comfortable room on location: you don't want them wandering.
- In what order do you communicate crisis information internally? It is suggested this order: executive leadership, the board, key physicians, the leadership team at large, employees, and then media (including a possible press release).

- Give staff the time to process and mentally prepare for the situation. Staff will be asked questions by colleagues, family, friends, etc. You may want to distribute a list of key talking points to staff if they will be receiving questions externally.
- Develop a crisis communication plan, policy, and procedure well in advance of needing it. This is part of emergency preparedness and risk management for institutional marketing.

HANDLING A PRESS CONFERENCE

A press conference should be a well-organized activity that is prepared for in advance.

- Prepare your SOCO and key talking points/statement in advance.
- Control the setting/environment.
- You may want to proactively address key questions the media and others may have with your talking points—in advance of them being asked. Think through what questions will be asked and how to best respond. Role play and practice beforehand.
- Decide, in advance, if you will be taking questions at a press conference and how many you will respond to, etc. If you aren't taking questions, be prepared to walk away after making your presentation: this will take discipline.
- If appropriate, indicate that this is all we know at this point, and we will be providing further information or updates (on the hour, every three hours, etc.). Do not speculate!

DISCUSSION QUESTIONS

1. Identify a few of the factors driving the public and media scrutiny of hospitals and health service providers today.
2. List a few of the action steps to take to build a positive relationship with local news media.
3. Describe why internal marketing and communication is an important function that should not be overlooked in a health service organization's media relations plan.
4. List two or three criteria that should be assessed when determining whether an internal news story might be newsworthy.
5. What does the phrase "There is no such thing as off the record" mean, and why is it important to always remember?
6. Describe two or three important points to remember when conducting an interview with the media.
7. What is meant by the SOCO?
8. What are a few general guidelines to follow for dealing with local media on an ongoing basis?
9. What are one or two objectives for media releases?
10. What are the two primary questions the audience has about the person being interviewed?

FIGURTE CREDITS

Figure 20.1: Copyright © Ezzex (CC BY-SA 3.0) at http://commons.wikimedia.org/wiki/File:Tv_camera2.png.
Figure 20.2: Patsy Lynch / FEMA, "Woman Being Interviewed," http://commons.wikimedia.org/wiki/File:FEMA_-_44946_-_FEMA_public_affairs_offcer_giving_interview_with_media_in_IL.jpg. Copyright in the Public Domain.

21

The Difference Between Good and Great

What's the difference between good and great in healthcare leadership? Can the difference be identified and described? Does it really matter? Yes, I think it does matter: a lot. The effectiveness, impact, and difference a healthcare leader can make results in the legacy he creates and that legacy can have impact on countless lives. This chapter explores the difference between healthcare leadership that's good and healthcare leadership that's great; what constitutes or creates the difference between the two; thoughts about why the difference in the two matters; and related perspective and thoughts for healthcare leaders.

OBJECTIVES

1. Explore how the intangible characteristics of a healthcare leader's drive to succeed, commitment to learn, commitment to serve, and willingness to work hard can lead to a successful career.
2. Explore how the fear of failure can freeze a leader out of success.
3. Examine the difference between good and great.

Most healthcare leaders want to do a great job. Most healthcare leaders would like to make a real difference in the work they do and the lives they touch. Most healthcare leaders would like to be thought of as not just "average," but great in terms of the impact their leadership makes. But what does it mean for a healthcare leader to be great in terms of the work he does and his impact on the lives of others? It may mean more or less than one might think. Let's explore.

A DRIVE TO BE SUCCESSFUL

Although it is a broad generalization to make, it stands to reason that most successful healthcare leaders have an innate, inner drive to be successful. Most healthcare leaders who have enjoyed great careers and been very successful began their careers with the thought and intent of being great. Not necessarily in a self-centered or boastful way, but one that drove them to be successful. This shouldn't really come as any surprise. Most anything in life (and in business, for that matter) that has been accomplished, first began with a person's desire to achieve or accomplish the goal, objective, or task, followed by thoughts about what that achievement or accomplishment means, and so on. The key point here is for a healthcare leader to be great/successful, he or she must first have the desire and the drive to make it happen. It is that inner drive to be successful and achieve that keeps a healthcare leader going through all the challenges, adversity, and set-backs most experience. There is a poster series with motivational leadership sayings featuring one that says "***Obstacles are those things you see when you take your eyes off your goal.***" Sam Odle says that it is motivating when you think about the importance of the work you do as a healthcare leader. The lesson here for healthcare leaders is to not lose sight of the bigger picture: why you got into healthcare leadership in the first place; the difference you want to make; and the difference you are making for all the lives that you touch.

Gary Player is a former Professional Golf Association professional golfer and winner of 24 PGA golf tournaments, including nine majors over a career where he was actively competing at the professional level for almost 30 years. Player was featured in an issue of Sports Illustrated in 2014, while in his early 70s, as one of the fittest mature athletes of all time. A story is told of Player practicing one day on the driving range, where he practiced hitting golf balls on a regular, routine basis. Player hit hundreds—countless—practice shots every day. Player's hands were blistered and sore, feeling the effects of a relentless practice routine and drive to be great. One day, a spectator who was observing Player said to him "***I'd give anything to hit the golf ball like you.***" To which Player immediately responded "***No you wouldn't.***" And with that, Player showed the spectator his swollen and blistered hands from all the practicing he'd been doing and said "***If you did, your hands would look just like this.***" I can only image the spectator was taken aback a bit by Player's actions and response. Gary Player had probably heard that comment or expression from many other golf fans and spectators during his professional golfing career and probably didn't—although he probably wanted to—make that same statement to others. Nevertheless, the point was clearly made by Player: success and greatness is never automatic and requires a lot of desire, hard work, sacrifice, and effort. Being successful and great at what you do requires many things, but it begins with the true desire to be successful or great. It also requires an incredible amount of sacrifice and hard work along the way, as well.

SUCCESS VERSUS FAILURE

Every person—and every leader—will make mistakes from time to time. The real question is what does the leader do as a result of the mistake he makes? Does he learn from them, or will history repeat itself? Mr. Sam Odle states that "***I can't remember who said it, but if you haven't made any mistakes you probably haven't done much. I think I made mistakes along the way. Fortunately I was given the opportunity to recover from those. Not all my negotiations always went: some of them went off track and had to be re-established and fixed along the way. One thing (a leader should do) is try to forget your failures: you learn whatever the lesson is, but you forget the real act. If you are afraid of failure then you won't succeed. It will make you timid; it will make you less likely to take risks; less likely to expand your scope of responsibility; you won't take on new challenges because you might fail. So you freeze yourself out of success. It's not that you don't have fear, but you have to overcome that by focusing on the importance of the work you are doing and the result you hope to achieve along the way.***"

> The fear of failure can freeze you out of success.

COMMITMENT TO LEARNING

Experience is a great teacher; however, the lesson experience teaches always comes after the experience. Therefore, learning through experience requires: 1) the healthcare leader to pay attention. Just like in a didactic classroom setting, learning through on-the-job experiences requires the leader/learner pay attention in order to observe and understand the lesson experience is teaching; 2) reflection about the experience, the lesson learned, and leadership strategy or action to change, improve, or otherwise do differently the next time; 3) the desire and commitment to learn, change, grow, develop and improve as a leader; 4) the mindset, belief, or attitude that every experience, event, moment, or interaction with others is an opportunity to learn, grow, develop, and improve; 5) being present in the moment—not just physically, but mentally present.

Lifelong learners are committed to learning; they enjoy and want to learn as much as they can from a variety of sources, including journal articles, books, conferences and seminars, observation, experiences, formal courses or instruction, self-study, or mentors. Best practices in leadership evolve; however, much of the fundamentals of effective leadership don't. It becomes a question of ongoing learning and its application to constantly improve and perfect leadership style and practices with the goal to improve overall leadership effectiveness.

COMMITMENT TO SERVE

The business of healthcare is service: people serving people. Most healthcare leaders typically aren't involved in the provision of direct patient care; however, they serve the people who are involved in the provision of direct patient care. Healthcare leaders are in a role of serving others: employees, physicians, other leaders, trustees, and volunteers, as well as patients and their families. Being in such a service role takes a real commitment to serve others. The servant leader philosophy takes this commitment to serve others to an even a higher level; one that is increasingly being recognized as what is expected from a healthcare leader. A commitment to serve often starts with a mindset, philosophy, or belief or attitude towards your role as a leader serving others; what matters most; and what healthcare leadership is about.

WINNERS DON'T QUIT AT QUITTING TIME

Success and greatness are not typically free—there is usually a price to be paid. This payment isn't one that can be made on credit with the bill coming due later. This is a payment that has to be paid up front with no assurances or guarantees whatsoever. In most cases, for healthcare leaders that price is paid in the form of extra time, hard work, and sacrifice. That translates into long hours with early morning meetings; meetings in the evenings; paperwork and recruitment visits on weekends; and paperwork at home after hours. But when you love the work you do, it doesn't feel so much like work.

In 2004 or thereabouts, I attended an all-day seminar with several different speakers, including Peyton Manning, the great NFL quarterback who played for the Indianapolis Colts at the time. One thing Peyton said, in particular, during his presentation that stuck with me was: "***Quitters don't win, and winners don't quit at quitting time.***" Manning's work ethic—both on and off the football field—is legendary. It can be argued that nobody in the history of the NFL has studied the playbook—and his opponent; practiced his craft; and been any more prepared for each game than Peyton Manning. He has an insatiable drive to be successful and great. By any criteria to measure success and greatness, Manning is one of the greatest quarterbacks in NFL history. His drive to be great and his work ethic have played significant roles in his journey to greatness—as much as any other element or characteristic. Of course, other factors, such as his God-given natural skills, abilities, and aptitude have a lot to do with his success, as well. But the point is this: whether you want to be a great quarterback in the NFL or a great leader in healthcare, it's not a 40-hour-a-week proposition—it takes much more than that—including a real dedication to your job, your profession, and your career.

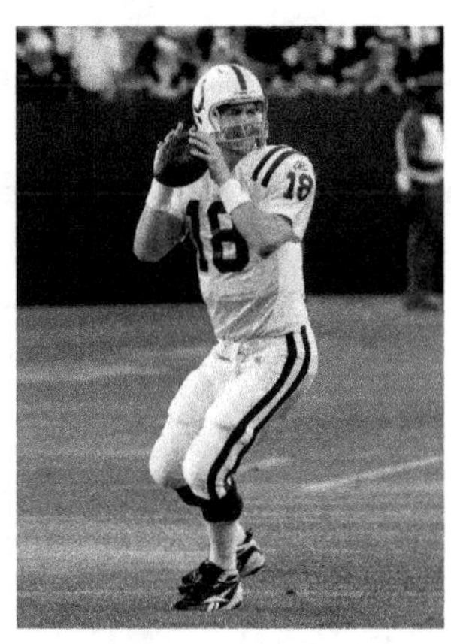

FIGURE 21.1 Peyton Manning

DEFINING SUCCESS: DEFINING GREATNESS

Every person wants to be successful. Every hospital and health service administrator wants to be successful as a leader. How should success be defined for a healthcare leader? What does success really look like? Of course, different healthcare leaders are going to define success differently. However, for any hospital success is going include some measurement of financial performance, service performance, quality outcomes, employee satisfaction, physician satisfaction, and other metrics. Evaluation criteria to measure success can include quantitative measurements, as well as qualitative measurements. For an individual healthcare administrator to define his own success in his career, it is more a matter of personal perspective as to how that person goes about defining his own success. But the impact that a leader has on the other lives he touches is certainly an important criteria.

According to Sam Odle ***"Success should be the number of people you were able to positively impact. Even if you can't count them, if you can look at the things that you did and say 'all the things that I did were all directed towards having a positive impact on as many people as possible.' That's what I wanted to do."*** In healthcare, sometimes that positive impact can't be found in the financial statement or other quantitative assessment. Healthcare is the business of people serving people. Sometimes, the positive impact made by a healthcare leader may be hard for him to really see or distinguish, even though it is clear, evident, and even heartfelt for the person he made a difference for.

Mr. Odle tells of a story that occurred in Methodist Hospital where he worked as President. ***"There was a woman who I knew because her kids went to the same school as our kids did. I happened to see her in the hallway [of the hospital] one day, and she, and her mother and sister were visiting her father [who was a patient] in the hospital ICU. She said he was stable, doing better and they were optimistic. I remember telling her 'If there is anything I can do, let me know.' I didn't see them anymore and it was about six months later when I received a letter from her written on behalf of her mother who just wanted to tell us how compassionate all the people were. And she remembered me, the President of the hospital, stopping in the hall just to ask how things were going and all the compassion she felt. Even though her***

husband ended up dying, she thought the hospital was a wonderful place." This type of story—and other similar stories—are repeated throughout the U.S. on a daily basis by conscientious healthcare leaders with a commitment to serving others in their time of need through their humanness and compassion. Many times, serving others and making a difference is taking the time to offer a helping hand or provide the caring, understanding, compassion or reassurance the person needs in the moment. Sometimes what, to the healthcare leader, doesn't really seem like doing much means all the difference in the world to the person he or she is interacting with.

In healthcare, many would call a healthcare leader who serves others and makes a difference in their lives as being successful. When a healthcare leader can serve others and provide the leadership his organization needs to foster efficient, effective operations that provide high-quality care, deliver great customer service, and generate the type of financial performance that allows them to generate the capital funds needed to grow, expand, and be sustainable in its mission of service to the community, he may be called great and successful.

GREATNESS: STATISTICALLY SPEAKING

In some instances, great results or performance can be quantified and measured statistically. Let's examine the results and performances attained by Peyton Manning over his career and during his record-setting season in 2013 as an NFL quarterback.

Over 16 NFL seasons—14 with the Indianapolis Colts beginning in 1998 (Manning did not play in the 2011 season due to a neck injury) and 2 with the Denver Broncos in 2012 and 2013 as of this writing—Manning has put up some impressive numbers. He has a career quarterback rating of 97.2; made 8,452 pass attempts and completed 5,532 for a career completion percentage of 65.5 percent; thrown for 64,964 yards for an average of 4,331 passing yards per season and 271 passing yards per game; and thrown for 491 touchdowns for an average of 33 touchdown passes per season and 2 touchdown passes per game. Manning has also thrown 219 interceptions in 240 games played for an average of almost 1 per game.

Compare his career statistics to his record-breaking season in 2013 when he had a quarterback rating of 115.1; attempted 659 passes and completed 450 for a completion percentage of 68.3 percent; and passed for a total of 5,477 yards and 55 touchdowns, both NFL records. But notice one thing here. Manning's completion percentage in his record setting year of 2013 was only 2.8 percent higher than what he has averaged for the 15 seasons he played in the NFL. Actually, his 68.3 percent completion percentage in 2013 ranks as his third highest in his career. And, compare his record-setting season to 2010, the last season he played in Indianapolis when he attempted 679 passes and completed 450 for a passing completion percentage of 66.3 percent. Yards-per-catch in 2010 were 10.44 yards, versus 12.17 in 2013. Two points to highlight here are 1) there are numerous other factors coming together with Manning's record setting 2013 season, which aren't reflected in any of his statistics, including the performance of his teammates and the team chemistry, and 2) his yards-per-catch in 2013 were only 1.73 yards more per catch than in 2010; however, Manning threw for 777 more passing yards in 2013 than in 2010 on the same number of completions—450! Talk about an incremental difference!

Michael Phelps is one of the most celebrated swimmers in Olympic history. Phelps has won a record 22 medals in 3 Olympics: 18 gold, 2 silver, and 2 bronze. Granted: Phelps has freakish athletic ability in a swimming pool, along with a grueling training regimen and a will to win. But, if we were to examine the margin of many of his victories, they would be a matter of no more than a few seconds or even a fraction of a second. On August 16, 2008, Phelps won his seventh gold medal at the Beijing Games in the men's 100-meter butterfly, setting an Olympic record for the event with a time of 50.58 seconds and edging out his nearest competitor, Milorad Čavić, by only one hundredth (0.01) of a second. That time is way less than what it takes to blink your eye! A total of 7 of the 8 gold medals Phelps won in 2008 were world records. The point is that the difference between winning gold versus silver versus bronze—or sometimes even last place in the event—can be the difference of the slimmest of margins. The real difference between athletes of comparable skill and talent can come down to the practice regimen and training: one that can provide the slimmest of margins of victory in the final analysis. Practice, training, hard work, effort, long hours, not quitting at quitting time. These are some of the very same qualities that result in greatness and success in healthcare leadership, just like life, in general.

In most instances, when greatness is measured statistically, it identifies something very revealing: greatness usually comes about through an incremental difference consistently applied on a repetitive basis. A deeper dive into this point suggests that greatness is based on a consistent incremental difference that is generated by incrementally more effort and hard work. In other words, it is a healthcare leader going the extra mile every day that generates the level of performance and success that most people would refer to as "great."

DISCUSSION QUESTIONS

1. Most healthcare leaders want to do a great job. Describe the difference between good and great in the context of healthcare leadership.
2. Describe what the following statement means: "Obstacles are those things you see when you take your eyes off your goal."
3. Identify two or three things that are required in order for a healthcare leader to learn through his experience.
4. What does Sam Odle mean when he talks about how the fear of failure can freeze you out of success?
5. How would you define success for a hospital or health service leader?
6. How does Sam Odle define success as a hospital or health service leader?
7. Can incrementally more effort and hard work result in greatness? Please describe how this might/might not be true.
8. What role does a commitment to learning play in the quest for great leadership performance?
9. Describe what is meant by the phrase "Best Practices"?
10. Describe the philosophy of "Servant Leadership."

FIGURE CREDIT

22

Transformational Leadership

The challenges faced by U.S. health service organizations today may be greater than any other time in the history of health service administration. With the expectations for health service organizations' results and performance increasing on the part of all stakeholders and the complexities associated with operating a business ever increasing, as well, the challenges for healthcare administrators are significant. At the same time, the opportunity to make a real difference in the lives of countless numbers of people has also never been greater. Healthcare leadership has now entered the era where transformational leadership is sought out, highly desired, and virtually expected from all leaders. The days of healthcare administrative stewardship are over. Health service boards, leadership teams, physicians, employees, community leaders, government officials and regulators, and even patients are no longer satisfied with leaders who are caretakers or stewards. Stakeholders are any persons or groups who have a legitimate interest or "stake" in an organization and its actions. Stakeholders, today, want healthcare leaders who can provide transformational leadership to their organizations to significantly improve their quality of care and delivery of service, reduce costs, provide greater value, and lead the organization into a new era of healthcare reform.

OBJECTIVES

1. Understand what transformational leadership is and how it affects a health service organization, its performance, and all its stakeholders.
2. Learn about several methods, techniques, characteristics, and examples of transformational leadership.
3. Appreciate the importance of transformational leadership in today's demanding healthcare environment focused on reform and value.

TRANSACTIONAL VERSUS TRANSFORMATIONAL LEADERSHIP

Healthcare leaders today—especially those at higher levels of management—must be more transformational than transactional in their role and approach to leadership. One primary question for transformational leadership is how, as a healthcare leader, can you help to engender higher levels of effort and performance from employees and physicians, both individually and as teams or work groups? What can you do as a healthcare leader to provide more effective leadership that will result in higher levels of performance within the organization?

Transformational leadership is leadership that generates awareness and acceptance of a group or organization's purpose and mission, as well as its vision for the future, and inspires employees to reach beyond their own personal needs and self-interests with effort and performance that is for the good of the group or organization. Visionary leadership is leadership that creates a positive image of the future that motivates organizational employees and provides direction for future planning and goal setting. Visionary leadership is a requirement for transformational leadership. Transformational leadership differs from transactional leadership, which is leadership style based on an exchange process, in which leaders use more of a command-and-control style. This style typically features followers being rewarded for good performance and reprimanded for poor performance. Therefore, one of the biggest differences of transformational leadership versus transactional leadership has also to do with tapping into employee discretionary effort by motivating and inspiring employees to be fully engaged, to give more effort and attain a higher level of performance for the good of the group or organization. Implicit in this difference is an employee focus on the group or organization, and not each employee's own individual circumstances or situation. Also implicit with transformational leadership is teamwork with each employee willing to help, support, and assist others in any way appropriate for the good of the group or organization. Individual recognition and reward are secondary to that of the group or organization.

One of the biggest differences of transformational leadership versus transactional leadership has to do with tapping into employee discretionary effort by motivating and inspiring employees to be fully engaged, to give more effort and attain a higher level of performance for the good of the group or organization.

Sam Odle says, ***"Talking about the difference between management and leadership, I look at as it is all leadership. But management is more focused on the transactional leadership. If you are a unit leader, you're managing a section; you're managing the buyers; you're managing the technicians. There are incremental transactions that have to be done, whether they are patient care, business, or whatever. There are some people who are good transactional leaders. What hopefully happens over time is that people [(leaders)] master the transactional skills and then they get up to the vision and strategy. That's where transformational leadership comes in. You don't lose your transactional skills, but you develop those transformational leadership skills which are all about the 5th discipline principles and those kinds of things."*** In essence, Mr. Odle is saying that transactional leadership skills are important, and healthcare leaders must be effective in exercising their transactional skills on a daily basis. However, it is the transformational skills that more experienced and seasoned healthcare leaders learn and apply that can make the biggest difference for driving a healthcare workforce to make big strides in the results that it achieves and the performance that it attains.

Visionaries are able to create a shared vision with others so that everyone in the group or organization knows and understands the direction they are headed and the path they will follow to achieve the shared vision.

As previously stated, visionary leadership is part of transformational leadership. Visionary leadership requires the healthcare leader to have the foresight, imagination, and the ability to form mental images of the future in a specific way and effectively articulate and communicate that vision to others. Visionaries are able to create a shared vision with others so that everyone in the group or organization knows and understands the direction they are headed and the path they will follow to achieve the shared vision. But the vision has to be a shared vision. As Mr. Sam Odle states, ***"If you have a vision, and no one else shares it, then it might as well be a nightmare because you [(the leader)] are going to try and get there but these other people [(employees)] don't share your vision and they're not marching or following you."***

THE CRITICAL INTANGIBLES OF LEADERSHIP

Transformational leadership primarily involves the use of the critical intangible skills of leadership. David Handel talks about the difference between tangible, or content skills of leadership and the intangible skills of leadership. "*One has to assume a healthcare leader has a certain level of content skills or tangible skills, and that is sort of a given. That doesn't mean you have to be a content expert in everything, but it means the leader has to have a certain level of content expertise. I think the intangibles are really what you do and how you do it. For example, what kind of role model do you serve for the people who work with you? To me it is emphasizing values, integrity, or doing the right thing. I think the intangibles include creating an environment—or being part of creating an environment because no one person does that by themselves—that people are happy in; that they feel it is professionally rewarding and challenging; that it is an open environment, and people can say what they think; that you really focus on a team environment. Healthcare is a team sport, and occasionally it involves teams coming together. So healthcare leaders need to create or be part of creating an environment that people are comfortable with all that. It is really modeling by what you do that you are open to hear people's opinions. It doesn't matter if they agree with you or not; what is their opinion? Why do you think that? It is also creating an environment where you try to reach consensus. Now consensus doesn't mean if there are 15 people in the room that every one of the 15 is willing to say 'Yes, I agree'. But it means basically there is pretty good unanimity [around a strategy or decision] that it is the right way to go. And then moving forward with it: deciding something, taking action, and then holding people accountable. To me the intangible is that people look at you [(the leader)] and what you do.*"

Ken Stella talks about using the critical intangibles of leadership by "*encouraging others to work to their maximum. You encourage other people and support them and assist them in getting their LPN license, or getting that RN license. You show people, you demonstrate to people that you care about them. For example, going to a funeral. A person that worked at the hospital in dietary or one of the service department positions, and they lose a sister or they lose a brother, or they lose a parent and guess what? Stella shows up at the calling and goes to the funeral because you care about them. They are part of the family. So you can support them and help them and encourage them to help themselves and improve themselves. You are there also when there is a loss. And you're there when there are celebrations: the weddings, the baptisms. You just constantly try to show your support for others.*"

When asked about techniques, methods, or thoughts in general he had as they relate to encouraging others and inspiring others to achieve, Mr. Ken Stella states that "*In my mind, there are three things that you have to be cognizant of, aware of, as you [(the leader)] move through a professional career. My mother and father really taught me that you have to be academically prepared. So I've always stressed [to others] you have to be academically prepared. The first examples I can remember really pushing that was in Martinsville [(Morgan County Hospital)] as the Personnel Director. We had a number of good, good nurse aides. And given the right opportunity they could have been nurses. But they didn't have that opportunity. And that was right at the time Indiana was starting Ivy Tech State College, and Ivy Tech had an LPN program. I encourage the hospital board to establish a fund. I encouraged the hospital*

board to support these aides that they would become LPNs. At the same time, I was hiring LPNs. But I was looking at some of them saying 'You could be a two year RN. With just a little more you could have become a two year RN.' So one of the things I am the most pleased with is this: I had a lot of people where aides became LPNs; LPNs became RNs. We just had a tremendous success in that."

Healthcare leaders showing their support for others, encouraging others, demonstrating their confidence and belief in others, being there for employees when they need you, celebrating the moments in life that are important to others—all of these are intangibles but show tangible, visible signs that demonstrate the leader cares about people. The old axiom that succinctly summarizes this is: ***People don't care about what you know until they first know that you care***. And, when employees believe their leaders care about them, they will, in turn, be willing to support their leader. This is a big part of developing followership, which is the capacity of an individual or group of individuals to actively follow a leader.

EMPATHETIC LEADERSHIP

Empathetic leadership is being compassionate, sympathetic, and understanding of employees and other stakeholders. Sam Odle says, "***An empathetic leader is not just being around your listening but it is in everything you do. It is about understanding that the decisions you make do affect people. Even when you are making the most difficult decisions such as a layoff or cutting back on jobs; not giving a pay increase or as much of a pay increase; changing the employee's contribution to health insurance; and other things that impact people, I think you have to be empathetic on all those kinds of decisions. [You have to] make sure you are thinking about how this [decision] affects the people, and making sure you are doing it in an empathetic way. A leader can do anything in a managerial way, but it may not necessarily be empathetic. I remember this story about this drill sergeant who was very competent and one of the best drill sergeants but he wasn't very empathetic. In the morning after revile played all the soldiers are standing out on the line and the sergeant is giving the orders of the day. The sergeant then says 'And Smith, your mother died.' The general was going by at the time and he heard the sergeant and says 'Sergeant, come here. That's not the way to handle that situation. You've got to be more empathetic. You've got to show some feelings to these soldiers when something serious like that happens.' So the sergeant says 'Ok, general.' A couple of weeks later the sergeant got a notice that one of the other soldier's father had died. When the soldiers were together the sergeant says 'Men, all you men that have a father step forward! Not so fast Jones!' So with anything you do as a leader, you need to have empathy.***"

EMOTIONAL INTELLIGENCE

Emotional intelligence has received increasing attention as a key intangible skill of an effective leader. With the tremendous diversity in healthcare at all levels—race, culture, socioeconomic, education, income, perceived power, control and influence, and knowledge and understanding of the healthcare system and its components—emotional intelligence has become more challenging, as well as more vital as an effective leadership skill. Healthcare leadership involves working with people at all levels and interests.

In discussing emotional intelligence with Mr. Abel, he was asked what he has seen as a real strength of emotional intelligence with Ken Stella, Dave Windley, and John Render—all three recipients of the Indiana Hospital Association Award of Merit—and how they had applied it respectively in their healthcare leadership roles. Mr. Abel states, "***The biggest aspect of that is I can't ever remember seeing any of the three lose their temper: in any public or private meeting, and I've had both with all three. That's a pretty tough thing to do. For them to not lose their temper and not say something you would regret later: that's a pretty key attribute to somebody in such a public position. But I haven't seen it. Actually, quite the opposite when they would hear things that might be foolish and said by other people; they would, in a very kind way, go through and dissect it and say 'Is this really what we want to do?' That's a talent that a lot of people don't have. To be able to bring somebody back to seeing the impact of what they are saying and re-evaluating whether it was the right thing to say or not. All three of them could do that very professionally and very effectively.***"

FORMAL AND INFORMAL POWER AND INFLUENCE

Another critical intangible is the ability to influence and persuade others in a positive and appropriate way. A healthcare leadership position comes with a certain level of power inherent with the formal position held and its role and responsibilities in the organization. However, the power and influence of a healthcare leader can go far beyond the title or position he or she holds. Ed Abel talks about how informal power was exercised by Bill Hall, one of the founders of the Hall Render Law Firm headquartered in Indianapolis, Indiana. "***He preferred to work directly one-on-one with folks. Instead of power by position, he had more power by acceptance and persuasion. That was a trait that he had that was outstanding.***" Formal power is that authority which is inherent with the title, role, or position. Informal power, however, is the capacity to influence others without resorting to formal authority. An important point to note about formal power is about coercion. Coercion is the use of formal power and authority to force others to change. Coercion has a very limited role in leadership today and is no longer considered an effective strategy or style as it once was. Moreover, coercion is not advised and should not be used in other than the rarest occasions. In today's world, coercion is seen as manipulative and overbearing and will likely backfire on the leader who uses this style.

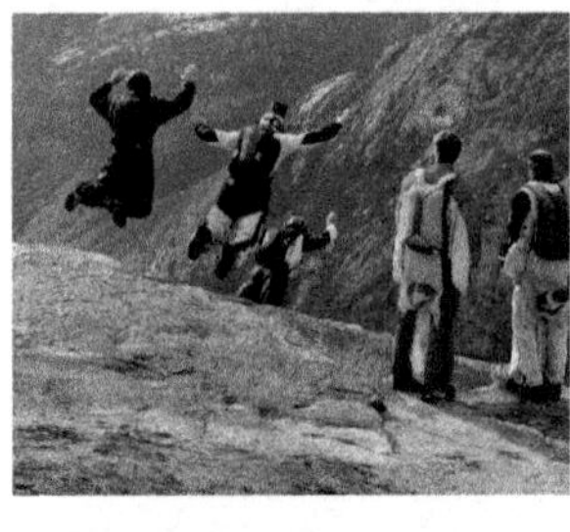

FIGURE 22.1 Base Jumping
Copyright © Håkon Thingstad (CC BY-SA 2.0) at http://commons.wikimedia.org/wiki/File:Kjerag_BASE_jumping.jpg.

RESULTS-DRIVEN CHANGE

Creating transformational leadership includes the application of a number of leadership elements, techniques, and methods to create a shared vision that others can clearly identify with, embrace, and support; move the focus and effort of the work towards the things that matter most and that will have the greatest positive impact on results and performance; and engage employees. As discussed in more detail in Chapter 15 on Results-Driven Change, focusing on the desired outcomes to be achieved is critical to creating transformational leadership. The process starts with having the end in mind, or the desired future state the organization wants to create, and then involves developing and implementing a plan and processes to achieve that shared vision or future state. Employee buy-in and emotional ownership is critical, so they will support the shared vision and goals, work to align what they do daily with that shared vision, and work hard to help achieve it.

IT'S A MATTER OF TRUST

Trust is everything. Without trust, a leader has no real power to create transformational change. Without trust, there won't be a shared vision, strong collaboration, or teamwork at the highest levels, nor will there be engaged employees. An absence of trust in the leader creates a culture where employee engagement, caring, and accountability are lacking—sometimes to a great degree. When trust is lacking in leadership, there is a sense of inequity, politics, and hidden agendas. Communication messages from leaders are perceived as suspect. Leadership decisions are second-guessed. Simply put, why would people follow a leader they don't trust or believe?

A common expression that speaks to this is does the leader ***"Walk the walk"*** In other words, does the leader's actions back up or support his or her words? Are his or her actions and words congruent and consistent? Judy Monroe, MD, says that ***"I don't think there is anything more powerful than a leader in a top leadership role to admit when they're wrong. To humble themselves: that is incredibly powerful. Or to change their own behavior when it hasn't been as productive as it could be. People are very forgiving. If the leader has started down a path that isn't very productive—and could even be the demise of the leader—but the leader has folks around him or is wise enough to alter that behavior; people are not only forgiving but that builds trust in the leader."***

Ed Abel says that ***"The absolute most important intangible has got to be honesty/trust. You can't lead if people don't believe what you are saying or don't trust you.***

> The absolute most important intangible has got to be honesty/trust. You can't lead if people don't believe what you are saying or don't trust you.

Everything that follows that is double, triple, or quadruple checked if they don't believe you or if they think you can't be honest with them. You can have all the vision in the world, but if they don't trust you or trust what you are saying, the organization is going to have a difficult time. Some leaders are visionary, some are sociable. You can look at a number of different leaders who have survived without having some other intangible (besides honesty/trust). In the book **The Economics of Trust,** ***the author talks about if we could trust***

everything that is given to us, we wouldn't have to double check it. He alludes to the fact that so much of our systems are built around (the premise) that we aren't sure if that's right or not. If you could eliminate that (the need to double-check because we don't trust) how much more productive our society would be. If you can't believe what the hospital CEO is telling you, how are you going to get to the next step? I can't describe in enough detail the number of conversations I've had with people where they have said 'We'll this is what he said, but we aren't sure that is what he meant.' They weren't saying they didn't understand the question, they were saying we don't believe it. So how do you lead in that kind of a vacuum? It is impossible. I think it's also safe to say with just about any leader for any significant period of time, there are going to be certain things that somebody is going to say 'We're not sure they are being totally honest.' There is the truth and the whole truth as it is said when [a witness is] sworn in to testify in front of a jury or court of law. Everybody has their days when maybe they don't give the whole truth, or maybe they kind of hedge a little bit on the facts. That's when you see [leaders] lose their effectiveness. Ultimately there is a price to pay for that. That attribute, I will tell people early in their career, it is the one thing—honesty—that nobody can take away from you: you have to give it up. If you can stay true to that you'll be fine. If you don't, there are going to be consequences and be prepared. Nobody can make you tell a lie. Nobody can make you be dishonest. Only you give that up."

> I will tell people early in their career, it is the one thing—honesty—that nobody can take away from you: you have to give it up.

DISCUSSION QUESTIONS

1. Describe one method or technique a leader can use to help drive transformational leadership.
2. What is meant by the term "Shared vision"?
3. What does the term empathetic leadership mean, and what might it look like in the organization?
4. Describe the difference between transactional and transformational leadership.
5. Describe how transformational leadership affects the organization and all stakeholders.
6. What is visionary leadership, and how does it relate to transformational leadership?
7. What does David Handel say about the critical intangibles of leadership?
8. What is emotional intelligence, and why is it important in healthcare leadership?
9. How is results-driven change important to transformational leadership?
10. Describe how a lack of trust in a leader impacts employee and organizational performance.

FIGURE CREDIT

Figure 22.1: Copyright © Håkon Thingstad (CC BY-SA 2.0) at http://commons.wikimedia.org/wiki/File:Kjerag_BASE_jumping.jpg.

23

The Role of Consultant

A consultant can be a valuable asset to a health service organization for a specific project or need or for ongoing counsel and advice. Many times, a consultant is engaged to help address or solve a problem; define or improve a process; provide guidance, support, technical assistance or other expertise with the planning or implementation of a new strategy, system, or technology; complete a project, activity, or function; provide advice or counsel; perform an evaluation or assessment of a defined function, process, outcome, or database; or other functions or services. These are general examples of what a consultant might be engaged to do. However, just like the different types of services and functions a consultant may provide, there are a myriad of reasons why a consultant might be engaged, including the need for an extra pair of hands, given existing workloads and schedules; needed technical or other expertise or experience; requirement for a set approach, process, or method; or outside advice or opinion from an independent, third-party who is perceived as being objective, unbiased, and impartial.

OBJECTIVES

1. Explore some of the roles and functions of consultants and consulting engagements.
2. Examine some of the important and practical aspects involved in rendering consulting services effectively to a health service organization client.
3. Understand the critical role that emotional intelligence plays in rendering effective consulting services to clients.

INTERNAL OR EXTERNAL CONSULTANT

A consultant can be either external to the organization or someone from the inside. The role of a consultant can be anything, but it is best when the role, as well as scope of the work to be completed, is clearly defined, along with the goals or objectives to be achieved. Can the role of the consultant change? Yes, and so can the scope of the work. However, it is important that clarity be maintained, should the consultant's role or project scope change.

Many times the consultant is internal, and someone with extensive experience, expertise or time, energy, and focus being given to one subject matter area or project, allowing him or her to concentrate on and devote all or much of his or her time and attention in one area. Engaging a consultant to dedicate significant time, energy, and expertise on a given project, task, or assignment typically allows or produces a more rapid or expedient attainment of the objective and improvement to performance. In healthcare, there are so many different functions and services that are connected—even interconnected—that an improved process, procedure or performance in one area can lead to or support an improvement in another. Moreover, performance improvement can be infectious. Performance improvement in one area can help spur momentum toward improvements being made in others. This is the type of action that can change an organization's culture to one where change, innovation, and performance improvement becomes more entrenched, more pervasive, and increasingly part of what occurs and what is expected on a daily basis in all areas.

THE LETTER OF ENGAGEMENT

When a health service organization uses an outside consultant, it's good practice to have a letter of engagement between the parties that outlines and summarizes the roles and responsibilities of the parties, the objectives to be achieved, and scope of work to be performed, along with other key terms, like compensation and payment terms, timeframe with milestones, and final deliverables. The process of discussing and agreeing to a letter of engagement helps both parties work towards a clearer and more complete understanding of the engagement and associated expectations of the parties. Moreover, it also allows/provides an important reference in the future regarding the engagement, expectations and obligations that, many times, prove helpful for the working relationship and business terms as changes evolve. It is customary for the letter of engagement to be prepared and proposed by the consultant, but it can be drafted by either party.

UNWRITTEN COURTESIES

An external consultant is an invited guest; however, sometimes not many people in the organization are aware the consultant has been engaged by the organization or that the consultant is coming into the organization for an on-site visit or extended fieldwork. In certain situations, only the CEO or other senior leader who has contracted the consultant is aware. Ideally, it is good for all those leaders and staffs who will be working and interacting with the consultant to know about the engagement and when the consultant is planning to be on site; however, sometimes situations occur that are less than ideal. The point is, sometimes people in the organization don't know the consultant is coming or has been engaged; what his or her role or scope of work may be; or what to expect. Quite simply, the consultant may not be welcomed by everyone; some people may feel anxious or threatened, for whatever reason. Nevertheless, the consultant should always be mindful that he is a guest and extend common courtesies to others. This means, of course, being polite and courteous, even if the same has not been extended to the consultant by all. It also means providing clear, open, ongoing communication to one or more people in the health service organization who the consultant is working with and that needs to be kept informed and up to date. This communication includes providing advance notice if a milestone, deadline, or other component of the project or schedule is not going to be achieved on time or as previously contemplate—and why. How can the health service organization's process or project owner help the consultant in this regard? What other support, resources, data, or availability of personnel are needed? Is there a logical work-around to maneuver around an unanticipated roadblock or barrier? How critical will a delay be overall, and what other steps can be taken to get back on track? The consultant should always keep the primary contact or process owner informed and not make that person have to seek out the consultant.

CLARITY OF EXPECTATIONS

In every leadership or consulting engagement, it is important to clearly define, discuss, and understand expectations—for all parties involved and concerned. One of the biggest mistakes made in the beginning of a project, engagement, or even a committee meeting for that matter, is to not discuss, outline, and clearly understand expectations. What are the expectations for how the consultant and the organization will collaborate, interact, and work together on the engagement? What does the organization expect with regard to the final deliverables—for example, the final presentation and/or report to leadership? How much detail is desired and expected with the final deliverables? What are the consultant's expectations regarding the submission of requested data he or she may need and the format it is desired to be submitted in? Has this been discussed? What about the consultant's expectations towards key background information provided, input received, insight shared, feedback given, and support and assistance the process owner or others in the organization may provide during the engagement? However, clarity of expectations goes far beyond the identified roles and responsibilities of the parties and helps those involved visualize how they will work together; what they are truly trying to achieve; what's important in the process, and what success looks like; and what the work and work product should look like along the way. Moreover, maybe above all, clarity of expectations builds trust.

Maybe above all, clarity of expectations builds trust.

THE UNDERLYING PROBLEM

Many times, the consultant is brought in to help address or solve a problem that may lie on the surface of an underlying problem. The problem may be symptomatic of a deeper-rooted issue or one that may be unrelated. When this occurs, communication with the process owner is paramount. What is the process owner's knowledge, understanding, and perspective on the underlying problem or issue? Has there been any previous attempt to acknowledge, discuss, or address it? If so, what were the results? What insight can this provide to the consultant regarding the engagement at hand? What change in objective or scope, if any, does this create with the existing engagement? Here again, open communication and clarity of expectations is critical. As Peter Block states, ***"Every problem has layers, like an onion. The deeper you go, the closer you get to causes and actionable items"*** (*Flawless Consulting*, by Peter Block).

Many times, the problem and associated solutions are clear and obvious to an outside consultant—even in the very initial stages of the engagement. Regardless, it is neither the consultant's role nor professional prerogative to start casting blame or criticism regarding the problem. It isn't a good practice nor acceptable client relations or business practice to blame or criticize. Blaming and complaining is also counterproductive to fostering a positive, healthy working relationship based upon trust. However, it is good practice for the consultant to be intellectually curious and inquisitive while asking insightful questions to reveal the current state and foster clear understanding about it. Gaining different insights and perspectives about an issue, problem, or objective during an engagement is important in order for the consultant to truly grasp the reality of the situation, its impact, contributing factors, areas of resistance, and obstacles or even "hot spots" or "land minds" to avoid. In addition, many times, strong conceptual skills are needed to clearly see how different departments, functions, services, or processes are affected, contribute to the situation, or are dependent on an improved process or outcome.

EMOTIONAL INTELLIGENCE (EQ)

How does the client feel about the project or engagement? How visible, contentious, or political is the problem, issue, or challenge at hand? Is there history with this that has created anger, animosity, apathy, or other strong feelings or emotions? What are the different views, opinions, and perspectives that exist, and are there sides that have been taken? What might be politically incorrect to say or ask? These and many other questions and matters will need to be assessed—through observation, interviews, conversations, and written documents—in order to gain a good perspective on the current psychological and emotional state of the organization and its key people. This type of qualitative assessment—discovered through good listening, observation, and emotional intelligence—is critical in order to have a good feeling and sense about how to maneuver throughout the engagement. Emotional intelligence is the ability to recognize one's own strengths and weaknesses, see the linkage between feelings and behaviors, manage impulsive feelings and distressing emotions, be attentive to emotional cues, show sensitivity and respect for others, be an open communicator, and be able to handle conflict, difficult people, and tense situations effectively.

An example of this is the client's unspoken desire to control all aspects of the engagement, including the final deliverables. If there is both a presentation and written report made as the final deliverables of the engagement, how much input and control does the client want over these? In most cases, participatory management and close collaboration is the right style to practice; however, this can vary by client or engagement. How is the client reacting to this approach and the consultant's style and process? What's not being said by the client verbally that is telling about how they perceive the consultant's approach? What can be observed by the consultant? What is the question behind the question being asked, or the real point behind what the client is saying? What are the messages and vibes being sent? How is the client reacting and responding emotionally to what is being said or discussed? These all provide clues as to how the consultant should maneuver, interact, create the most positive working relationship, and best meet the needs and expectations of the client. This is about emotional intelligence and the consultant's skill and effectiveness in this leadership competency.

> **What is the question behind the question being asked, or the real point behind what the client is saying?**

Emotional intelligence is also about being aware of and controlling your own emotions. Mr. Ed Abel talks about ***"Trying to stay balanced and not letting your own emotions dictate the issue can sometimes be pretty difficult. You can get excited about things, and sometime you can get so excited you can say something pretty stupid. The number one thing that is important if you are trying to have a pretty candid discussion is to understand what—if they are available—the facts are. Because if you don't understand and you are trying to consult or move to a position in some area, and you say something that isn't***

accurate, it is going to throw a monkey wrench into things. I've seen instances where somebody says something that is stupid and it immediately raises the temperature in the room pretty quickly and all of a sudden there is no collaboration; its finger-pointing, we—they, and it escalates pretty quickly if people don't know what they are talking about. Having said that, I am not afraid to say something to get people to talk about a topic and draw them out of their comfort level to talk about it and get the real issues on the table. Too often people don't always want to give you what their real position [on an issue] is, so they will talk around the edges. The quicker you get to the heart of issue the more likely you're going to be able to come to some resolution."

Another important aspect regarding expectations is for the consultant to seek feedback periodically throughout the engagement. Asking for feedback is a matter of good timing. A consultant must realize when the appropriate time and place is to ask for feedback and know what, exactly, he or she is asking for feedback on. Clarity and specificity are important here. Use of EQ is important here also. As a consultant, it is imperative to know how you are performing in the eyes of the client and whether expectations are being met. In addition, at the risk of using a couple of somewhat worn out phrases, what can the consultant do to "exceed expectations" and "add more value"? Is there anything else that the consultant can do to be of greater service?

A PRODUCTIVE WORK ENVIRONMENT

Just like in hospitals or health service organizations, fostering a productive work environment in a health-care consulting organization is important. Mr. Abel states, "***To be able to attract some of the talent we have attracted is a tough thing to do. I've seen in so many other organizations, including some we consult for as well as some we compete with, as well as others you read about in books: they have this organizational hierarchy that promotes things being done that are anti-productive. Our approach is simply 'What can I do to make it easier for you to do your job?' Organizations can build a hierarchy and an infrastructure that is ridiculous. What I want people to do is to spend their time on potential clients, existing clients, and the people we have working here: that's it. If people can stay focused on that, we can do some awfully good things.***"

ADVISING AND COACHING

Many times, a consulting engagement includes coaching and advising the client. Sometimes the coaching and advising may be part and parcel with the engagement or solicited from the client. However, sometimes the consultant identifies opportunities for improvement outside the scope of the engagement and is faced with a decision about whether to provide unsolicited suggestions and advice or not. This can be tricky. Most consultants want to help and assist their client in any way they can; however, overstepping the boundaries of what is expected or even sought by the client should be done only if it is felt the client would

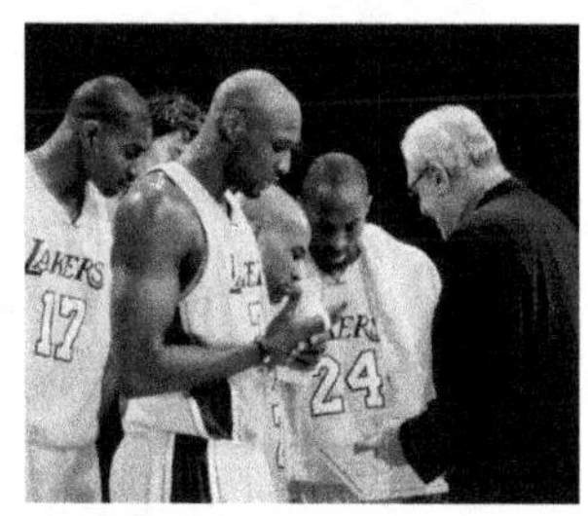

FIGURE 23.1 Basketball Team with Coach
Copyright © Bridget Samuels (CC BY-SA 2.0) at http://commons.wikimedia.org/wiki/File:Phil_Jackson_coaching_LAL.jpg.

be open, interested, and amenable to the suggestions or advice the consultant has to offer. Again, this determination should be made principally using the consultant's EQ. How will the client react? Will the client welcome the suggestions or advice or be turned-off? How will the suggestions or advice impact the client relationship if offered? What are the downsides of offering the suggestions or advice, as well as the possible upside? Clearly the decision on this must be made thoughtfully and carefully, as a mistake in judgment in this area could prove very deleterious.

Mr. Ed Able is Director of the healthcare consulting practice of Blue and Co., LLC, a medium size accounting and consulting firm with headquarters in Indianapolis, Indiana, and whose primary clients are hospitals and health service organizations. Ed Able describes how to go about advising and helping clients achieve their goals and objectives: ***"I think it's important to have regular dialogue (with clients) and ask them 'What are you doing during your normal work hours? Who are you touching? How are you improving what other people are doing? It forces clients to think about what I am helping or suggesting them to do; are they doing it with their folks? A lot of it is having basic interaction, and being blunt and appropriately honest with folks about what they can do differently to improve. Everybody wants to hear about the good stuff, but not the bad stuff. I don't think it's fair to not tell a client something you, as a consultant, see and feel strongly about. Being appropriately honest with clients, whether it's about them doing the right thing or something they can do better, goes a long way towards getting them to move to a behavior that everybody has agreed on the front end it is the appropriate thing to do. We always agree it's important to develop people in back of you. We agree it's important to go try and establish new relationships so you can do new business with folks, or just to have referral sources. These are all things we have agreed to. When people aren't doing these things and you start to have dialogue about it, I think it's a healthy thing."***

One piece of advice that Mr. Abel shares with healthcare leaders is to work to help advance the performance and careers of those around them. Mr. Abel says, ***"People's leadership styles—to the extent they are advancing the people around them—increases the likelihood their success is going to be far greater."***

DISCUSSION QUESTIONS

1. Describe the difference between an internal versus external consultant.
2. Explain what is meant by Peter Block's quote "Every problem has layers, like an onion."
3. Explain what is meant by "The question behind the question".
4. What are some of the general functions or services a consultant might-provide to a health service organization?
5. Describe two or three of the reasons why a health service organization-might hire a consultant.
6. Describe one or two advantages that an external consultant might offer over using an existing staff person for the given project or engagement.
7. What type of dialogue does Mr. Ed Able say can help an external consultant direct clients towards doing the right thing or something they can do better?
8. Describe two or three common courtesies a consultant should extend to clients.
9. How can clarity of expectations help the consultant–client relationship go beyond just creating a clear understanding of the roles and responsibilities?
10. Describe the role that emotional intelligence plays in developing a positive working relationship between a consultant and client.

FIGURE CREDIT

24

Leading Healthcare Operations

More than ever, hospitals and other health service organizations are being forced to operate in a more business-like manner, making strategic and judicious use of resources in order to perform well financially. Regardless of their tax-paying status, health service organizations must generate a positive net income consistently over time to be financially self-sustaining. Some experts, such as Uwe Reinhardt or Ed Abel, suggest a hospital or health service organization must generate an operating margin of 3% to 5% at a minimum over time to remain financially viable and sustainable. As healthcare third party reimbursement shrinks on a per-unit basis, financial performance is becoming increasingly challenging to obtain on a consistent, ongoing basis. Healthcare leaders must have basic knowledge and skills in operations and financial management, including budgeting and managing resources, to be effective and succeed. Prudent fiscal management includes the fundamentals of staffing, productivity, and full-time equivalent (FTE) management; effective supply chain management; judicious allocation of resources; revenue cycle management; budgeting, monitoring, managing, and reporting regarding actual operating performance versus budget and identifying budget variances; spotting undesirable trends and managing proactively to minimize or eliminate negative variances to budget; and all the while, creating a culture that fosters employee engagement, commitment, and satisfaction.

OBJECTIVES

1. Understand and appreciate the important role of leading operations in a hospital or health service organization.
2. Learn and apply some basics of managing budgets, productivity, and other resources.
3. Appreciate the leadership skill of assessing potential in others.

MANAGING THE OPERATING BUDGET

A budget is a financial plan. There are two basic types of budgets used by hospitals and health service organizations: an operating budget and a capital budget. An operating budget is a financial plan of revenue as well as expenses incurred in the daily operations of the business for a set period of time. A capital budget is a financial plan that outlines a company's future expected expenditures on new assets, such as land, physical plant and facilities, and equipment. Operating budgets are typically developed and managed at the department and cost-center level. For example, the diagnostic imaging departments in most hospitals today offer a variety of different modalities, such as general radiology and fluoroscopy, mammography, ultrasound, computerized axial tomography (CT) scanning, magnetic resonance imaging (MRI), nuclear medicine, positron emission tomography (PET) scanning, or invasive diagnostic imaging procedures. Each modality will typically be designated in the budget as a separate cost center and have its own operating budget with actual ongoing financial results reported. This financial detail of revenue and expenses at the cost-center level provides leaders the ability to see how each modality or service is performing and spot variances or emerging trends, allowing for the insight and understanding necessary to manage effectively. For example, if CT isn't tracked and reported as a separate cost center from other modalities, and its staffing, volume, and other costs are lumped in with those from the other diagnostic imaging service modalities, a department manager or senior vice president wouldn't know how that modality or service is performing financially and if any changes are warranted. Budgeting at the cost center level provides the data leaders need to effectively manage the allocation of resources and other related factors involved with managing budgets and performing fiscally.

For the Director of Diagnostic Imaging and other senior leaders to see how the department of diagnostic imaging is performing overall, all the cost centers for the department will be "rolled-up" into a consolidated financial statement for the department that shows volume, staffing, gross revenue generated, and operating expenses incurred for the entire department for the reporting time period—typically on a month and fiscal-year basis. Most financial reports include a column that computes the variance for each line item on an actual-to-budget basis. In addition, most financial reports include a comparison of results from the same time period compared to the prior year.

Revenue is money generated by the hospital or health service organization's reimbursable activities. Gross revenue is full charge or 100% of charge. Net revenue is the money the organization projects it will receive after accounting for discounts off charges and contractual allowance. Discounts off charges are pre-negotiated discounts contractually given to a third-party payer or preferred provider organization by the hospital or health service organization in exchange for being a network provider. Contractual allowance is the difference between full charges and what Medicare or Medicaid reimburses a hospital or physician. Direct costs are expenses associated with a specific activity provided by a department or cost center. Indirect costs are expenses that are not directly associated with a specific activity provided by a department or cost center, such as the salaries, wages, and benefits of top management or general liability insurance for the organization such as utilities. Fixed costs are expenses that will be incurred regardless of volume. Variable costs are expenses that will change as the associated volume changes, such as supplies.

PRODUCTIVITY, STAFFING, AND FTE MANAGEMENT

Healthcare is considered, by many, to be the ultimate people business; it is people taking care of people in their time of need. The biggest expense in any hospital, and in most other health service organizations, is the cost of people in the form of salaries, wages and benefits. Therefore, productivity, staffing and FTE management is crucial. Productivity is the amount of input needed to produce a desired outcome. In regards to staffing, productivity is the number of full time equivalent (FTE) staff or man hours needed to generate the respective units of service produced in the given department or service. For example, productivity in the CT scanning cost center would be measured by the number of FTEs required to generate the number of CT scans being produced for the time period being measured. For example, if the CT scanning cost center takes 3.50 FTEs to generate 240 CT scans for a given month, the productivity factor would be represented by either FTEs/CT scan or 68.57 or manhours/CT scan or 0.394. There are approximately 2,080 manhours in an FTE in a year. In an average month, 1.0 FTE = 174 manhours. Converting between FTEs and manhours is a fairly simple process and one frequently done in healthcare.

Manpower expenses—salaries, wages, and benefits—are the single largest expense in a hospital or other health services organization delivering patient care. As such, the efficient and effective management of staffing is critical for two primary reasons: 1) meeting the ongoing, ever-changing needs of patients in the delivery of care, many times with highly specialized services requiring highly trained, licensed specialists; and 2) expense control and subsequent financial performance of the organization. Not surprisingly, these two goals are frequently at odds: opposing forces that must be thoughtfully and expertly negotiated and balanced—at any given moment and consistently, on an ongoing basis.

AREAS IMPACTING STAFFING AND LABOR COSTS

Overtime policy and practice—Overtime is expensive. Overtime is calculated at 1.5 times the employee's base hourly rate of pay. Therefore, a hospital or health service organization should monitor and manage the use of overtime. While overtime can't be completely eliminated, an organization's policy toward the use of overtime and its practice regarding eliminating "incidental" overtime (overtime worked in small quantities that could be avoided without any negative consequences for patient care or operations) greatly impact the overtime it incurs.

Skill mix—Skill mix refers to the number and percentage of registered nurses (RNs) who work in a given unit or department versus the number of non-RNs, such as licensed practical nurses, certified nurse assistants (CNAs), and nurses' aides. In general, the greater mix or percentage of RNs compared to non-RNs, the higher the salary and wage expenses will be.

PRN pool and policies—PRN stands for the Latin phrase *pro re nata*, which means "as needed." PRN is a category of employee who basically works as needed. PRN employees can provide an organization with greater staffing flexibility, particularly when acuity or volume increases and additional staffing is needed on a short-term, temporary basis. In general, the larger the organization's PRN pool, the more PRN employees it has access to for temporary staffing needs. In addition, policies that impact PRN compensation and the amount of usage of PRN employees also impact the size of the pool and PRN employee availability.

Discharge policy—Many hospitals don't have an actual policy and procedure as it relates to patient discharges. While a discharge can't occur without a physician or midlevel provider's order, patient discharges are somewhat time intensive; therefore, the timing of discharges can impact staffing. For example, without a target time for patient discharges during the day or evening, discharges can and do occur at any time; therefore, this unpredictability negatively impacts the ability to plan for discharges, thereby potentially impacting staffing.

"Working manager" model—This refers to department managers or supervisors who routinely work some hours as hourly, rank-and-file employees in the department. For example, if the director of environmental services in a small hospital works the equivalent of one eight-hour shift per week in the department (where the job being done would otherwise be done by another employee paid an hourly rate of $15.00/hour), the annual savings to the department would be $6,240 (8 hours × $15.00/hour × 52 weeks/year = $6,240).

Surgery department policies and practices—Surgery is a department where both the patient and the surgeons are the hospital's customers, and many policies exist to better serve each customer type; however, these same policies and practices can have a significant impact on staffing and productivity. The scheduling of cases impacts both patients and surgeons alike. When a surgery department experiences large gaps/blocks of open time between cases during a typical day, it creates a tremendous challenge for efficiently scheduling staff. As a general rule, the majority of patients as well as surgeons prefer scheduling cases in the morning. In addition, both patients and surgeons are interested in cases starting on or around their scheduled times. While it is unavoidable for some cases to run longer than scheduled, assessing the percentage of time that cases start on time and making any reasonable changes accordingly can help create greater efficiencies in staffing. Also, evaluating the utilization of block time—reoccurring times reserved for selected surgeons based on their typical case volume (for example, Wednesdays from 7:30 a.m. to 11:30 a.m. weekly for a given surgeon)—can identify whether block time is being used as intended and its resulting impact on staffing. Turnover time of the operating rooms is another process that impacts staffing and involves the length of time it takes to get a given operating room cleaned and ready to accept the next case.

Process for review and approval of open positions—Any time a position becomes vacant, there is a possible opportunity to reduce staffing in some way, including by not refilling the position. The process used for reviewing, evaluating, and approving open positions is very important. Although not easy to do and many times not appropriate to do, improving productivity by not replacing part of a position—or an entire position—when it becomes vacant should be thoughtfully and carefully evaluated when turnover occurs.

Ongoing monitoring of staffing and FTEs—The ongoing monitoring of staffing and FTEs is vital to operating at an appropriate staffing level—in all areas. Without this constant, ongoing monitoring of staffing and FTEs, "FTE creep" will most likely occur. FTE creep is simply a gradual increase in staffing and overtime over time: a common occurrence when the necessary monitoring is not happening with any real rigor or vigilance. This monitoring is simply exercising the basic management function of control.

Setting FTE/productivity goals and budget—Goal-setting theory supports the fact that setting goals for FTEs and productivity, along with an operating budget that targets these same goals by department or cost center, is critical for achieving a staffing level in an efficient manner. Like the saying "A goal without a plan is simply a wish," without goals for FTEs, there are no targets to strive to attain. The absence of FTE and productivity goals creates a situation echoed by another old saying: "If you don't know where you're going, any path will get you there."

Ongoing training of department managers—Ongoing training of department managers regarding staffing, productivity, and FTE management is important to be sure the entire management team is working in concert, collaboratively, and in the same direction to attain the staffing, productivity, and FTE goals desired throughout the entire organization.

Use of contract labor—Should the organization use contract labor for positions that could otherwise be filled by employees, the worked hours of contract labor positions should be included in any staffing or productivity analysis; otherwise, the analysis will be skewed and not entirely accurate.

Working relationship between nursing and environmental services—This working relationship is important, as it relates to the proper, efficient, and timely cleaning of clinical areas, especially patient beds and inpatient rooms, so these areas and services can be used for new patients coming into the service or organization in a timely manner and without unnecessary delay. A lack of collaboration between nursing and environmental services can create inefficiencies and negatively impact staffing in both areas.

DETERMINING AN APPROPRIATE FTE LEVEL

So how does a hospital executive or other healthcare leader determine how many FTEs the organization should consistently operate with? While a multitude of variables and factors impact this, two that will be explored here are trending the organization against itself and using that trending analysis to benchmark against other similar hospitals or health services organizations of similar size, with similar service offerings, and with similar patient volumes. However, while a comparison of a hospital's total FTEs and trending analysis to another similar hospital or group of similar hospitals in a combined database is beneficial, there are shortcomings as well. A main shortcoming is that even if the hospital or hospitals in the database are similar to the hospital being compared, there will be some differences in important factors within given service lines, with the type or level of acuity of patients seen, or even volume. Differences in physical space and technology can play a role in any comparison as well.

One total hospital FTE measurement commonly used is hospital net revenue per FTE, where the annual net revenue of the organization is divided by total FTEs. While this analysis helps to compare the actual money being generated by the organization (in the form of net revenue) to a function of its payroll (total FTEs), it too has shortcomings. One variable that can significantly impact this analysis—particularly when it comes to comparisons with other similar hospitals—is payer mix. If the hospital has a lower mix of commercial patients as compared to other similar hospitals, it will skew this comparison toward a lower figure of net revenue per FTE. Conversely, a hospital with a high percentage of commercial patients will typically skew this analysis toward a higher figure of net revenue per FTE.

Another total hospital FTE measurement commonly used is hospital salary and wage expense as a percentage of total operating expenses. This percentage can range anywhere from 45 percent in highly productive hospitals to 65 percent in hospitals that aren't nearly as productive. Again, limitations in this analysis exist. For example, this analysis is impacted by expense control overall (total operating expenses) as well as salary and wage rates. A rural hospital located in close proximity to a large urban area may have higher salaries and wages when compared to most other rural hospitals due to the fact it has to compete for highly skilled manpower against the adjacent urban area and its corresponding wage rates.

With these limitations, is there value in completing a total hospital analysis of FTEs? The short answer: "Yes." However, the shortcomings just need to be considered so the analysis has greater meaning and value. Moreover, it is recommended that multiple approaches be used and different "slices" of the overall spectrum of staffing and FTE management be analyzed from multiple approaches or perspectives to provide the most comprehensive and insightful analysis possible. This includes analyzing a hospital or other health services delivery organization by department, service, or cost center.

So how does a hospital or healthcare manager know how many FTEs should be used to staff a given department, service, or cost center? Using several approaches, analysis of staffing and FTEs in a given area should include trending against historical staffing (by total FTEs and productivity) as well as comparison against hospitals with similar areas. Productivity is the effectiveness of productive effort as measured in terms of the rate of output per unit of input. In hospitals, productivity is measured by man-hours per relevant statistic.

Productivity is the effectiveness of productive effort as measured in terms of the rate of output per unit of input.

Sometimes referred to as "efficiency," "output," "work rate," or "yield," productivity in hospitals or other health services delivery organizations is a function of man-hours per the volume or statistics that represents work rate/yield/output. For example, how many nursing man-hours or FTEs does it require to provide care to a twenty-four-bed hospital medical/surgical unit with an average daily census (ADC) of sixteen patients and total annual patient days of 5,840? What if observation patients are also treated on that same unit and are included in the ADC of sixteen patients?

Here is an example of productivity analysis for a hypothetical twenty-four-bed hospital medical/surgical nursing unit with the following statistics:

- Beds – twenty-four
- ADC – sixteen patients (includes observation patients)
- Occupancy rate – 66.67 percent
- Patient days – 5,840 (includes observation patients)
- FTEs – 32.23
- Man-hours – 67,043

Productivity calculation $\frac{67{,}043}{5{,}840} = 11.48$

Keep in mind: a lower productivity factor (represented in the productivity calculation above as 11.48) represents greater productivity, which correlates to fewer man-hours per unit of output—in this case, patient days.

Below is a table representing an example of a trending analysis for productivity for this same hypothetical nursing unit over a three-year period.

STATISTIC	YEAR 1	YEAR 2	YEAR 3
ADC	16.5	16.0	15.5
Patient days	6,032	5,840	5,658
FTEs	32.78	32.23	31.47
Man-hours	68,180	67,043	65,463
Productivity	11.32	11.48	11.57

At first glance, man-hours and FTEs are going down over the three-year period, which appears to indicate a good job by nursing management of managing staffing for the unit over this three-year time period. While this may be true, analysis of productivity—which accounts for the volume being experienced during this three-year period in the form of patient days—shows a different observation: productivity has gotten slightly worse over this three-year term. While there may be—and usually are—many factors at play impacting the staffing, patient care, and volume on the unit over any three-year period, one quantitative fact exists: productivity has gotten worse during this same time period. It stands to reason that a nursing unit will need less staffing if it experiences fewer patients on average than during a previous time period; however, how many fewer man-hours is the question. Productivity analysis can help answer this question.

Therefore, a productivity analysis at the department, service, or cost center level is the most effective way to analyze staffing, productivity, and FTE management performance. While there are probably a multitude of qualitative factors that must be accounted for in any analysis (many of which are addressed previously in this chapter), a quantitative analysis of productivity by cost center promises to be the most effective, meaningful, insightful, and appropriate way to analyze an organization's efficiency in staffing and FTE management.

Below is a table offering a framework for productivity analysis and trending by cost center.

COST CENTER	VOLUME/ STATISTIC	PROD. YEAR 1	PROD. YEAR 2	PROD. YEAR 3	DELTA
Accounting/Finance	Adj. Disch.				
Administration	Adj. Disch.				
Business Office	Registrations				
Cardiac Rehabilitation	Visits				
Education	Adj. Disch.				
Environmental Services	Square Feet				
Food Service/Dietary	Meals				
Foundation	Adj. Disch.				
Human Resources	Adj. Disch.				
Imaging/Radiology (consolidated)	Procedures				
Infection Control	Adj. Disch.				
Information Technology (IT)	Adj. Disch.				
Intensive Care Unit (ICU)	Patient Days				
Labor/Delivery/Recovery	Patient Days				
Laboratory	Tests				
Maintenance/Plant Operations	Square Feet				
Materials Management	Adj. Disch.				
Marketing & Public Relations (PR)	Adj. Disch.				
Occupational Health	Visits				
Oncology/Infusion Center	Visits				
Patient Access/Registration	Registrations				
Pharmacy	Prescriptions				
Physical Therapy	Visits				
Quality Assurance/Improvement	Adj. Disch.				
Respiratory Therapy	Procedures				
Sleep Lab/EEG	Procedures				
Social Services	Adj. Disch.				
Speech Therapy	Visits				
Surgery/Recovery/Anesthesia/Sterile	Cases				
Total Opportunity in FTEs					

Using this framework, an administrator can complete an analysis of productivity by cost center by year and then analyze for trends and corresponding opportunities for improvement going forward. Moreover, this framework can be used to compare or benchmark against similar-sized hospitals as well, looking for opportunities where improvements in productivity can be made. This type of analysis, featuring benchmarking against a best-practice hospital for productivity, can be enlightening.

Benchmarking productivity is used to compare the organization's productivity with other organizations that are similar in size and scope of services. Benchmarking can also be used to compare the organization's staffing and productivity to best practices, helping to identify areas of opportunity for improvement.

MONTHLY REVIEW OF OPERATIONS

Consistent monitoring and review of actual-to-budget performance at the cost center level is central to the management function of controlling—monitoring progress towards goal achievement and taking corrective action, when needed, to get back on track towards goal attainment. It is highly recommended that every hospital and health service organization create an organized process for this type of monitoring and review to occur. Moreover, in order to foster a culture of accountability, this process should include department managers and senior leaders meeting monthly or, at a minimum, quarterly to review and discuss operations, financial performance, and action plans and steps being taken to meet the budget/financial plan.

MANAGING THE CAPITAL BUDGET

A capital budget is a financial plan that outline's a company's expected expenditures on new assets, such as land, physical plant and facilities, and equipment. Each organization can tailor its capital budget policy according to generally accepted accounting principles; however, a general guideline for defining a capital item is typically a tangible item or asset with a useful life greater than one year and a purchase cost of $1,500.00 or more. Capital budgets are typically prepared on an annual basis; however, some organizations may prepare capital budgets over three years or longer when major capital improvements to the facility are involved. A key to managing the capital budget is planning for the required capital needed to make the proposed capital purchases at the point in time the items are needed.

SUPPLY CHAIN AND MATERIALS MANAGEMENT

The function of purchasing, receiving, storing, inventorying, and distributing supplies and minor equipment is typically performed through the central department of materials management. In most cases, routine supplies are purchased through a contract that stipulates all the terms, conditions, and pricing for those purchases. Most healthcare organizations are part of a group purchasing organization (GPO) in order to pool their purchases of routine, ongoing supplies, such as syringes, gauze, pharmaceuticals, IV solutions, implants, office supplies, food, etc. Group purchasing power can help a hospital or other health service organization save significant money on its supply costs. Many GPOs also can save organizations on the cost of capital items, in addition to providing other value-added services.

All supplies cost money—whether used for clinical or non-clinical purposes—and in most cases, significant money. The cost of supplies that are sitting in unused inventory can be viewed as idle capital that is not generating revenue, not being used for support services or administration, and therefore, working capital that is providing no benefit to patients or staff and yet can't be used for anything else. The goal here is to have all the necessary supplies needed and available when and where needed at the point of service, but no more than is needed. "Just-in-time inventory" is the phrase used for a system or process that provides for necessary and needed supplies to be available when needed at the point of service but with minimal shelf time in the organization. Systems or processes that include computerized inventory, par levels, and ordering; contracting and vendor relationships that promote regular, consistent, and timely deliveries; capturing of supply charges; and the efficient and effective management of supplies throughout the entire process is called supply chain management.

REVENUE CYCLE

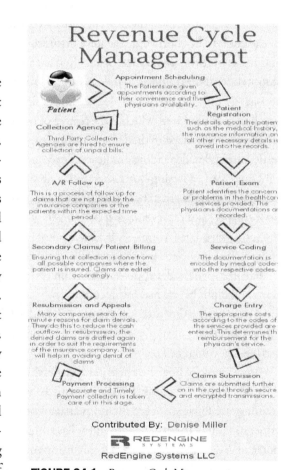

FIGURE 24.1 Revenue Cycle Management

Copyright © DeniseMiller (CC BY-SA 3.0) at http://commons.wikimedia.org/wiki/File:Revenue_Cycle_Management(3).jpg.

The revenue cycle begins with the scheduling of the patient. Next, the patient is registered as a patient when he or she checks in to the health service organization and respective department or service. When clinical services are rendered, documentation is recorded by the clinical staff in the patient's medical record regarding his or her diagnosis, tests and results, care and treatment rendered, and related supplies used. These services are then translated in various codes that are applied to the respective bill, either a UB-04 bill for institutional or facility charges or a CMS-1500 for professional charges. The bill(s) are then presented/billed to the patient or to the respective third-party payer for payment. The bill is reviewed and processed by the third party payer and either paid or rejected. If rejected, the provider is typically required to clarify or correct an error identified in billing. The tracking of patient and third-party payments and their accuracy is an important provider function to verify payments are being made accurately. Finally, follow-up and recovery of payments that are not made occurs, sometimes with the assistance of outside collection agencies. Managed care contracting is also a key component in the revenue cycle and includes provider contracting with different insurance carriers, health plans, preferred provider organizations, or even directly with employers. Managed care contracting also includes the periodic auditing of payments received for accuracy and compliance with pre-negotiated contract terms. All this patient account and payment information connects into the health system's financial system so that accurate and timely financial statements can be produced and relied upon by management and others.

SITUATIONAL LEADERSHIP AND PATH–GOAL LEADERSHIP THEORY

Leading healthcare operations means working with a diverse workforce in a multitude of different situations and environments. A healthcare leader must be skilled and adept at maximizing productivity and efficiency in the quest to be effective and achieve organizational goals given this diversity and variations of situations and environments. Situational leadership is a leadership model where the leader matches his or her leadership style with the readiness of followers. Follower readiness involves two components: job readiness, which consists of the amount of knowledge, skill, ability, and experience people have to perform their jobs, and psychological readiness, which is the feeling of self-confidence or willingness to perform their jobs.

Path–goal leadership theory is a contingency theory of leadership based on using one of four different leadership styles, depending on the employee and situational contingencies.

Directive Leadership—A leadership style in which the leader lets employees know precisely what is expected of them, gives them specific guidelines for performing tasks, schedules work, sets standards of performance, and makes sure that people follow standard rules and regulations.

Supportive Leadership—A leadership style in which the leader is friendly and approachable, shows concern for employees and their welfare, treats them as equals, and creates a friendly climate.

Participative Leadership—A leadership style in which the leader consults employees for their suggestions and input before making decisions.

Achievement-Oriented Leadership—A leadership style in which the leader sets challenging goals, has high expectations of employees, and displays confidence that employees will assume responsibility and put forth extraordinary effort.

An example of how this theory and leadership model might be applied is with the management of two different registered nurses (RNs): one with 10 years of patient care experience and one just out of nurse's training. A nurse manager should manage both employees fairly and consistently, but not exactly the same. Assuming the experienced nurse has a high degree of psychological readiness and job readiness, the nurse manager might use an achievement-oriented leadership style with her. Assuming the nurse just out of training has a high degree of psychological readiness, but low degree of job readiness, the nurse manager might use a combination of a directive leadership and a supportive leadership style.

ASSESSING POTENTIAL

Putting the right people in the right place is a leadership skill that requires leaders to know the skill, talent, ability, and potential of employees. In order to effectively lead operations, a healthcare leader must become adept at assessing potential and putting the right people in the right place. The first step, and maybe the most critical element to assessing leadership potential, is being aware of and cognizant of an employee or other leader's skill, talent, ability, and potential. Being aware of and paying attention to the potential in others is critical in order to be able to assess and evaluate those who might be able to accept more responsibility or even be promoted. So, how does a healthcare leader go about assessing the potential of an employee or the leadership potential in another leader? Clearly, one important aspect is to be able to accurately evaluate and assess a leader's current set of skills, talents, and abilities. Then make an assessment for what his or her potential is to achieve a higher level—above his or her current level of skills, talents, abilities, and performance. This type of assessment is mostly qualitative and intuitive; however, assessing the current level of skills, talents, abilities, and performance can include some quantitative factors and criteria, as well.

For a senior healthcare leader, assessing the potential of another leader might include asking others: is he or she doing a good job, what is he or she doing effectively, and what potential exists in this person to take on more responsibility? Getting the input and perspective of others is important in knowing how another leader or employee is seen through the eyes of others. Knowing who has the potential to take on additional responsibilities also begs the question: how can the organization assist him in learning, growing, and developing into his potential? Two topics that are part and parcel with this are mentoring and performance evaluation/appraisal.

One area that has received much attention lately is succession planning. Succession planning requires leadership's ability to accurately assess for potential. A lot has been written recently on succession planning, which typically refers to the planning for top leadership positions; however, succession planning can relate to just about any type of position in any level of a hospital or health service organization.

RISK MANAGEMENT

Risk management is an organized effort to identify, assess, and reduce, where appropriate, risks to patients, visitors, staff, and organizational assets. In a hospital, risk management is typically a program designed to reduce the incidence of preventable accidents and injuries in order to promote safety and minimize the financial loss to the institution, should an injury or accident occur. General areas of potential risk in a hospital include medical malpractice, general liability, automobile or vehicle operations, mechanical equipment failure, clinical equipment malfunction, drugs, emergency preparedness, employment, directors and officers, and public relations. More specific areas of risk in a hospital includes the dispensing of drugs; clinical variability stemming from unstandardized clinical practices; use of agency or contract clinical personnel; high turnover or low employee satisfaction; credentialing and privileging of physicians;

patient falls; hospital-acquired infections; equipment or drug recalls; drug shortages; employment policies and procedures; back injuries; needle sticks; and emergency or disaster preparedness, including dealing with the media.

A typical approach to managing risk in a hospital is the use of a five-step process: 1) risk identification, 2) risk analysis, 3) risk treatment and control, 4) risk transfer, and 5) risk financing. Anticipating what can go wrong and working to prevent it, minimize it, control it, or manage it is a fundamental strategy to risk management. Identifying risk on an ongoing basis is typically done through a combination of qualitative and quantitative methods. Evaluating and analyzing past experiences and current or future exposures is required so that action steps can be developed and implemented to reduce or eliminate risk and its potential effects. Therefore, a structured and organized risk management program is necessary in order to systematically identify, assess, and reduce risk to patients and employees through daily operations.

DISCUSSION QUESTIONS

1. What is meant by the phrase "Operations management"?
2. How does reporting revenue and expenses at a cost-center level aid leaders as an important management tool?
3. Describe the difference between gross revenue and net revenue?
4. What is a budget, and how is it used in healthcare leadership?
5. Define productivity and why it is important in healthcare.
6. Describe two or three key components of the supply chain.
7. Describe two or three key components of the revenue cycle.
8. What are situational leadership and the path–goal leadership theory, and how do they connect or relate to one another?
9. Why is it important that healthcare leaders accurately assess the potential of others?
10. What is risk management, and what are a few of the components typically involved with the risk management process in a hospital?

FIGURE CREDIT

Figure 24.1: Copyright © DeniseMiller (CC BY-SA 3.0) at http://commons.wikimedia.org/wiki/File:Revenue_Cycle_Management(3).jpg.

25

Enterprise Risk Management

The delivery of patient care and the operation of a hospital or health service organization is not devoid of risk. The typical community hospital offers a multitude of specialty services using a myriad of different sophisticated medical technologies, drugs, supplies, and surgical equipment that are delivered by highly trained and skilled physicians and other healthcare personnel. At a macro level, there are hundreds—if not thousands—of systems, processes, procedures, and clinical protocols that go into the delivery of patient care. Simply put, there is virtually an unlimited number of ways in which a system or process can break down, thereby creating risk. Add in the element of human error, and it's not difficult to see how a comprehensive, well-planned and coordinated Enterprise Risk Management (ERM) program is essential in today's modern hospital. Clinical risk can manifest as a clinical mistake or mishap that may or may not affect the quality of care being provided or clinical outcomes. A significant clinical mishap could result in a significant untoward event, also called a sentinel event or "never" event—something that should never happen.

OBJECTIVES

1. Learn about the various areas and types of risk exposure in a hospital or health service organization.
2. Learn several approaches to identifying risk exposure.
3. Understand how to apply cost-benefit analysis in analyzing risk exposure.

Administrative or business risk can manifest as an event or situation in which the organization is out of compliance with a law, regulation, or standard; a loss in an area referred to as general liability, such as an accident with a hospital-owned vehicle; a natural disaster that interrupts the business and its ability to generate revenue; or even a financial or strategic risk to the organization.

Stepping back and taking a panoramic view of the organization can reveal risks at all levels and areas across the entire enterprise, therefore calling for an enterprise-wide approach to risk management, or ERM. This is particularly true with hospital and health systems in which multiple hospitals and other health service business lines operate under one corporate umbrella, suggesting an even greater need for coordination or risk management processes across a larger, diverse, multifaceted organization.

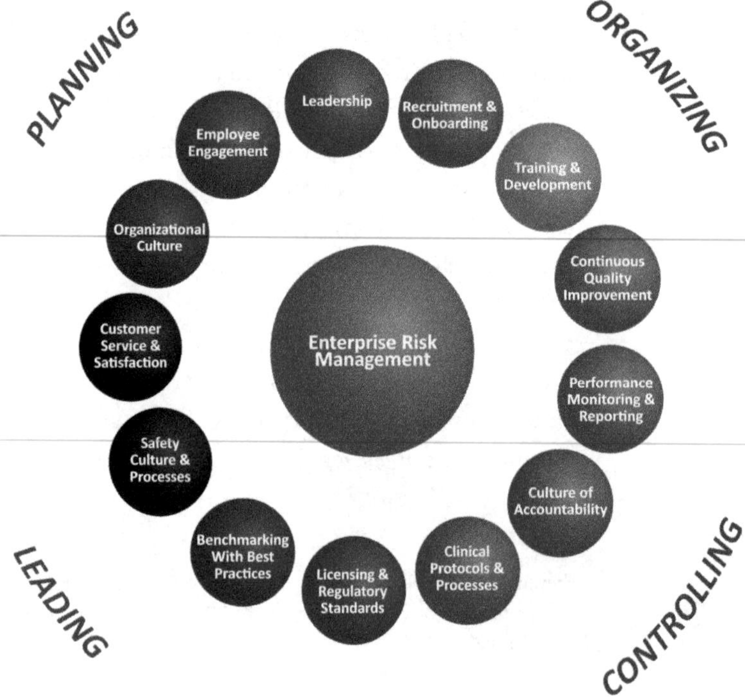

FIGURE 25.1 Enterprise Risk Managment

SCOPE

The scope of ERM should include all departments, functions, services, facilities, and communication provided to clients and families designed to diagnose, evaluate, assess, stabilize, and improve the care, treatment, service, safety, and medical care rendered to clients and families. Moreover, the scope of ERM also includes communication and service rendered to customers and referral sources. Components of ERM include leadership; management and staff accountability and evaluation; physical facilities and the environment of care and treatment, including areas of daily living and recreation; the delivery and documentation of care, clinical treatment and medical care provided in a safe and efficacious manner; and the monitoring, review, assessment, evaluation, improvement, and documentation of the inputs and outcome measures that provide for a quantified method of performance measurement for continuous improvement and problem-solving through corrective action as needed.

KEY FUNCTIONS & TASKS OF ERM

Assess the efficiency, effectiveness, and/or performance of systems, processes, policies, procedures, practices, risk management strategies, quality improvement interventions, and action steps that have been implemented, along with the severity of risk and opportunities for improvement.
Anticipate possible mishaps, events, possibilities, emergencies, situations, outcomes, and risks that may be mitigated, avoided, or managed.
Avoid mishaps, mistakes, sentinel events, never events, lawsuits, negative public relations, unwanted outcomes, and repeated failures in systems or processes.
Control the level of quality, safety, and security provided by **measuring** and **monitoring** actual results compared to established standards and goals and take corrective action as necessary for goal achievement.
Investigate and **verify** the proper functioning of systems, processes, policies, procedures, and practices; **validate** the implementation of previous actions taken and causes and effects.
Identify areas of risk, possible alternative solutions, and other opportunities for improvement.
Rounding throughout the organization and its facilities to conduct visual inspections and complete assessments regarding the environment of care and the effectiveness of safety and security measures.
Evaluate data, outcomes, and results and compare to preestablished standards, benchmarks, and goals while **analyzing** for patterns and trends.
Integrate the quality improvement, client safety and security, and risk management functions through organized and coordinated processes and reporting.
Coordinate tasks, functions, reporting, and communication to provide a seamless, gap-free approach that promotes efficiency and effectiveness.
Document a plan and program along with outcomes, results, goals, measures, processes, standards, benchmarks, risks, concerns, patterns, trends, opportunities, and achievements.

Report findings and results through a structured, organized reporting process that highlights problems and accomplishments and fosters **communication** and ongoing engagement of management and staff for action that results in continuous quality improvement.

ENTERPRISE RISK MANAGEMENT PLAN DOCUMENT

A fundamental component of an ERM program is a written enterprise risk management plan. The goal of a written ERM plan is to identify the key elements and processes for the program, including such things as its organization and structure; personnel; how it fits into the organization chart as a whole; key functions and tasks and various processes utilized; definitions; evaluation criteria and metrics, objectives, and target outcomes; reporting; scope and key interconnections within the organization; and overall philosophy and approach and alignment with the organization's mission. A written ERM plan can help provide clarity around the purpose, goals, and objectives; foster greater understanding about risk management and its implementation enterprise-wide; and promote goal identification and evaluation, allowing a performance-improvement approach to be taken for enterprise risk management.

The overarching goals and objectives for the ERM plan and program are to promote and foster:

1. The greatest possible care experience for patients and working environment for employees.
2. The highest quality of care and treatment in an environment of care that is safe and secure for patients, families, and employees.
3. Minimizing and preventing accidents, incidents, injuries, occurrences, and financial outlays of the health services organization.
4. The efficiency of operations and the effectiveness of care, service, and treatment overall.
5. Ongoing, continuous improvement in quality outcomes, care and treatment, service, operations, and financial performance of the health services organization.

RISK MANAGEMENT COMMITTEE

The Risk Management Committee (RMC) should consist of a number of designated management and staff and should be led by the facility risk manager or other administrator as committee chairperson. Committee members shall be appointed by administration in collaboration with the facility risk manager. Members can be appointed for a specified or unspecified length of time. The RMC should meet monthly. The charter of the RMC shall be to assist and support the organization and its ERM initiative with overall guidance and direction; engagement and analysis; advice and support; education and communication; planning, assessment, and evaluation; and input and feedback. The facility risk manager should compile, distribute, and review the monthly Risk Management Report (RMR) at committee meetings for discussion, analysis, input, and overall review and acceptance. Moreover, through this process, the RMC should provide input and feedback as to ERM issues, trends, challenges, problems, initiatives, strategies, goals, objectives, activities, opportunities, and accomplishments that can help to structure and organize the most effective ERM plan and program possible in a culture supportive of CQI.

QUALITY IMPROVEMENT & PATIENT SAFETY CULTURE

An emerging philosophy is to incorporate the patient safety and quality improvement functions and initiatives into a comprehensive ERM plan and program. This is logical and makes good sense, given the significant overlap and required integration of risk management, quality, and safety. A coordinated initiative and program that includes ERM, quality improvement, and patient safety offers a more efficient, comprehensive approach versus one that is more fragmented and disparate. Here is an example of an organizational structure with the various ERM functions, depicting a comprehensive organizational structure and approach.

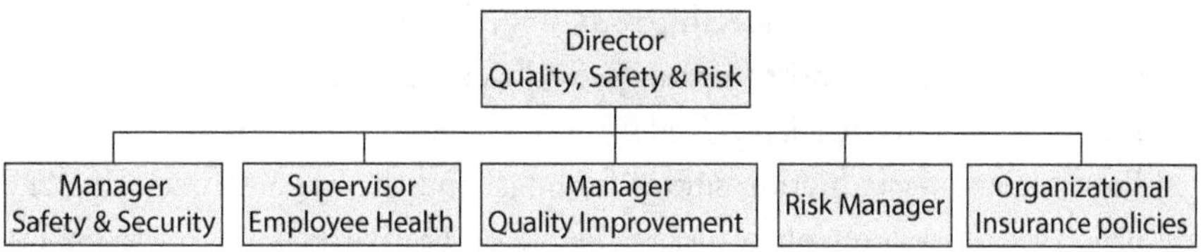

FIGURE 25.2 Hierarchy

The organizational structure will vary depending on the size, scope, and resources of the organization. However, the concept has merit: consolidate these key functions under one leader to promote coordination, efficiency, communication, reporting, and overall effectiveness.

In a multi-hospital system, enterprise risk management may be organized corporately, with leadership of the enterprise risk management function centralized. Alternatively, the enterprise risk management function can remain decentralized, with some level of coordination at the central corporate office level. The third alternative is for enterprise risk management to be totally decentralized and therefore fragmented. This latter option is not recommended, as it fails to take advantage of possible economies of scale, the transfer of knowledge and best practices, and benchmarking.

PATIENT SAFETY ROUNDS

The environment of care refers to the physical plant/facility and surroundings in which the delivery of patient care occurs. Elements of the environment of care include: proper heating, ventilation, and air conditioning (HVAC) systems; quality control procedures to continually monitor the HVAC systems to validate the quality of their outputs and proper operating controls; preventive maintenance and repair; proper conditions of the interior finishes, including the floors, walls, and other surfaces; proper cleaning of the facility, equipment, and reusable medical and surgical supplies to prevent infection; and related aspects. Administration and risk managers routinely make rounds to observe, assess, and inspect the environment of care, documenting the results of these rounds; taking proactive steps to improve or correct deficiencies observed or noted is important and a powerful tool and approach to risk management. In addition, interaction with staff and physicians during patient safety rounds is an effective way to gather input from those on the front line—where the work occurs and care is being provided—and to see and hear firsthand how things are really going.

DATA & INFORMATION GATHERING FOR ERM

Methods for data and information gathering for ERM shall include, but not be limited to: incident reports; medical record and treatment reviews; personnel file reviews; patient and family surveys; customer surveys; staff surveys; observations from leadership rounding; documentation made from routine management and staff committees, teams, and other meetings; feedback received from managers, staff, and clients; feedback received from families; feedback received from customers and referral sources; formal grievances and complaints; licensing and accreditation survey findings; and the ongoing gathering and analysis of data that reflects processes, procedures, outcomes, incidents, and activities pertinent to quality, safety, and risk management.

On the surface, developing a patient safety culture in a hospital or other health service organization delivering patient care seems logical and straightforward; however, to do so is anything but simple. Why? Because developing a patient safety culture takes a comprehensive, multifaceted approach that encompasses all aspects of the operation, from consistent adherence to checklists and important policies and procedures to hiring, training, engaging, and retaining the right people. At the heart of a patient safety culture is the culture itself, which is represented by the values, beliefs, and attitudes of leadership and employees—everyone. The organizational culture is how things are done and is manifested as what actually gets valued, appreciated, rewarded, measured, monitored, reported, tolerated, permitted, encouraged, and reinforced. The organizational culture is not what we say we believe or do; it is represented by what we actually do and how we do it.

Organizations change and evolve, and so does the external environment in which hospitals and other health service organizations operate. Therefore, it is good practice to complete a comprehensive review and assessment of the ERM plan and program annually. An evaluation should include assessment of the strengths, weaknesses, opportunities for improvements, and other issues that should be addressed.

- What have been the major accomplishments of the risk management program the past year?
- What level of goal achievement was attained?
- What evaluation metrics were met, and which ones weren't?
- What evaluation metrics should be continued, modified, or eliminated?
- Are there new service or business lines that have recently been implemented or that are being planned, and should they be part of the ERM plan and program?
- How will these new service offerings be included in the risk management plan?

An annual evaluation and assessment of the ERM plan and program should include documentation of the findings of the evaluation and assessment, along with modifications to the risk management plan document as appropriate.

A good place to start in developing a patient safety culture is with the administration of a patient safety culture survey throughout the organization. A patient safety culture survey can help identify the perceptions that the board of directors, leadership team, medical staff, and employees have regarding the organization's existing patient safety culture. It is not uncommon for such a survey to show a difference of opinion and perception between leadership and the board, medical staff, and employees. The survey can help leaders better understand the current state of the patient safety culture and gain insight into strengths, weaknesses, opportunities, and issues for action planning to strengthen the patient safety culture.

Developing a stronger patient safety culture can be part of an overall ERM that is effective in anticipating risk, identifying risk, assessing risk, avoiding risk, and mitigating risk as appropriate. A strong patient safety culture translates into an environment of care that is patient centered, with a greater emphasis and focus on patient safety in all areas and levels of patient care delivery and support.

QUALITY IMPROVEMENT

Quality improvement is a formal approach to the analysis of performance and systematic efforts to improve it. Quality improvement is a philosophy and process aimed at improving the performance, efficiency, effectiveness, or outcome of a clinical intervention or process. Quality improvement can also incorporate other administrative, support, and nonclinical processes as well. These nonclinical functions and processes are typically referred to as areas for performance improvement, while quality improvement refers more specifically to clinical areas.

Total Quality Management (TQM) is a management philosophy that integrates all aspects of operations toward the goal of long-term organizational success through the strengthening of a culture that continuously improves quality and performance; meets or exceeds customer expectations and promotes their satisfaction; and engages management and employees in the continuous process of improvement. Foundational elements of TQM include:

- Commitment by senior leadership and all employees
- Meeting customer requirements, expectations, and needs
- Reducing improvement cycle times
- Use of improvement processes, including lean improvement teams and benchmarking
- Improving efficiencies and reducing service delivery costs
- Systems and processes to facilitate improvement
- Line management ownership, engagement, and accountability
- Employee involvement and empowerment
- Recognition and celebration
- Challenging quantified goals and benchmarking against best practices
- Focus on processes/improvement plans using measurable inputs and outcomes
- Incorporation into strategic initiatives and operational performance dashboards

Quality control, quality assurance, and quality assessment have been concepts/functions to control and improve quality throughout history by identifying, assessing, evaluating, and validating the inputs and outcomes around processes that generate efficiency, effectiveness, and performance for improved results. These concepts/functions have their own unique strengths, weaknesses, and limitations. Various aspects of these functions still have application today in healthcare. However, conventional thinking and practice revolve around performance improvement/quality improvement.

DETERMINING APPROPRIATE RISK EXPOSURE

Rendering or receiving healthcare service—like life in general—is not risk free. Operating a hospital or health service organization is replete with different types and levels of risk exposure. Various types of risk involved with the delivery of healthcare services include such areas as malpractice and omissions or commissions involved in patient care; general liability such as a visitor falling down a flight of stairs; medication errors or failure of medical technology or clinical equipment; wrong-site surgery or other surgical mishaps; employment of staff, including wrongful discharge and on-the-job injuries; the operation of boilers, chillers, or other equipment, including motor vehicles; management of legal documents, including contracts; and regulatory compliance. Identifying and understanding these risks is the first step in determining appropriate risk exposure and developing a plan and process to better identify and understand, as well as minimize and manage, risk exposure.

GENERAL RISK AREA CATEGORIES

Areas of risk in a hospital or health service organization can be categorized into three general categories: 1) business or general risk, 2) clinical risk, and 3) corporate risk. Examples of business or general risk are support service areas such as plant operations, mechanical, maintenance, and environmental; operation of company vehicles; and administrative services such as contract management. Examples of clinical risk are clinical and ancillary service areas such as surgical procedures in surgery, deliveries, invasive diagnostic procedures, inpatient care delivered on units, and emergency services. Examples of corporate risk are governance and management areas at the board, senior management, middle management, and front-line management levels involving the application of policy, procedures, and rules, along with compliance with various pertinent standards, laws, and regulations.

IDENTIFYING RISK

Identifying risk exposure in a hospital or health service organization is the first step, and can be done by a manager internal to the organization or by contracting with an outside consultant. Commonly referred to as a "Risk Management Audit," this process involves identifying risk exposure throughout the various departments, functions, and operations of the organization, and making a determination as to the significance of risk exposure in identified areas. The determination of risk exposure along with an evaluation of whether the risk is preventable or can be appropriately minimized is a judgment call based upon both qualitative and quantitative data.

The table below provides an outline/overview that can be followed to identify risk exposure. This table is intended to be an example or illustration and by no means should be considered comprehensive or complete. These areas and others can be assessed and analyzed for key findings, patterns, and trends relating to deviations from desired procedures, practices, outcomes, and risk exposures. When analyzing risk exposures in various areas, are there common threads between any findings or trends in these areas? What clinical functions, services, or activities have the greatest variability in practice and outcomes indicating a need for greater use of evidenced-based, standardized processes and protocol? What areas appear to pose the greatest current overall risk to the organization?

AREA/DEPARTMENT	PRACTICES/DOCUMENTS	KEY AREAS OF ASSESSMENT
Nursing & patient care	Trends in patient incidents/occurrences by department, service, and shift; malpractice claims by service, shift, and physician; key clinical outcomes by department, service, and shift; clinical variability in practice, protocols, and outcomes; complaints and satisfaction scores by department or service.	Focus on high-risk, high-volume patient care functions and activities. Policies, procedures, processes, practices, and standardization of clinical protocols. Training, communication, and reinforcement of standard clinical policies and protocols. Use of checklists.
Medical records & documentation	Problems of non-compliance and variability from policy and procedure. Inadequate or incomplete documentation.	Adequate documentation for accurate and timely coding. Malpractice issues with documentation variability. Documentation policy and procedures. Training with policy and procedures, and compliance with same.
General liability	Housekeeping policies, procedures, and practices. Patient, visitor, and employee incidents/occurrences by department, service, and shift.	Patterns and trends of problems or incidents. Visual inspection of public entrances and other general/visitor areas.
Mechanical & clinical equipment	Preventive maintenance policies, procedures, and practices. Policy and procedure when equipment failure or device recall occurs.	Age, identification, performance, and tracking of mechanical and clinical equipment. Utility consumption tracking and benchmarking.
Infection control	Policies, procedures, and practices.	Training and enforcement of proper hand washing. Management of contagious or high-risk patients. Emergency preparedness.
Employee health	Policies, procedures, and practices. Tracking, assessing, and reporting of employee health incidents and problems. Workers' compensation plan, policies, procedures, and practices.	Patterns and trends of problems or incidents in employee health or on-the-job injuries or exposures. Training for injury prevention such as low back injuries or needle sticks; wellness programs based upon health claims or health appraisals.
Vehicles	Policies, procedures, and practices regarding employee use of organization-owned vehicles.	Vehicle preventive maintenance and service records.
Directors & Officers (D&O)	D&O insurance policy coverage; board orientation, education, and training practices; conflict-of-interest policies.	Ongoing board development practices.
Disaster preparedness & media relations plan	Disaster preparedness planning and training; crisis media plan and policy.	Training and assessment of internal drills and role-playing; policies and procedures.
Insurance coverages	Boiler, professional liability, general liability, automobile, D&O, business interruption, workers' compensation, employee health, property and casualty, or equipment.	Outlays vs. potential losses and premiums.

Credentialing	Policies, procedures, and practices; malpractice claims, patient complaints, and variability by physician.	Physician quality, cost and variability trending, and benchmarking.
Business practices	Contract accountability, policies, practices, and management; joint-venture practices; debt-covenant compliance; regulatory reporting; formal succession planning.	Key business policies, procedures, and practices.
Corporate ethics & compliance	Ethics and compliance policies, procedures, and practices.	Identified and/or reported violations or issues.

COST-BENEFIT ANALYSIS

In general, the concept of evaluating costs versus benefits can be applied to help determine the significance of a given risk exposure, actions that can be taken to mitigate risk, and associated costs (time, money, effort, or negative impact on efficiency or effectiveness). By weighing the costs associated with actions, changes, or interventions, and comparing that to the possible reduction or mitigation of the risk exposure—along with considering all of the other pertinent factors and variables—a determination can be made as to the appropriate steps to take. Organizational priorities, culture, and experience should also be considered when making such a determination. Again, the determination of risk exposure along with an evaluation of whether the risk is preventable or can be appropriately minimized is a judgment call based upon both qualitative and quantitative data.

FUNCTIONAL COLLABORATION AND INTEGRATION

There are a number of clinical and administrative functions that overlap or connect with the function of risk management, as previously highlighted, and include, but are not limited to, quality improvement and patient safety; medical staff credentialing; hiring and employment; safety and security management; infection control; employee health and workers' compensation; regulatory reporting; corporate ethics and compliance; business practices; disaster preparedness; and media relations. It is important for the designated Risk Manager to have timely access to the flow of data and information from these areas that have implications for risk exposure identification, trending, and pattern discovery. Moreover, these are functions where collaboration should occur on perceptions, understandings, ideas, strategies, and plans to address issues and opportunities for prevention, improvement, and problem resolution of risk. It is important that risk management not be allowed to function in a silo, as collaboration and integration of risk management with these other important functions is critical to foster and promote improved efficiency and effectiveness overall for the success of the risk management initiative and the organization as a whole.

In small hospitals or health service organizations, the designated Risk Manager may wear multiple other hats, having responsibility for one or more other functions that overlap or connect with risk management. This is entirely appropriate and can facilitate a cost-effective approach. In larger organizations, there may be several employees working together in a risk management department with responsibilities that extend on an enterprise-wide basis. Regardless, a collaborative and coordinated approach includes risk management's participation on key standing committees with ongoing access to the flow and reporting of important data and information impacting risk exposure, identification, mitigation, and management.

SUMMARY

Risk exposures continue to increase as various environmental forces are exerted on hospitals. Identifying risk exposures in a hospital is the first step toward creating a risk management plan, program, and structured process to effectively identify, mitigate, and manage risk. Determining the extent and significance of various risk exposures and what actions might be the most appropriate for the organization to take includes the prudent judgment of management and the ability to weigh costs vs. benefits.. Clearly that judgment includes overall administrative acumen, conceptual skills, participatory leadership, and decision making.

DISCUSSION QUESTIONS

1. Define the term "Enterprise risk management"?
2. What does the term "Root cause analysis" mean? Explain.
3. Describe the rationale behind integrating quality, safety, and risk into one department.
4. Describe several areas in a hospital where there is risk exposure.
5. Once identified, should risk exposure be eliminated at whatever cost is required? Why/why not?
6. What is corporate compliance and what does it involve or encompass?
7. Describe, in general, several risks associated with corporate ethics and compliance.
8. How might one determine if insurance coverage is appropriate to purchase in a given area of operation?
9. Identify the three general categories of risk in a hospital or health service organization.
10. The management of various contracts is considered an example of risk in what general risk category?

26

Mentoring

A central theme emphasized in this book is that becoming a healthcare leader is a journey of learning, growth, and development. One of the most effective ways to learn about healthcare leadership is from a mentor. A mentor can help you access wisdom, lessons learned, and insight from someone who has progressed along the journey of becoming a healthcare leader before them. A mentor can support the growth and development of a developing leader to reach more of his potential to become the most effective leader he can become. Mentoring is somewhat akin to apprenticeship, where a trainee—works under a skilled professional in order to learn an art, craft, or trade and become qualified in it (*Encarta World Dictionary*). However, in a mentorship, there is no supervisor–subordinate relationship: there is a mentor, a mentee, and the relationship they create together. A mentor is somebody, usually older and more experienced, who provides advice and support to and watches over and fosters the progress of a younger, less experienced person (*Encarta World Dictionary*). In healthcare, this is typically when a more experienced healthcare leader becomes a mentor to a less experienced healthcare leader, maybe even to an aspiring healthcare leader, such as a health administrative student who does not yet have any healthcare leadership experience.

OBJECTIVES

1. Appreciate the role mentorship can play in helping a healthcare leader learn, grow, develop, and advance in his career.
2. Compare and contrast the roles of mentor and mentee.
3. Learn about 10 key principles for an effective mentorship.

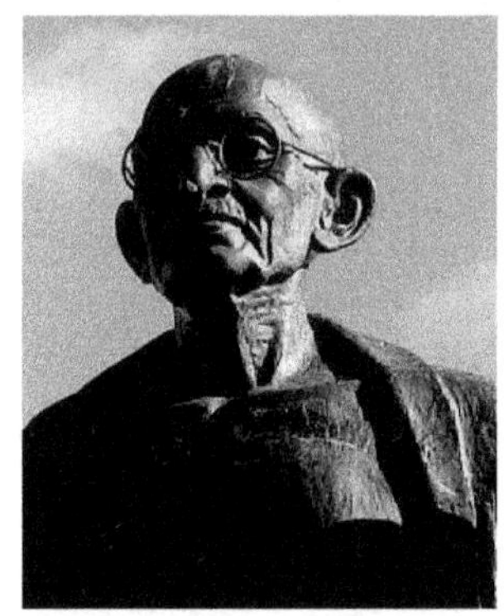

FIGURE 26.1 Ghandi Statue
Copyright © Vitor Oliveira (CC BY-SA 2.5) at http://commons.wikimedia.org/wiki/File:Monumento_ghandi_seccion.jpg.

Mentoring can be an effective method for learning, growing, developing, and advancing in a healthcare leadership career. Being a mentee can be an effective way to learn from a healthcare leader who has ***"Been there, done that."*** A survey whose results were published in a USA Today snapshots article several years ago, asked the question ***"How much of an impact does coaching and mentoring have on career success?"*** A total of 46 percent of the 4,561 respondents said it had a "Great" impact, while 45 percent said it had a "Moderate" deal of impact on career success. That is a total of 91 percent of survey respondents saying mentoring has a moderate to great impact on career success! The source sited was the Development Dimension International (DDI) Global Leadership Forecast from 42 different countries. (*USA Today*)

Leadership is a set of skills that can be learned, developed, and put into action. Having a mentor can assist the mentee in both learning and acquiring knowledge and insight and developing the skills needed to put the learning into action or practice. And, being a mentor is an important process, as well. Phil Jackson, the record-setting NBA coach and current general manager of the New York Nicks NBA basketball team, is quoted as saying "***The sign of a great player is not how much he scores but how much he lifted his teammates' performance.***" A mentor is someone who clearly has the opportunity to lift the performance—and even level of career success—of a mentee.

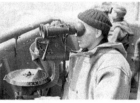

FIGURE 26.2 Man with Binoculars
R.G.G. Coote / Crown Copyright, "Man With Binoculars," http://commons.wikimedia.org/wiki/File:Bismarck-spotted.jpg. Copyright in the Public Domain.

LOOKING FOR A MENTOR

It is wise for healthcare leaders, no-matter how experienced in the field they may be, to have a mentor. It is also a good rule of thumb to be on the lookout for a good mentor. Who can you learn from? Who do you respect and trust? Who can teach, coach, and support you in areas that will aid in your growth and development? Who can provide you with solid career advice? Who can help you expand your professional network? Who will be willing to give you the honest, constructive feedback that you need to gain valuable outside insight? Is there someone in the organization you currently work in that could mentor you? Would any of your friends and colleagues have recommendations for a possible mentor? What healthcare leader have you met or seen in action that comes to mind?

WHY BECOME A MENTOR?

There are a myriad of reasons why a healthcare leader might consider becoming a mentor, but here are five important ones:

1. Teaching is a great way to learn. Being a mentor can help create greater understanding for the mentor about leadership, as the old saying ***"If you really want to learn something, teach it"*** comes alive.
2. Being a good mentor is certainly not required; however, it is somewhat increasingly expected in today's world of healthcare leadership.
3. Mentoring can help the mentor stay current with different generations of leaders and their thinking and perspectives, along with new changes and thoughts about healthcare leadership taking place in the field.
4. Mentoring is a great way of giving back to the healthcare profession.
5. Mentoring is a wonderful opportunity to make a positive impact on the life and career of someone, and subsequently, an organization. It is also a way to create an impactful, sustainable legacy as a healthcare leader.

For the mentor, a mentorship is about sharing yourself in a supportive, creative, loving way using the skills, knowledge, abilities and experience that you've gained in your career for the betterment of another. What qualities, attributes, skills, knowledge, abilities, and experiences could you offer to a prospective protégé or mentee? For many healthcare leaders, they feel more on purpose when they are giving away their time and attention in the service of others through activities, such as mentoring. And, being on purpose to help make life better for others is what many self-actualized healthcare leaders strive to accomplish in their leadership journey.

For many healthcare leaders, they feel more on purpose when they are giving away their time and attention in the service of others through activities, such as mentoring.

A mentor's overall purpose or goal for a mentorship is to help the mentee learn, grow, and develop as a professional healthcare leader. Typically, this includes seeking to help achieve the mentee's objectives in the mentorship, such as providing the mentee with needed emotional support and encouragement; providing perspective, advice, insight, and understanding about healthcare leadership and the profession; passing on lessons learned, including leadership methods and techniques acquired through experience; thoughts and ideas about effective leadership and a leadership style the mentor may have learned or observed through experience; career advice and support, including building a professional network; and other matters of professional development. In some cases, the objectives of the mentorship may be lofty, while in others, they are smaller and more incremental. But, don't forget about the concept of boiling water and steam.

At 211 degrees, water is very, very hot. However, water at 211 degrees is still—well—hot water. But, water at 212 degrees becomes something totally different: steam. Decades ago, locomotive engines that most trains used to operate were powered by steam. Think about it. Steam has the power to pull or push a train weighing hundreds of tons! The metaphor here is clear: sometimes, an incremental improvement in leadership effectiveness generates the type of force that can move careers and organizations forward. Sometimes a mentoring relationship is exactly what is needed to propel a healthcare leader/mentee forward to being much more of an effective leader (*212: The Extra Degree*, by Sam Parker).

MENTORING

A productive mentoring relationship can help leaders tap into what they don't know or haven't experienced through the outside insight provided by a trusted and respected mentor. Every healthcare leader should have at least one mentor at any given time. Mentoring is a philosophy that is based on a belief that one leader can learn from the knowledge and experience of another who's **"been there, done that"** and willing to share. The primary objective in a typical mentorship is to create a relationship based upon caring, sharing, listening, advising, and advocacy. Mentoring is about one leader helping another reach more of his or her leadership potential by providing learning, insight, professional development, career counseling, professional networking and professional coaching that can result in enrichment for both the mentor and the mentee.

Mentoring is one of the highest callings in leadership—to help develop others in the field—and it is an act of servant leadership. Moreover, helping others reach more of their leadership potential may be one of the greatest gifts that can be given from one leader to another, making a real and lasting impact on both careers and leadership legacies. A healthcare leader should be both a mentor and a mentee. Why? Being a mentor for another leader or aspiring leader can not only provide support, insight, and learning for the mentee, but for the mentor, as well. An old saying about that is apropos here: ***"If you really want to learn something then teach it to someone else."*** From the mentee's perspective, having a mentor is a great way to learn from someone who has already experienced some of healthcare leadership's lessons the mentee hasn't and gain valuable insight into the practice of effective healthcare leadership.

Having a mentor who can serve as a role model for leadership growth and development is both an asset and a blessing to the mentee. At the same time, there are many benefits to the mentor, including application and enhancement of coaching and counseling skills; satisfaction with enhancing the values and leadership style of a developing leader; gaining insight and perspective from a developing leader; exploring experiences and challenges that can lead to greater insight into alternative methods, techniques, and leadership strategies for the mentor's own work.

A FEW PRINCIPALS FOR AN EFFECTIVE MENTORSHIP

Here are 10 principals for creating a positive, healthy, vibrant mentorship.

- Acknowledge mutual interest for the mentorship. A mentoring relationship can be created in several ways; however, there should always be recognition and acknowledgement by both parties that mutual interest and intent to create a mentorship exists, and there is common interest shared by both the prospective mentor and mentee.
- Set the tone for trust. Like any good relationship, there must be honesty and trust at its center. It has been said that results in leadership are attained by fostering and maintaining relationships: the same can also be said of an effective mentorship. Set the tone for honesty and trust early in the mentorship.
- Clarify expectations. Ideally there should be some discussion regarding goals and objectives for the mentorship. What do the mentee and mentor want to get out of the experience? If the mentorship is successful, what will that look like? What is important for both parties to achieve? What are the expectations of both parties for the relationship?
- Validate understandings. There should be discussion and learning, as well as validation, about the strengths, weaknesses, interests, and passions of the mentee. It is important for the mentor to gain a good grasp of the mentee's self-confidence, self-esteem, and potential.
- Determine structure. There should be some discussion and agreement regarding communication frequency and methods, including some face-to-face time for the mentor and mentee to share and discuss things together. What is the optimum structure and process for the mentor and mentee to develop the relationship and work together moving forward?
- Create a safe learning environment. Discussions should feature open dialogue and not be about persuasion or influence, with an emphasis on the presentation and discussion of thoughts, ideas, suggestions, and stories. The mentee's role in discussions should center around posing questions on important topics for learning, growth, and development. The environment created should be cooperative, respectful, and nurturing for sharing experiences, opinions, perceptions, preferences, critical thinking, and related information. The environment can even be reflective. However, the idea for the mentor is to inform—not to sell or persuade.
- Mentee as process owner. The mentee should learn from the mentor's knowledge, experiences, judgment, and leadership style; however, the mentee must create his or her own learning path and leadership style that is ultimately his or her own.
- Provide outsight insight. Mentor's should look for opportunities to provide outside insight to the mentee and discuss important topics of leadership and leadership style the mentee may not know about himself—otherwise referred to as a "blind spot." This can include asking insightful questions or providing examples, illustrations, or stories about key points the mentor learned from someone else—maybe a hero, role model, or mentor—that can serve as an example of learning for

the mentee. Effective mentors look for valuable teaching moments. This can also help to increase the mentee's own self-awareness—an extremely important and necessary attribute to becoming as effective of a leader as possible.

- Create clear understanding. The "why" must be explored and discussed as much as the "what" regarding advice, suggestions, lessons learned, etc. It is critical for the mentee to understand the "why," as well as the "what," so he or she can develop the critical thinking skills and insight needed to put a strategy or method of leadership style into action. Mentees should be encouraged to ask questions, and mentors should ask insightful questions of mentees to reveal perspectives and understandings.
- Put learning into action. Ideally, the mentee may want to take notes of key points learned in discussions with the mentee and follow-up on key points, suggestions, and ideas that resonate with the mentee in order to put the good advice and perspective into action. Moreover, there should be some discussion about how the mentee might go about applying some of the things learned and putting them into action. Learning isn't complete until it is put into action.

DISCUSSION QUESTIONS

1. Describe how being a mentor can help a healthcare leader feel more on purpose.
2. Why do some consider mentoring one of the highest callings for a healthcare leader? Explain.
3. What is meant by the term "Outside insight", and how might it help a mentee identify a blind spot in his leadership?
4. Compare and contrast apprenticeship with mentorship.
5. Describe two or three reasons to consider becoming a mentee.
6. Describe two or three reasons to consider becoming a mentor.
7. What is the overall purpose for a healthcare leader and protégé entering into a mentoring relationship?
8. Describe the metaphor for the difference in water being at 211 degrees Fahrenheit versus 212 degrees Fahrenheit, and explain how it applies to mentoring.
9. Identify two or three principals for creating a positive, healthy, vibrant mentorship.
10. Describe how mentoring can positively impact a healthcare leader's effectiveness and his career, along with the organization's performance.

FIGURE CREDITS

27

Healthcare Leadership Distinctions

Distinctions are how we see the world around us, including the world inside us. Distinctions are formed based on experiences and events and what we've learned through those experiences and events; what we've been taught and what we've learned from family, friends, and others; and our attitudes, values, and beliefs. How we distinguish—or interpret and understand, what we see, feel, hear, and experience—create the distinctions that bring us meaning about our world.

This chapter discusses distinctions, their power to structure a healthcare leader's behavior, why it is important for healthcare leaders to be cognizant of their distinctions, and how they can change. This chapter also provides a few stories of how a hospital CEO Mr. Allen Hicks positively impacted the lives of countless other people given the resources available and his philosophy of servant leadership, the view that leaders serve followers, rather than vice versa. Servant leaders are always on the lookout for ways to help employees and others fulfill their needs and are coaches, stewards, and facilitators of employee performance.

OBJECTIVES

1. To understand the power of distinctions and how they impact a healthcare leader's philosophy, style, and actions.
2. To appreciate the power of walking in someone else's shoes.
3. To appreciate how healthcare leaders are in a position to help a lot of people, even those they aren't responsible for.

WALKING IN SOMEONE ELSE'S SHOES

The following illustrates the power of distinctions that leaders and nurses can make in healthcare. There could literally be thousands of other examples that could be used, but the following is one of a personal nature.

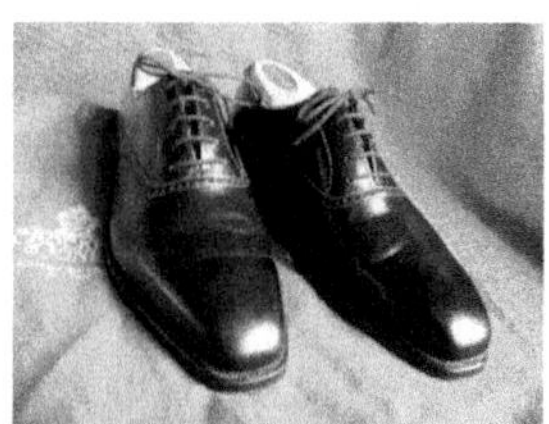

FIGURE 27.1 Dress Shoes
Copyright © OlafJanssen (CC BY-SA 3.0) at http://commons.wikimedia.org/wiki/File:Crockett_%26_Jones_men%27s_dress_shoes,_type_Dalton,_black_calf_leather_01.JPG.

It is 6:30 PM in the evening; I am in my office trying to get through the day's emails before heading home. As the COO of a 345-bed not-for-profit private community hospital, I get many, many emails every day—some of them important and time sensitive, but not all. On this particular evening I notice the next email is from a surgical intensive care unit (SICU) nurse who periodically sends me emails with suggestions. As a senior-level hospital administrator, I like receiving suggestions about ideas for making improvements. However, in the case of this particular nurse, by the name of Carla, most of her emails are complaints with accompanying unrealistic or impractical suggestions. As a rule, I always acknowledge and respond to her suggestions, providing rationale why her suggestion might not be practical, feasible, or possible. I do respect Carla—she's really a very good nurse. It seems she understands and, at least to a degree, accepts my explanations and rationale when I respond to her suggestions. Moreover, she is always approachable but, usually, very direct in face-to-face dialogue and likes to put me on the spot occasionally, as well. Overall though, I feel she means well.

Carla's email is there waiting in my inbox. It's late. I want to finish up responding to all emails before going home; otherwise, the emails just pile up, and it will become increasingly difficult to respond timely given my demanding schedule. Should I open the email and take the time to respond right now? Will it be a waste of time? Will it spoil my evening? These thoughts are distinctions I was making from my past experiences with Carla. I decide to go ahead and open the email.

As I begin reading the email, I quickly realize it's not the typical one that she sends: it's an invitation. Carla, on behalf of her SICU unit, is inviting me to spend the day with her on the SICU unit shadowing her, observing unit operations, and "working," doing whatever might be appropriate for me to do given my lack of clinical experience or training. The email says the SICU won the United Way contest in the hospital by having the highest level of pledge contributions made on average on a per-employee basis. The units reward? To invite one hospital administrator to work on their unit for a day and they were inviting me. My first thought was "Oh no! I'm so busy I don't have time to spend the day on SICU!" My second thought was "I might as well look at my calendar and send her a possible date to schedule for my day observing and working on the unit—I have to/need to do this." My third thought was "This will be real interesting—I hope it won't be a bad experience."

Well, the day finally arrives that I am to spend a shift with Carla and her colleagues on SICU. I spent most of the eight-hour shift on SICU with Carla, shadowing her; observing the nursing care and clinical operations occurring on the unit; watching Carla and other nurses and staff interact with patients, families, physicians, and one another; and pitching in just a little where I could to help out. What an incredible experience! I was able to see Carla in action, and she was amazing! She was on top of everything, providing great patient care; anticipating her patient's needs; handling dozens of interactions with a smile; teaching, coaching, and mentoring several of the younger nurses who clearly liked and respected her; and explaining what she was doing and thinking to me as she worked throughout the day. She answered every question that I asked. She even put me to work changing a patient bed—it was great! I was so impressed. I even got to see an open-heart surgery patient, who had recently undergone a Coronary Artery Bypass Graft (CABG) procedure, being admitted to SICU from the post anesthesia recovery room. This patient had more tubes hanging out than I could count. I witnessed the anesthesiologist who had accompanied the patient from the post anesthesia recovery room to the SICU ask JJ, the SICU nurse who was receiving the CABG patient as a new admission to the unit, if he needed any medications ordered for the patient. JJ responded with some jargon I didn't really understand. I was amazed; here was the physician asking the nurse what medications he needed for the patient! The collaboration and teamwork I observed was nothing less than fantastic.

What a great day of learning. I had witnessed the process of clinical care, collaboration, and quality patient care in a way I had never seen before, and it was truly impressive. I remember feeling this strong sense of pride to be part of a hospital organization where the staff was working together as a team and providing such great care for patients. They were truly making a profound difference for patients. My distinctions about Carla and her job and role had changed dramatically and forever. I would never see her in the same light again—ever. That experience changed me and compelled me to think for change (i.e., think about an idea to create a positive change). This next thought would have seemed crazy just the day before that SICU experience occurred, but now, it seemed like a great idea: invite Carla to shadow me for the day in my role as COO!

Walking in Carla's shoes was a powerful experience. My thought was to ask her to walk with me—in my shoes—and hope that it might somehow have an impact on her. I asked Carla if she would shadow me, and she agreed to spend a day with me. We scheduled it for a Wednesday, and not by accident. At that time, Wednesdays included weekly management meetings: a 7:30 A.M. Hospital Council meeting and the 10:00 a.m. managers meeting. The Hospital Council meeting was attended by the senior management team—about eight administrators. I typically organized the agenda and facilitated this meeting. The managers meeting consisted of approximately 75 managers from all levels throughout the organization. I also organized the agenda and facilitated this meeting (with the help of my wonderful administrative assistant Michelle, I might add). In addition, I asked my assistant, Michelle, to "load up my schedule" that day with meetings, so that my day would be jam packed with discussions that included physicians and physician issues; budgets and financial issues; and performance, policy and procedure development, and administration issues; and strategy-related matters. My goal was for Carla to hear about and observe a variety of the challenges, issues, goals, and strategies being discussed at the senior management level.

During her day shadowing me, Carla asked questions and seemed to take it all in just like I had done on the SICU unit a few weeks before. The day was a typical Wednesday—full of activity and important topics of discussion. Carla was able to hear and observe a lot. The day seemed to go well, but the next day things got even better.

The next day, I received a short but really wonderful email from Carla. She thanked me for allowing her shadow me for the day, then she stated "***I now realize that we can achieve anything we set our minds to when we work together as a team***!" That experience was so very powerful and made a lasting impression on me.

From that experience, I now distinguish a number of things, including Carla, much differently than I had in the past. It seemed as though the experience had a similar impact on Carla, as well. Distinctions are very powerful. They structure how we see our world. As healthcare leaders, we must be cognizant of our distinctions and how they are structuring our impressions, perceptions, attitudes, actions, and behaviors—and, sometimes, not really for the better.

THE BIRTH OF A NEW DISTINCTION

The birth of a new distinction—or how physicians and others viewed the viability of premature babies being delivered several months ahead of full term—occurred one day while I was a CEO of a 145-bed proprietary specialty women's hospital that was owned and operated by HCA—the largest hospital company in the world at that time. It was a typical day in the hospital delivery room in many ways, except for one; a pregnant mother was giving birth to a newborn that was more than two months premature because of medical complications. The attending obstetrician didn't even call to arrange for the Neonatal Intensive Care Unit (NICU) team to be present during the delivery because, well, it wouldn't be needed, as it was felt the baby would not be viable. But the doctor—who was an excellent obstetrician and well respected by her peers—was wrong. The newborn baby was delivered weighing 13 ounces at birth and was clearly viable. Immediately after delivery, the NICU team was contacted, and the baby was taken to the NICU. Four months later, a healthy newborn left the hospital NICU. Was it a miracle? Many of the clinicians said it was. And, if it was a miracle, then it was proof that miracles happen. Needless to say, it changed the minds and distinctions of most every physician on the hospital's medical staff towards the minimum number of week's gestation needed for a viable baby to be delivered. Moreover, it changed minds and distinctions about the minimum number of weeks gestation needed for a healthy baby to be born. I'll never forget the picture of the baby's left upper arm with her daddy's wedding ring on it, and loosely fitting at that. How incredibly tiny she was! One of the reasons I won't forget that picture is that I had it enlarged and framed and hanging in my office for several years as a reminder of the miracles that hospital and staff produced and the incredible opportunity we had every day to change lives for the better. Healthcare is a higher calling for most of the caregivers who join its ranks.

Distinctions in healthcare leadership impact how a leaders see what they believe is important, including perceptions of their roles and responsibilities, as well as the impact they are having and the difference they are making. In turn, these distinctions have a tremendous impact on healthcare leaders' sense of satisfaction and fulfillment with their work and their job. This sense of fulfillment and satisfaction helps healthcare leaders to: 1) stay focused on their own mission of servant leadership, 2) stay focused on the big picture of the impact they can and do make, and 3) stay focused on the "little things" they can do to positively impact others and make a difference for them, whatever that is.

As a healthcare leader, do you distinguish your primary role as a business manager/leader, a steward of resources, or a caregiver? There isn't necessarily a right or wrong answer to this question; however, how you see your role and the impact you can, and want to, have will strongly influence where you put your limited time and energies and how you distinguish the results or impact of your efforts.

Vince Caponi talks about modeling the way for what you want to see in the hospital. ***"We expect our employees to be efficient. We have all the cost pressures and other things that are driving that (expectation). What we can't allow is [our employees to ever forget] their reason for being—the patient. We can't take the patient out of the equation. We need that relationship piece. Quite frankly, we can be very efficient with some of our patients and a gentle hand, a kind word is all they need. If I am enthusiastic, I'm smiling, I'm concerned, I'm really focused on the patient, so when I talk to the patient—first and foremost—I look them in the eyes. I explain to the patient what I am going to do and why I am here. There are things that we can do to allay the fears of patients and their families that do not go against any efficiency. [Taking good care of patients] and being efficient are not mutually exclusive. We have to be about the business of allaying those fears."***

ALLEN HICKS: HEALTHCARE LEADER AND HUMANITARIAN

Allen Hicks was asked if he considered himself a caregiver as a hospital CEO, and he replied, "***I considered myself a humanitarian.***"

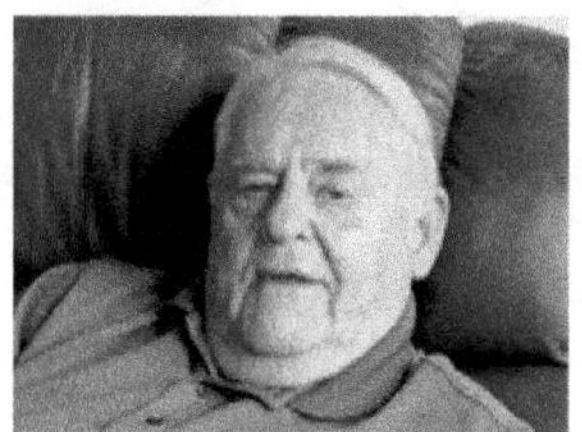

FIGURE 27.2 Allen Hicks

Allen was asked if he always considered himself as a humanitarian when working as a hospital CEO. Allen replied, ***"I think I really geared into that during my administrative residency in Davenport [Iowa]. That really was where I think it all started. Then in Beardstown [(his first CEO position)] there were only 5,000 people. The town ranked fourth in the State***

of Illinois for welfare per capita. I became a JC there, and I remember going out there with two trucks: we had turkeys, we had clothing [at Christmas time]. I remember one house with nine kids right before Christmas—they didn't have a stitch of clothes on! They didn't have a stitch! You see people so desperate: you'd like to do a lot more than you can do. I think that helped mold me, when I saw those people [in need] and what they had to go through."

Allen went on to say "***I had this great physician leader at my hospital in Pekin, Illinois, who dropped dead at age 41 in front of the refrigerator on Thanksgiving morning. He had delivered my baby—my youngest daughter. I used to think about this doctor and his wife, Tex, as having the perfect marriage; I would think, 'Man, his marriage is so wonderful.' However, after he had died suddenly that Thanksgiving morning, it was discovered that Tex's marriage had been a total disaster.***" Then later, after Allen took a hospital CEO job in Chicago, he heard from Tex out of the clear blue: this was after 10 years of no contact with her. ***"I had not heard from her in 10 years. I don't know how she knew I was in Chicago. Maybe she got my number from a mutual friend, I don't know. This lady [Tex,] called me around midnight one night. She said, 'Mr. Hicks, I have a lady standing at my door naked. She told me if I called you that you could help her. But I tell you, Mr. Hicks, she is really loaded. I think I could take her down and tuck her in, and if you come down tomorrow morning, you could come then."*** Allen said, ***"Well that would be wonderful."*** Unfortunately, the lady at Tex's door that night—who she had called Allen about coming to help her and said he could wait to come in the morning—committed suicide that night. ***"That one I always remember, because I didn't go. I don't give a damn what it was, I would always go. But that night I didn't go. When you are running a big place, you just always had access to help people. A lot of times it was little, and you really couldn't do much about their situation. But at least you tried. People know you tried."*** Allen went on to say, ***"I had a lot of these [different situations where I could help someone]."***

"***When I was at Community, one of the cardiologists came to my office one time and said, 'Allen, we've got a problem.'***" This was a case involving a hospital employee who needed hospital care beyond the scope of what Community Hospital could provide. The cardiologist said, ***"The only place I think that can help him is Stanford."*** Allen responded ***"'Well, Ok.'*** *And the doctor said,* ***'Yeh, but they won't take him unless we send $50,000 in advance.'"*** So Allen spoke with Rex Smith, his hospital CFO, about this case and the need to send $50,000 in advance to Stanford for the hospital employee, and Rex said, ***"Oh God, do we have the authority to do that?"*** To which Allen said, ***"Send it Rex."*** Allen went on to say ***"Two years later, the employee came back to Community Hospital with a little baby. The case was written-up in several medical journals, too. At Stanford, they had done a cardiac procedure on this employee involving some type of component from a pig heart.***"

"When I was in Chicago, an Auxiliary member called me at 4 p.m. on a Friday afternoon and said, 'I'm on the corner of Grand and Illinois. I've been evicted from my apartment. I am using my last dime to call you, because you can probably help me.' There were so many things over the years. People would come to you with all kinds of problems. You could always do something. Maybe you couldn't solve their problem, but you could always help in some way."

"I used to feel sorry for the employee that had cancer, yet had to come to work every day. They would just never feel good. One time, I had this little old lady—a volunteer—in Chicago. She was working in

the emergency room. She fell down. So she came in to see me and she said, 'Mr. Hicks, I just fell in the emergency room and I think that nurse there is going to fire me. You know, I get one free meal a day at the hospital for being a volunteer here and I really need that meal. I don't know what I am going to do if I lose that meal.'" Allen went on to say, "The nurse [Sue] happened to end up my wife later in life. So I called the emergency room and said, 'Sue, take care of that lady. Don't fire her. 'Sue said' I'm not going to fire her!' Allen said, "Well she thinks you're going to fire her, and she needs that free meal every day!"

Allen was asked how he compares helping someone at a time of desperate need versus being the visionary and creating the vision and plan for the development and construction of Community Hospital North—a brand new hospital that was built in 1983—that included the planning for a new hospital campus in a new location from the ground up, where only a field of grass stood before. How do you compare these two things? "***Well, those individual things are so personal. Some of these people are just desperate, some of them. I remember a guy sitting in my office at 7 a.m. in Chicago. They had brought his wife into the hospital at 2 a.m., and she died on the operating room table.***" He said, "'***You know I am a truck driver. I have nine kids at home. What am I going to do?' I used to get more than my fair share of these types of situations. Maybe I referred him to the minister, I don't know. I just tried to get them whatever help they needed.***"

When Mr. Hicks was asked which one of these types of situations is more important: being the visionary for Community Hospital North or helping someone during his or her time of need? For Mr. Allen Hicks, his career as a hospital administrator included many tremendous accomplishments, including being one of the founders of Voluntary Hospitals of America (VHA). But when he was asked what he liked most about being a hospital administrator he stated: "***They both are important. I don't know how to put one ahead of the other. It's what happens in the moment.***"

"The thing I really liked about being a hospital CEO was I could always help in some way when people came to me."

DISCUSSION QUESTIONS

1. Why can leadership distinctions be such a power force?
2. Describe one way Vince Caponi says a healthcare leader can model the way for others.
3. What does Allen Hicks say is more important: being a visionary or helping someone in their time of need? Explain.
4. What is a distinction?
5. How do we form distinctions?
6. How do distinctions affect the philosophies, management style, and actions of a healthcare leader?
7. What does it mean to walk in someone else's shoes?
8. Provide a few examples of how walking in someone else's shoes might be used in healthcare leadership setting.
9. What was the one thing Allen Hicks always liked about being a hospital CEO?
10. Discuss a distinction you have about healthcare leadership that you may not be sure is accurate and that you would like more information about to increase your understanding and perspective.

FIGURE CREDIT

28

A Plan to Develop Your Leadership

Leadership is a journey. Leaders are always becoming the leader they are through their own experiences, growth, and development. What leaders learn along their journey and apply in their leadership is critical to becoming more effective leaders. It isn't always easy to go through an extended learning process where part of the learning includes making mistakes and learning from them; however, learning through your own experiences requires a willingness to do just that. Moreover, for a leaders to become the most effective leaders they can be, they should have a plan for learning and developing their leadership philosophy and style.

OBJECTIVES

1. Learn about how outside insight can provide a leader with learning he can't access on his own.
2. Learn about the importance of having a mentor and how a mentorship relationship can benefit both the mentor and the mentee.
3. Create your own plan for developing your leadership using the leadership development pyramid.

Are you making the type of progress you want in your current leadership position or career? Are you looking for a way to attain a higher level of leadership performance and effectiveness? The performance expectations for leaders today have never been greater. The pressures, demands, and expectations on leaders come from a myriad of sources, including shareholders, boards, colleagues, customers, regulatory agencies, and even community organizations and their constituents. Given the pivotal role most leaders play in their respective organizations—and with so much at stake—is it really any wonder many leaders feel their performance is perpetually under the microscope of judgment and scrutiny by so many? Consequently, many leaders today are looking for effective ways to improve their performance through further development of their leadership style, knowledge, and skills. What about a leader with aspirations of assuming new leadership responsibilities someday? How can he become better prepared to face new and unknown challenges at the next level? As a leader, have you ever wondered: ***What don't I see in myself and my leadership style that, if I could see it, would make a positive impact on my effectiveness and career? What are others around me seeing in my leadership style that I don't?*** The answer can be found through outside insight.

OUTSIDE INSIGHT

Outside insight can provide a clearer picture of how a leader's style is being perceived and how his or her actions are impacting those around him or her. How? By providing a leader with insight about his or her leadership style outside his or her realm of knowing, also referred to as a "blind spot." This type of knowledge can create new and powerful understanding by identifying strengths, weaknesses, and pitfalls in leadership style a leader never new existed. Outside insight can be pivotal in unlocking a leader's peak leadership performance potential. Why? Because how will a leader know or discover certain weaknesses in his leadership style that are perceived by others unless he is informed about them, or in other words, receives outside insight.

Outside insight can be pivotal in unlocking a leader's peak leadership performance potential.

Sometimes leadership can be a lonely endeavor. Most people around you are reluctant to offer you honest, constructive feedback that can provide you with valuable knowledge and understanding about how others are receiving and reacting to your leadership style and actions. Is this type of feedback really important? Absolutely! How can a leader who isn't receiving honest, constructive feedback from those around him—the people directly impacted by his leadership style and actions—really know and understand his strengths and weaknesses as a leader with respect to those he is leading? There may be no more fertile ground of discovery for a leader to develop his leadership style than through outside insight. Moreover, when it comes to assessing and evaluating your leadership in action, there is no substitute for the discovery of outsight insight from those around you who are most directly impacted by your leadership.

Leadership development is not a goal or destination; it is an ongoing process that can involve a variety of different resources and mediums. Most leaders have attended leadership seminars and conferences, read books and articles on various topics and strategies of leadership, and even tried incorporating changes into their leadership style to be more effective. Sometimes these changes work—sometimes they don't. But, seeking outsight insight is about seeing your leadership style and actions through the eyes—the perception and judgment—of those around you, those most affected by your leadership. Why is this so important? Without outside insight a leader won't discover what others see in his leadership that he doesn't. We all see, react to, and interact with the world differently. The saying "reality is whatever you make it" is true; a leader's own perception, or reality, about his leadership style is whatever he thinks it is. But, what do others think?

Without outside insight, a leader won't discover what others see in his leadership that he doesn't.

Consequently, a leader may be unintentionally misled, uninformed, or unaware of key aspects of his leadership style and actions if he relies solely on the limited perceptions, viewpoint, and judgment of himself or even just his boss. With respect to this limited assessment of the strengths, weaknesses, and opportunities for improvement in a leader's style, erroneous conclusions may easily be drawn. So how does a leader go about getting outside insight?

DESIRE TO LEARN, GROW, AND DEVELOP

Leadership development is a process of ongoing learning, growing, and developing the knowledge, skills, and abilities that will make a leader more effective and perform at a higher level. The process is about working towards becoming a better leader tomorrow than you are today. In the quality assurance arena, this is called performance improvement. It is the quest to continually improve and perform at a higher level, and it first takes the desire to do so. Without desire, it simply won't happen.

Like most things in life, gaining outside insight takes desire—a sincere interest by the leader to improve his or her leadership effectiveness and performance. Otherwise, without a true desire to improve, the notion will just become another passing thought or idea. Moreover, the desire must be strong enough for the leader to make a commitment to seek outside insight and put new knowledge and understanding into action.

Gaining outside insight isn't always easy or straightforward. A leader isn't always going to hear what he or she wants. He or she will, however, more than likely hear what he or she needs to. When you seek outside insight, be prepared by having the right mental outlook that allows you to maintain a positive and constructive attitude and disposition at all times. Maintaining a positive attitude requires commitment to the overall purpose for gaining outside insight in the first place—to learn, grow, and develop as a leader and to continuously improve your leadership style and performance.

In the sporting world, the phrase "no pain, no gain" refers to the sacrifice, hard work, and effort that it takes in practice and off-the-field workouts for an athlete to improve on-the-field performance. This phrase implies there are experiences along the journey to peak performance and goal achievement that will create discomfort. However, these experiences are prerequisites for an athlete wanting to reach the top. Any champion in sports knows exactly what his goals for success are. What are your goals for your leadership career? What are the significant achievements left to be pursued and realized in your career? What role can new knowledge and understanding about your leadership style play in facilitating the achievements and goals you've yet to realize in your career? As Brian Tracy states in his book *Maximum Achievement*, "***Goals are the fuel in the furnace of achievement.***" If you haven't already done so, commit your career goals and personal mission for your life's work to writing and keep these in front of you at all times. These goals should represent the significant achievements yet to be attained in your life's work, providing the driving force behind your leadership spirit and energy moving forward.

CONDUCIVE ATMOSPHERE FOR FEEDBACK

Creating the proper environmental space and context for outside insight is critical—both for you and the giver of feedback. Initial conversation should provide the right background, context, mood, and framing for a crucial conversation of constructive feedback.

Do you make suggestions and recommendations about possible organizational improvements to your boss on a regular basis? Does that involve leadership style and actions? If you answered "no" to these questions, then think about whether you are providing this type of constructive feedback and if you feel safe in doing so. Leaders who don't create an environment that is conducive to feedback won't get the valuable outside insight they need—it's that simple. Although there may be a few subordinates or co-workers who give the leader feedback regardless, chances are it won't be outside insight, but only what the giver of feedback thinks the leader wants to hear—not what he needs to hear. So, what does an environment that is conducive to feedback look like?

An environment conducive to feedback is one created through conversation around common background. It is also established by the leader's demeanor, mannerisms, countenance, gestures, innuendoes, facial expressions, tone of voice, words, and actions. Clearly, a leader's desire to gain outside insight must be sincere and genuine. Phony, contrived, and insincere actions will be easily recognized by others, injuring the leader's credibility and trustworthiness for honest feedback, as others perceive it unsafe. But, even if the leader is credible and trustworthy, why would someone provide him with outside insight? What's in it for them?

The reasons why someone might provide a leader with outside insight are as varied as they are hard to define. However, people typically provide feedback from the basis of their own personal concerns, or whether their own commitments and dignity are being honored. In many cases, people are willing to provide honest, constructive feedback when they believe it will benefit them in some way. Some people who give feedback may believe they will receive special favors, perks, or even a raise or promotion as a result. But, a leader's loving critics—those who provide constructive feedback as a way to benefit his leadership style and performance, the organization's performance, and themselves—are the true champions of outside insight and should be sought out, respected, and listened to in conversation. And, conversations to gain valuable outside insight are crucial and must be treated accordingly. So, how should a leader handle a crucial conversation where he is seeking Outside Insight?

A leader's loving critics—those who provide constructive feedback as a way to benefit his leadership style and performance, the organization's performance, and themselves—are the true champions of outside insight and should be sought out, respected, and listened to in conversation.

A CRUCIAL CONVERSATION

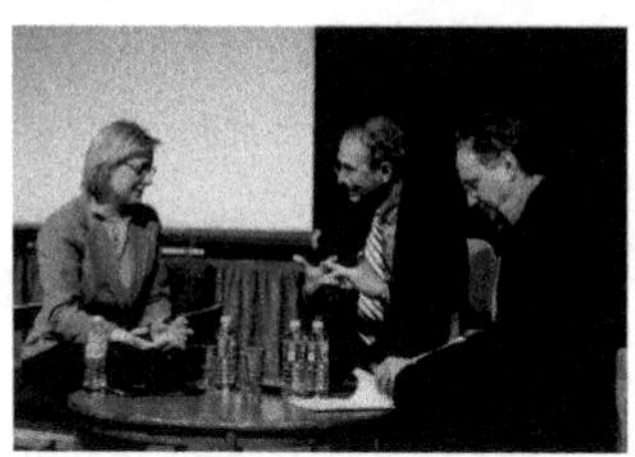

FIGURE 28.1 Panel Discussion
Copyright © David Bruce (CC BY-SA 2.0) at http://commons.wikimedia.org/wiki/File:Panel_Discussion_Close-up,_Science,_Faith,_and_Technology.jpg.

In the book *Crucial Conversations: Tools for Talking when Stakes are High*, the authors give various strategies and techniques for conducting and handling crucial conversations. An entire chapter is devoted to "How to make it safe to talk about almost anything." One key point the authors make is to look and pay attention to factors, situations, conversation, and body language that indicates safety may be an issue to the other person. Safety must first be interjected and managed before crucial conversations can effectively ensue. Any leader seeking valuable outside insight must first make it safe for the giver of constructive feedback—this is imperative. Furthermore, the leader must be mentally present; utilize his listening skills and intuition for important clues, inferences, and suggestions that can be revealing; and recognize, acknowledge, and demonstrate respect of the other person in an honest and sincere way. It is about seeking the value and merit that exists in the conversation and constructive feedback being received.

Ok, you've sought out and received feedback, some of which is conflicting and confusing. So, how do you filter through and determine what is truly real?

PROCESSING FEEDBACK

It's clear that not all constructive feedback is accurate or representative of reality. And, how could it be when every human being sees the world in a unique and different way? We perceive reality through our senses and our mind, including our memories, beliefs, experiences, etc. Differing views of reality makes processing the feedback we receive challenging and difficult. What's reality anyway? Is that really true? Is that just one person's perspective or is it representative of a broader, more accepted viewpoint?

There is no simple formula for processing feedback. It is prone to differences in development and values that exist in our thinking, our interactions, and relationships. And every leader has his "*already always way*" of how he sees himself, his leadership, and the world around him. This is exactly the reason why a leader needs outside insight—so he can see his world from a different perspective, orientation of development, or set of values—where other people are coming from. So, how does a leader know what is real in the feedback he receives?

In general, a leader should use his experiences in leadership and life to compare, contrast, and process outside insight. At the same time, the leader must be open and receptive to new possibilities, as well as other perspectives and viewpoints. The following offers a few key points to understand in this process.

Seek outside insight from a number of loving critics—not just one or two. Why? Because outside insight from a variety of sources will make you less susceptible to the individual biases, prejudices, or limited perspectives when you get feedback from more than a limited few. In other words, the more outside insight a leader gets (all other things considered equal), the easier it will be to discover and distinguish common assessments, viewpoints, or perspectives, giving greater credence to the truth—or what is reality. Secondly, you must be open to these different perspectives and viewpoints. Remind yourself that, regardless of how much you value your own perspective and self-assessment, it may contain one or more elements that are flawed, inaccurate, or simply of a different value system. Thirdly, and maybe most important, don't act defensive, offer excuses, or become agitated or irritated while receiving constructive feedback. Use your emotional intelligence to control your thoughts, emotions, words, and actions. Creating a hostile environment is self-defeating and can injure relationships, as well as disconnect you from a valuable source of outside insight. Be mentally present with the giver of feedback, and be open to new information. Listen to and use your intuition. What repeating themes are emerging from the feedback I am receiving from my loving critics? What does this mean for my leadership style? How might I "flex" my leadership style to more effectively lead this person or others in the organization?

DISCOVERY TAKES INITIATIVE

Can valuable outside insight come to a leader if he just sits back and waits? Why should a leader seek it? Unfortunately, unless a leader actively seeks outside insight his feedback will be more limited, selective, and potentially less beneficial. By actively seeking it, a leader will be able to choose those sources that are the most credible and insightful—his loving critics. For example, the loving critic who has the most valuable outside insight may never be open to or approach the leader with feedback, unless it is sought. And seeking it in private conversations behind closed doors is a simple and appropriate way to gain outside insight. There are, however, other appropriate avenues in which to purse the discovery of outside insight.

AVENUES FOR OUTSIDE INSIGHT

The formal performance review process is an opportunity to gain valuable outside insight. However, the leader will probably have to go beyond the typical routine aspects of a performance review and seek feedback on specifics aspects of his leadership style to gain valuable outside insight. Gaining valuable outside insight through the performance evaluation process will probably require the leader to have probing questions ready in advance of the actual session, to generate feedback on specific aspects of leadership style during the performance evaluation conversation.

Another avenue in which to seek valuable outside insight is with employee surveys. While most employee surveys don't typically contain specific feedback targeted at an individual leader's style, some do. However, for the majority, one can only draw general observations and themes that relate to the overall leadership culture as a whole. While use of employee surveys is certainly predicated around the amount of specificity they contain for an individual leader, their usefulness as a component or part of the overall picture can prove useful in some cases.

A "360" leadership assessment process is an excellent way to gain valuable outside insight. It is also an excellent way to determine what gaps exist between the leader's own personal assessment and perspective and how others assess his leadership style. A "360" can be quite revealing. Moreover, it can demonstrate how a leader's own perspective of his leadership style can be quite different from others' perspectives of his leadership style, highlighting the need for outside insight, not just overall, but in specific, targeted areas of his leadership.

Mentoring is another great way to obtain outside insight on an ongoing basis. This can be particularly true if the mentor works with the leader in the same organization and can provide valuable outside insight based upon direct observation. A mentor can be a loving critic who can also offer thoughts and ideas on how to put new knowledge and understanding into action. By developing a relationship with trust at the foundation, a mentoring relationship can prove to be invaluable to a leader's growth, development, and career, regardless of the leader's position or experience. But what about the leader with 20 years or more of leadership experience? John Wooden, the famous college basketball coach, addressed this issue succinctly when he stated "***It's what you learn after you know it all that counts.***" A leader is never too smart, too old, too wise, or too experienced to learn, grow, or develop his leadership style and effectiveness. Through the power of an effective mentoring relationship, a leader can gain valuable outside insight with a trusted and respected mentor.

Somewhat similar to mentoring, coaching is another avenue to gain outside insight. In coaching, the leader confers and discusses issues, problems, challenges, decisions, leadership philosophies, style and actions, specific situations, and other similar subject matter. A simple comment like "Have you ever thought of… "can provide valuable outside insight, helping the leader to see other perspectives, viewpoints, and possibilities.

TURN KNOWLEDGE INTO ACTION

Discovering valuable perspective through other viewpoints with outside insight is critical for any leader to reach peak leadership performance. Without outside insight, a leader doesn't have a clear or whole picture of his leadership style and how others perceive it or react to it. Furthermore, without outside insight, the leader continues to have blind spots that, if discovered, could be addressed and redeveloped. But that isn't the whole story. New knowledge, understanding, and perspective are of little value if not taken to heart and put into action.

Taking steps to incorporate outside insight into your leadership style and actions is a vital step, and one that relies on a commitment to execution. Frankly, this is where the ball gets dropped by many leaders. It's hard. You're busy with so many other priorities and demands. Who has time to work on leadership style? But, don't we usually make time for those things we believe are important? And, isn't your leadership style central to most everything you do as a leader? Leadership involves leading many things, including processes, functions, projects, and activities. But leading other people in a way that maximizes their productivity, performance, and contributions—individually and collectively—hinges upon your leadership style and actions. And, achieving peak leadership performance is all about the leadership style you exhibit and the actions you take. This is exactly why outside insight is a key ingredient to peak leadership performance. Are you thinking of colleagues and co-workers right now who just might see things that you don't in your leadership style? Could there be a few loving critics who can provide you with the key that could unlock your peak leadership performance potential through outside insight?

LEADERSHIP JOURNAL

Reflection upon events, stories, experiences, key interactions, presentations, leadership philosophy or style, leadership methods or techniques, mistakes, successes, or observations made of other leaders in action is essential for learning, growth, and development of a leader. A Leadership Journal can facilitate the capturing and documentation of these experiences and observations. The Leadership Journal at the end of this chapter provides a template that can be used as is or modified for this purpose.

10 QUESTIONS FOR LEADERS TO CONTEMPLATE

1. What is the number one reason you want to be or became a healthcare leader?
2. How do you define and describe your leadership philosophy and style?
3. How are you defining and measuring the success of your leadership?
4. How do you solicit and use feedback about:

    a. your leadership style?
    b. your leadership communication?
    c. your leadership performance?

5. Do you have a personal leadership development plan? If not, why not? If so, how are you going about implementing it, and what have been the results? Have you assessed your leadership development plan in the past twelve months and considered any needed changes?
6. What do you consider the major accomplishments of your leadership in the past twelve months?
7. How will you measure and define your leadership success in five years?
8. How do you describe your leadership contributions and impact on those around you?
9. What three things are you the proudest of about your leadership performance and success in your career to date?
10. What is your ultimate desired leadership legacy?

LEADERSHIP DEVELOPMENT ACTION PYRAMID

David Windley, one of the original founders of Blue and Co., LLC, a CPA firm specializing in healthcare, always said to "***Plan your work, and work your plan.***" The Leadership Development Action Pyramid is a tool to help a leader create a plan to identify his leadership development goals and a plan to achieve them. Complete the pyramid, found at the end of the chapter keep it in front of you, and implement it to develop your leadership effectiveness as you work to attain your career goals and create a desired leadership legacy

DISCUSSION QUESTIONS

1. Why should a healthcare leader have a plan to develop his leadership?
2. What role can outside insight play in leadership development?
3. What is important for a leader in processing feedback about his leadership style?
4. What does outside insight mean?
5. Describe one or two means in which outside insight can be received by the leader.
6. What is a loving critic and what roll can he or she play in providing a leader with outside insight?
7. Describe one or two characteristics of an atmosphere conducive fo constructive feedback to be given?
8. Why should a healthcare leader have at least one mentor?
9. Identify one or two steps that are part of a successful mentoring relationship.
10. Describe one or two benefits for the mentee and the mentor in a mentoring relationship.

LEADERSHIP JOURNAL

GOAL

Document key experiences, observations, stories, and lessons learned in order to foster and promote reflection for the purpose of leadership development.

KEY AREAS FOR JOURNAL ENTRY AND REFLECTION

1. Emotional intelligence and observation of situations and circumstances involving the need for or use of emotional intelligence.
2. Leadership style, actions, methods, techniques, and critical leadership intangibles observed or used.
3. Leadership distinctions or perceptions made, including the impact leaders have on others.
4. Methods and techniques observed or used for providing key leadership communication and feedback, as well as feedback received, including that designed to foster engagement and accountability for effort and performance.
5. Content skills and subject-matter competencies and expertise observed or used.

GAINING INSIGHT THROUGH REFLECTION

- What was ***observed or heard*** that worked well that ***should be emulated*** and/or continued/repeated?
- What was ***observed or heard*** that worked well but ***should be changed or adjusted*** in some fashion to improve upon its application and effectiveness?
- What was ***tried*** that worked well that ***should be emulated*** or continued/repeated?
- What was ***tried*** that worked well but ***should be changed or adjusted*** in some fashion to improve upon its application and effectiveness?
- What was ***experienced*** and what can be learned from it?
- Where are the ***gaps*** between desired intentions, actions, behaviors, or expressions, and actual action, effort, or performance?

ADDITIONAL NOTES ON JOURNAL ENTRIES

- Entries should be made with clarity, specificity, and complete thought.
- Entries can include anything pertinent and appropriate for leadership development and may focus on:
    - Stories involving strong emotions, associated emotional triggers, and challenges faced, as well as successes with controlling feelings and emotions.
    - Mistakes made and reflection regarding associated learning about those mistakes.
    - Lessons learned through observation or experience, and different actions, methods, or techniques that can be taken in the future.

  - Insight gained through feedback received from others and their perceptions of your leadership philosophy, actions, methods, words, behaviors, skills, style, or techniques.
  - Leadership decision-making styles and processes in different environments and at different levels of responsibility.
  - Leadership actions taken or presentations made and observations about presentation styles, methods, and techniques, along with words and behaviors that are motivating and inspiring, or demotivating and uninspiring.
- Where do gaps exist between your own leadership distinctions and perceptions of your leadership style and performance and how others may view you?
- Where do differences exist between your own leadership distinctions and perceptions of events, experiences, and trends and how non-leaders view these same things? What are the causes of these different distinctions and perceptions?
- Take time to periodically review your Leadership Journal to assess progress being made and reflect upon experiences and opportunities for growth and development, and lessons learned in order to formulate strategies and actions that can facilitate leadership growth, development, and performance effectiveness.

JOURNAL ENTRIES

KEY AREAS OF FOCUS, OBSERVATION, AND REFLECTION	EXPERIENCES, OBSERVATIONS, AND REFLECTION
1. Emotional Intelligence	
2. Leadership Style	
3. Leadership Distinctions/Perceptions	
4. Communication & Feedback	
5. Competencies & Expertise	
6. Other	
7. Other	

List key strategies and objectives for growth, development, and performance effectiveness.

List key tactics and action steps to apply and implement.

My Leadership Development Action Pyramid: ________

Build your Leadership Development Action Pyramid from the bottom up. Write the steps of your plan to develop your leadership philosophy and Leadership Legacy Statement and put it into action.

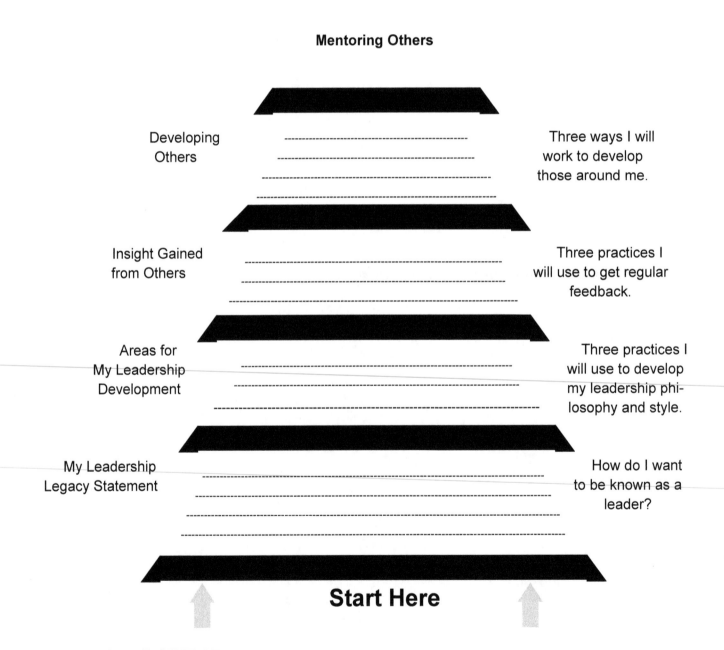

Mentoring Others

Developing Others	________ ________ ________ ________	Three ways I will work to develop those around me.
Insight Gained from Others	________ ________ ________	Three practices I will use to get regular feedback.
Areas for My Leadership Development	________ ________ ________	Three practices I will use to develop my leadership philosophy and style.
My Leadership Legacy Statement	________ ________ ________ ________	How do I want to be known as a leader?

Start Here

FIGURE CREDIT

Figure 28.1: Copyright © David Bruce (CC BY-SA 2.0) at http://commons.wikimedia.org/wiki/File:Panel_Discussion_Close-up,_Science,_Faith,_and_Technology.jpg.

29

From Leadership to Legacy

As previously stated, a career in healthcare leadership is a journey. There is nothing linear about a typical healthcare leader's journey. Many healthcare leaders experience twists, turns, setbacks, disappointments, and frustrations, along with achievements, successes, and rewarding experiences, during their healthcare journeys. But one thing is for certain with every healthcare leader's journey, he or she will create a legacy of leadership that impacts the lives around them.

OBJECTIVES

1. Learn what a healthcare leader's legacy is, and how it's created; why it is important for every leader to contemplate; and why a healthcare leader's legacy represents his or her own unique brand and impacts how he or she is thought of by others.
2. Appreciate the impact a healthcare leader's legacy can make on others.
3. Understand the importance of legacy thinking and developing a written leadership legacy statement.

LEADERSHIP LEGACY AND SCHEMA

What do you think of when you hear the phrase "leadership legacy?" Where does it take you? Below is a schema diagram on the phrase leadership legacy. The concept of schema relates to the fact that we draw meaning from words and phrases based on other words and phrases we associate or connect with—including visual pictures—and that quickly come to mind when we read or hear a word or phrase. This schema diagram identifies a partial listing of words and phrases that are commonly associated or connected with the phrase leadership legacy.

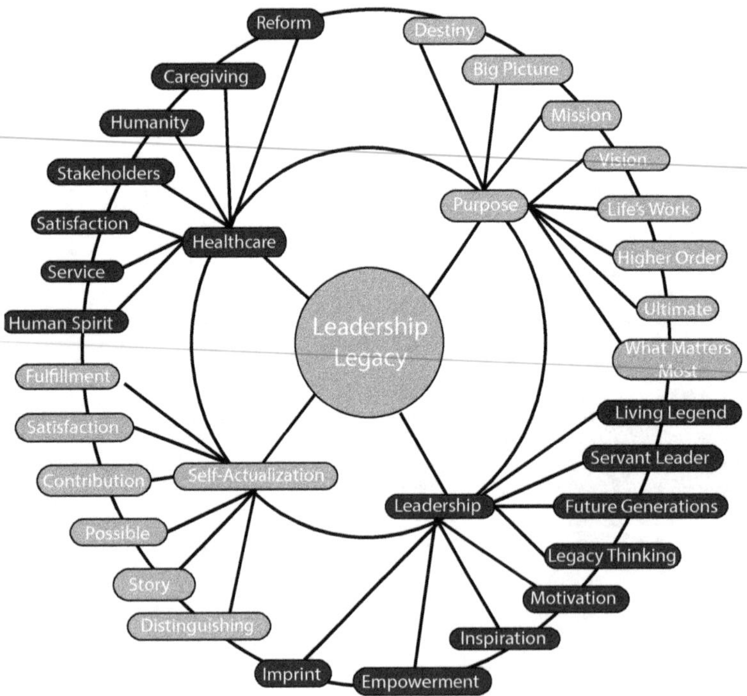

FIGURE 29.1 Leadership Legacy

Schema is a theory about how we interpret the world around us and how we bring meaning to our lives. When you think of a healthcare leader's legacy, do you think more about the human side of healthcare or the business side? Are you more interested or passionate about impacting other people's lives or the business aspects that serve them? As a healthcare leader, what do you want to be known for? A healthcare leader's philosophies, beliefs, values, and attitudes shape how he or she views the world, determines what is important, and to a large extent, affects the impact he or she wants to have with his or her healthcare leadership career. Give thought to and reflect about what words on this schema diagram resonate with you about your own healthcare leadership legacy. Are there any other words and phrases not represented on this schema diagram that come to mind when you think about a healthcare leader's legacy, and what do they represent to you?

A HEALTHCARE LEADER'S LEGACY

Legacy is the lasting impact of your presence and actions on the lives of others. Something that is handed down or remains from a previous generation or time.

Dave Windley, Founder and past Director of Blue and Co., LLC, a mid-sized accounting and consulting firm that specializes in healthcare, when asked about what he thinks of when he hears the term leadership legacy says ***"To be honest, I guess I really haven't thought of legacies a lot. The concept or phrase is a little bit new to me. I just think more of personalities and what people have accomplished. I think about legacies in terms of athletics and haven't really thought about it in terms of healthcare."***

John Render states that ***"I worry today that preoccupation with the challenges of today provide less opportunity for constructive legacy leadership. I don't want to sound like an old guy reminiscing about the way [healthcare] used to be because every time and period has their own challenges and leaders that emerge and so on. I think there are many fine healthcare leaders today and many legacy leaders. But it seems to me that the leaders of today spend more time putting out fires and dealing with operational and other crises than they do with other manifestations of leadership. And I understand that crisis management and dealing with day-to-day challenges require substantial leadership too. But in terms of strategic planning, and strategic legacy, and strategic thinking: [it seems that] younger leaders don't seem to have as much time."***

Healthcare leaders should be concerned with their own legacy. In a conversation with Dave Windley, he was asked to think about a broader definition or construct of a healthcare leader's legacy as being the imprint that it makes on other people's lives—to think about the impact that healthcare leaders have on the lives of their colleagues, employees, physicians, patients, families, and the communities they serve. Regardless of whether that leader works in a small, community-based hospital or health service organization; a large, multi-billion-dollar integrated healthcare delivery system; or even a healthcare consulting organization that works with hospitals and health service organization; the impact a healthcare leader can have on other lives is immeasurable. In response to whether a healthcare leader should be concerned with his or her own healthcare leadership legacy, Mr. Windley states that ***"In that context a healthcare leader*** *may be purposeful about a legacy, maybe even if they aren't thinking about it that way. Healthcare organizations are a significant part of [almost] every community. When you think about all [healthcare leaders] do and all they impact, they really are developing a legacy. I have the feeling they aren't thinking about that: they are thinking about doing their job and serving their institution as best they can. And maybe that's exactly what they should be doing. And in doing that well they are developing a legacy."*

"Healthcare has grown so much, and healthcare has been a very well thought of and good profession to be involved in. Today it has become expensive and causing some people and employers some difficulty in terms of cost. One hopes that healthcare goes forward with the same—almost reverence. Healthcare as a whole has been able to do some pretty phenomenal things through the years. And healthcare is still pretty well thought of, especially hospitals. In many communities the hospital is a big employer; they are involved in a lot of different charities; their people are active in community organizations; and they are very responsible citizens and thought of that way. For most [healthcare leaders] I would think that is rewarding, and you hope they will continue to operate in a manner that will allow them to be thought of that way. Hospitals have always been important parts of communities, but they've never been the kind of employer they are now because they are so much bigger, and provide so many more services, and have so many more employees."

DEFINING A LEGACY OF SUCCESS

When asked about what success is for a healthcare leader, Sam Odle says it ***"Should be the number of people you are able to positively impact. [As a healthcare leader,] if I can say that all the things that I did were directed towards having a positive impact on as many people as possible—that's what I wanted to do."***

"I don't think I consciously thought of [my legacy], at least not in the concept of a legacy. I did think of it from the standpoint that I wanted it to make a difference that I was here. I wanted my presence, the work that I did to make a difference. It was about making a difference in the community, and with our employees and their families. You get inspired by thinking the work you do is important, and it really was when you stop and think about providing a secure, safe place to work and they can count on it: whether they are the person receiving healthcare or the person delivering it. I used to tell our hospital directors all the time that the reason we manage and have to be good stewards of our resources is because we want to be an ongoing concern. We want our employees to know we are financially secure and they know that paycheck is going to be there every two weeks. It's not just about building a bigger health system or getting more patients. It really is about making the community a better place."

Dennis Dawes talks about how his ***"career, from a personal standpoint, has given me great satisfaction seeing lives being saved. Some lives literally being torn-up and torn-apart, being put back together. Some more minor things but still being helped. Thousands and thousands of people—it is incredible the number of lives that have been touched in over 40 years in my career. That's very satisfying when you think about it. It was that institution that I sat in the chair of President and had an impact on a lot of people's lives from a healthcare standpoint."***

When asked to think about what a healthcare leader's legacy is, David Handel states, ***"I never really thought in terms of the word 'legacy.' It wasn't something that I used to hear people discuss. As people got late in their careers, or in early retirement, there were more conversations on what they had accomplished. I think lately people are using the word legacy. I have to confess, I never really thought of myself and the word legacy. I thought more in terms was I a part of helping them become a little better than they were without me. I also had a peculiar test of [a healthcare leader's] success which is: when they leave the organization, does it get bigger and better after they left? Now you have to be pretty secure with that notion so you don't get the feeling 'Well David left now we can really fly and grow!' You have to be comfortable with the notion that perhaps one of the most important things you can be part of is making sure that the organization could grow and be more successful after you've gone."***

A HEALTHCARE LEADERSHIP LEGACY

When asked if he thought healthcare leaders think about their legacy, and if their legacy is something they are intentional about creating, Ken Stella states "***I don't think about it in terms of the word 'legacy.' I don't think [healthcare leaders] take a position with the idea they are going to leave a monumental legacy. I've always been taught to try to keep your name with honor; respect others; and leave the place a little better than it was when you showed up. I don't think today we see the long tenures anymore: the 25 or 30 year runs. We are seeing more of the 10 year runs [for CEO-level positions]. Legacies become more individual than they do institutional.***"

CREATING YOUR ULTIMATE LEADERSHIP LEGACY: CONNECTING HEAD WITH HEART

What's your ultimate desired leadership legacy? Creating your ultimate desired leadership legacy is about connecting your head with your heart. It's just as much a feeling thing as it is thinking thing.

The freelance writer Po Bronson is quoted as saying "***People thrive by focusing on who they really are and connecting that to work they truly love.***" For healthcare leaders to thrive in their leadership roles they must be able to connect who they are at their core essence; why they chose a career in healthcare leadership; and what their purpose or mission is for their healthcare leadership career. Those who are not able to recognize the connection between who they are and their passion and what they do every day as healthcare leader probably would not respond positively to the question, "*Are You thriving in your healthcare leadership career?*" Sometimes being able to make this head-to-heart connection means reflecting back to the very beginning of your career and your decision-making process for that career and identifying your real purpose and what your career choice meant to you then. In looking back, some questions for reflection can include: why did I really choose a career in healthcare leadership; who was the most influential person in my decision; what did I believe a career in healthcare leadership would do ...; what am I telling others about a career in healthcare leadership; and similar questions. As stated many times in this text, reflection plays a significant role in a healthcare leader's journey, including creating a legacy that is both significant, meaningful, and lasting.

There are many challenges in healthcare today—too many to list. However, a short list of challenges might include demand and capacity issues; staffing and manpower shortages; shortfalls in third party reimbursement; increasing government regulation and scrutiny; patient safety; clinical variability; increasing expectations on results and performance from all stakeholders; and healthcare reform. According to survey results by Press Ganey in 2010, 45 percent of hospital employees report being distanced from or discontent with their current work. This last challenge could be as big of a healthcare leadership challenge as any. So how will these as well as other challenges in healthcare impact the creation of your leadership legacy?

The creation of a healthcare leader's legacy is really an inside job. As stated above, clearly there are numerous challenges in healthcare, most of which are outside of the complete control of any healthcare leader or one individual. However, make no mistake, healthcare leaders can significantly shape and influence how health organizations react to and address these challenges. Moreover, how a healthcare leader goes about understanding these challenges, working with others to create strategies, tactics, and actions to address them, and the style and manner in which the healthcare leader does this is a big part of how he is creating a leadership legacy in action. Therefore, as previously stated, a healthcare leader's beliefs, values, attitudes, and distinctions toward these challenges and actions, and how he works with others to address them, plays a significant role toward the creation of his healthcare leadership legacy.

Thinking about the creation of your healthcare leadership legacy is similar to thinking about what success means to you: your desired legacy is really all about how you define success for your career and life's work. In John C. Maxwell's book entitled *Thinking for a Change*, he talks about the power of thinking and the role it plays when a person changes his or her way of thinking and, consequently, his or her attitudes, actions, and life. This is exactly the type of thinking required for a healthcare leader to contemplate the desired legacy he or she would like to create in his or her healthcare leadership career. This concept implies creating a healthcare leadership legacy with intention—and not by accident or default.

DISTINCTIONS

Distinctions are how we see ourselves and the world around us. There is a chapter in this book devoted to healthcare leadership distinctions. Distinctions are the observations, conclusions, and meaning we make about what we hear, see, feel, and experience in our lives. What does it mean or represent? Do we like it? Is it good? Distinctions are based on what we've learned and experienced; what we've been taught; and what we believe.

Think about how a healthcare leader's distinctions, attitudes and beliefs are interwoven to create his or her reality about the world around him or her, including his or her job and the challenges, concerns, priorities, and successes—even his or her passion as a healthcare leader.

We relate to others based on how we distinguish them. We lead based upon how we distinguish ourselves, our role, and our purpose.

We relate to others based upon how we distinguish them. We lead based upon how we distinguish ourselves, our role, and our purpose.

One opportunity that a healthcare leader has—that, in some ways, is unique to management and being a leader—is the ability to support and assist others in their quest to learn, grow, develop, and advance in his or her career. This opportunity is one that healthcare leaders should not take lightly—for a variety of reasons. One reason is that the function of management is getting work done through others. Therefore, the more a leader can support and assist his employees in his or her quest to learn, grow, develop, and advance in his or her career, the more he is being effective in his job. It is only logical that workers can be increasingly more efficient and effective in their work as they learn, grow, and develop, making bigger contributions to the organization. In turn, this learning, growth, and development can result in higher levels of patient safety and quality; customer service delivery and patient satisfaction; and financial performance for the organization so that it can sustain its ability to fulfill its mission as a central healthcare asset in the community.

The environment around us can impact the distinctions we make. However, as healthcare leaders, one of the qualities that our employees look for from us is consistency. That consistency includes our philosophy, beliefs, approach, words, behaviors, and actions. Think about it; do you want to work for a boss who does not have these consistent qualities? Probably not.

In creating the desired leadership legacy, in what ways might his or her work environment prevent a healthcare leader from creating or living his legacy of leadership? In what ways might his or her work environment support him or her in creating or living his or her legacy of leadership?

The following graphic summarizes this mental construct about a healthcare leader's legacy, the challenges in healthcare, and the fact that creating a healthcare leadership legacy is really an inside job.

DEVELOPING THOSE AROUND YOU

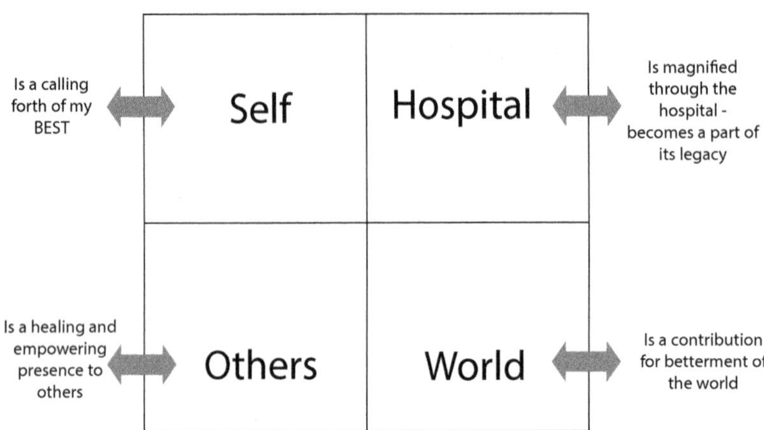

FIGURE 29.2 Quadrant Diagram

Another reason a healthcare leader may consider creating a legacy with intent—but which may get overlooked from time-to-time—is that a healthcare leader's impact on others is, in many ways, central to the creation of his legacy. In short, the difference that a healthcare leader makes is the legacy he creates, and that difference is typically thought of as the difference that leader has made for others—including employees.

The difference that a healthcare leader makes is the legacy he creates.

In his book, *Developing the Leaders Around You*, John C. Maxwell talks about a higher calling of leadership: developing those around you. This higher calling is for leaders to focus on developing those around them—including employees in leadership and non-leadership positions. It is a leadership philosophy about what a leader's job and role are, and what is important to others and the organization. It starts with the definition of how a leader defines his job, his role, and key ways he can make an impact and contribution to the organization and its people. Developing those around you is a leadership philosophy very much congruent with servant leadership: where a leader views his role more as serving others, versus a more traditional role of others serving the leader.

Maxwell talks about how recruiting, developing, and keeping good people is a leader's most important task. If you help grow and develop a leader, you are helping to grow an organization, and multiplying the effectiveness of others and their contributions. Maxwell talks about looking for the gold—not the dirt—when developing others. In other words, to analyze and understand their potential and work to help them develop it. As Maxwell says, great leaders share themselves and what they know and have learned with others: the sharing of leadership wisdom and lessons learned.

A leadership philosophy of developing others is about being in touch with the skills, abilities, and potential of others, including their passions, goals, and career objectives. Knowing this about others is vital to providing the type of coaching, teaching, and mentoring that will be the most helpful and effective in developing others. It means that, many times, a leader must choose spending his limited time with people and not with emails; with coaching and mentoring others more than completing or reviewing reports and paperwork; with communication that involves listening, encouraging, and inspiring, not just providing direction or instruction.

Developing those around you means the leader is treating employees more like volunteers than just employees, realizing they volunteer their best efforts and performance—it can't be mandated, legislated, or coerced. It is a leadership philosophy and style that translates into a leadership legacy that, in part, includes developing others and impacting their career opportunities and success. It is the kind of legacy that can have a deep and significant impact—for decades beyond the leader's own career.

When asked to think about what a healthcare leader's legacy is, Marilyn Custer-Mitchell states ***"To me what comes to mind is the people that you worked with and their thoughts, their impressions, and how they remember you. It's the impact you had on their lives and everything: the impact you had [as a healthcare leader] on the organization. Did you leave it in better shape than you started? Did you lead it through a tough time? The things you accomplished [during your tenure]. And sometimes you make an impact on someone's life that you don't even know you are making. From a legacy standpoint I think it's how you have impacted them directly or the organization. Or they may know how I've impacted somebody else and not them directly."***

LEGACY THINKING

Legacy thinking calls for you—the leader—to think about who impacted your life and career. Who provided you with the support you needed in your journey to date? What did you learn from this person? How did this person go about encouraging you or believing in you? What did this person make possible for you? Many people identify someone who impacted them and provided them with the human touch—encouraging them, supporting them, and believing in them—even when the person might not have believed in themselves. Rachel Naomi Remen, MD, says it this way: ***"It's not your expertise that blesses others, it's your humanness"*** (CD Care for the Journey). This is true about the opportunity that healthcare leaders have: to positively impact those around them and the lives of countless other people. It is the type of leadership legacy that impacts others through the leader's presence, words, and actions, and it fosters and supports the needs of others.

As Sam Walton once said, ***"Outstanding leaders go out of their way to boost the self-esteem of their personnel. If people believe in themselves, it's amazing what they can accomplish."*** Developing others means providing the support, belief, and encouragement they need—when they need it. One key theme of this book has been about reflection, including a leader reflecting on his or her leadership style. Here is a list of questions that can help foster reflection by a leader as he or she examines his or her leadership style.

- How am I tapping into the discretionary effort of my employees?
- How am I assessing talent and potential in others?
- How am I deciding on what to delegate to others? Am I providing opportunities for others to learn, grow, and develop?
- What am I doing to get top performance from my staff?
- What am I doing to recognize, support, and encourage others to take on new assignments and opportunities that stretch their skills and abilities and provide them with the experience they need to learn, grow, and develop?
- What am I doing to help others reach their potential and career goals?
- What type of guidance, coaching, and mentoring am I providing to others?
- Who am I becoming as a leader?
- What type of legacy am I creating in action?

Where are the gaps between your intentions and actions? This is something that a leader must give true, honest reflection to so that he or she can move to close the gap between his or her intentions and actions.

WRITING YOUR LEADERSHIP LEGACY STATEMENT

Every healthcare leader will create a leadership legacy; therefore, every healthcare leader should have a written statement of what they want their leadership legacy to be. This type of statement should be pretty short and succinct—from two or three sentences to a short paragraph, but no more. It is a statement that represents the type of impact or difference a healthcare leader wants to make and the legacy he wants to create through his life's work as a healthcare leader. It should be a high-level, big-picture statement but contain enough specificity to provide the needed guidance and direction for strategic leadership legacy thinking, direction, and action. A written leadership legacy statement acts, therefore, like a compass, and not a roadmap, to creating a desired leadership legacy.

Creating a desired leadership legacy with intent isn't about being narcissistic or myopic. Creating a desired leadership legacy with intent isn't about being singularly focused or closed-minded. To the contrary, setting out to create a desired leadership legacy as a healthcare leader is about making an impact—a difference—for the countless lives that each healthcare leader touches in his role and career as a healthcare leader. Creating a desired leadership legacy is a possibility, and it helps to push the healthcare leader beyond the world of survival, or just trying to get by, to a state or attitude of making a difference for others—every day. As Allen Hick's reflected on his career as a hospital administrator, he stated: ***"I [always] considered myself a humanitarian. The thing I really liked about being a hospital administrator was that you could always help [others] in some way."*** Mr. Hicks positively impacted the lives of thousands of people in his healthcare leadership career. Mr. Hicks was the consummate humanitarian. He was always there to help someone in need: from an employee who needed a new heart surgery procedure that only one hospital in the country at that time was performing to the volunteer who calls him at 4:30 p.m. on Friday afternoon with the last dime to her name; to all the patients who have received services at Community Hospital North in Indianapolis—created as a result of Mr. Hicks' vision—and the dozens of hospital administrators and administrative residents he coached and mentored; his legacy lives on in the lives he touched and impacted for the better. This is quite a legacy of leadership for any healthcare leader to aspire to.

DISCUSSION QUESTIONS

1. Describe some of the ways a leader's legacy impacts others.
2. Why is creating a leader's ultimate legacy about connecting head and heart? Explain.
3. How does focusing on the ultimate desired leadership legacy help a leader experience a greater sense of purpose and fulfillment in his career?
4. What comes to mind when you hear the phrase leadership legacy?
5. Describe what a leader's legacy is and how it is created.
6. Describe how success as a healthcare leader might be defined.
7. Is creating your desired leadership legacy more of a feeling or thinking thing? Please explain.
8. What are distinctions, and how do they impact how a healthcare leader might view his or her own desired leadership legacy?
9. What does the phrase **"Do you define your world, or does your world-define you?"** mean to you?
10. What is the purpose of writing your own leadership legacy statement?

Resumes and Bios

VINCENT C. CAPONI

Education
Masters in Science of Administration—Healthcare
Central Michigan University
Mt. Pleasant, Michigan

Selected Work Experience
Ministry Market Leader—Indiana/Wisconsin
Ascension Health

Chief Executive Officer
St. Vincent Health
Indianapolis, Indiana

President/CEO
St. Vincent Hospital
Birmingham, Alabama

President/CEO
St. Joseph Hospital
Augusta, Georgia

Community Service & Associations
Advantage Health Solutions, Inc.—Board Member
American College of Healthcare Executives—Fellow and Past Regent
American Heart Association—Midwest Affiliate Board Member
Archdiocese of Indianapolis—Investment Committee Member
Indiana Chamber of Commerce—Board Member
Indiana Health Information Exchange—Board Chair
Indiana Hospital Association—Past Chair and Board Member
Indianapolis Coalition for Patient Safety—Board member
Indianapolis Symphony Orchestra—Executive Committee
Legatus—Indiana Chapter
Midwest Healthcare Executive Summit—Member
United Way of Central Indiana—Past Chair and Board Member
Xavier University—Board Member
Saint Mary's College—Capital Campaign Committee and Past Board Member

DAVID J. HANDEL

Education
Master in Business Administration
University of Chicago
Chicago, Illinois

Selected Work Experience
Senior Vice President of Business Development and Strategy
Sisters of St. Francis Health Services, Inc.
Mishawaka, Indiana

Associate Director
Indiana University Center for Health Policy
Indianapolis, Indiana

Program Director & Executive-in-Residence
Master of Health Administration Program
Indiana University
Indianapolis, Indiana

Executive Vice President and Chief Operating Officer
Clarian Health
Indianapolis, Indiana

Director of Hospitals
Indiana University Medical Center
Indianapolis, Indiana

Administrator
Northwestern University Medical Clinics and Medical Associates
Chicago, Illinois

Selected Community Service & Associations: Past & Present
Indiana Hospital and Health Association Board of Directors—Member
University Health System Consortium Board of Directors—Member
VHA TriState Network Board of Directors—Member
Indiana Hospital and Health Association Government Relations Council—Chairperson
Indiana Hospital and Health Association Central District—President
Joint Hospital Association/State Medical Association Medicaid Task Force—Chairperson

MARILYN CUSTER-MITCHELL

Education
Master in Health Administration
Indiana University
Indianapolis, Indiana

Selected Work Experience
President
Parkview Wabash Hospital
Wabash, Indiana

President
Corning Hospital
Corning, New York

President & CEO
Washington County Memorial Hospital
Salem, Indiana

Administrator
West Central Community Hospital
Clinton, Indiana

Selected Community Service & Associations: Past & Present
American College of Healthcare Executives—Fellow
Indiana Hospital and Health Association Board of Directors—Member
Indiana Hospital and Health Association Council on Rural Health—Chairperson
Indiana Hospital and Health Association Governance Council—Chairperson
Indiana Rural Health Association Board of Directors—Member
Wabash Rotary Club Board of Directors—Member
Wabash Area Chamber of Commerce Board of Directors—Chairperson
Economic Development Group of Wabash County Board of Directors—Chairperson
85 Hope Healthcare Clinic Board of Directors—Secretary/Treasurer
Wabash First United Methodist Church Board of Directors—Administration Chairperson

JUDITH A. MONROE, MD

Education
Family Medicine Residency
University of Cincinnati
Cincinnati, Ohio

Selected Work Experience
Deputy Director for Office of State, Tribal, Local and Territorial Support
Centers For Disease Control and Prevention
Atlanta, Georgia

Indiana State Health Commissioner
Medical Director, Indiana State Medicaid
Indianapolis, Indiana

Director of Family Practice Residency
St. Vincent Hospital
Indianapolis, Indiana

Selected Community Service & Associations: Present & Past
Fellow, American Academy Family Practice
Institute of Medicine Roundtable on Population Health—Member
Institute of Medicine Forum on Medical and Public Health Preparedness for Catastrophic Events—Member
CDC, Global Health Leadership Council—Member
Robert Wood Johnson Foundation Roadmaps to Health Prize—Advisory Committee
Managed Emergency Surge for Healthcare Inc.—Board Member
Public Health Accreditation Board—Vice Chairperson
National Governors Association Healthcare Practice Taskforce—Member
Indiana Cancer Consortium Steering Committee—Member
Indiana Tobacco Prevention and Cessation Executive Board—Chairperson
Indiana Health Information Exchange—Board Member
Indiana State Department of Health Executive Board—Secretary
HRSA Peer Review National Panel—Member
Indianapolis Homeless Initiative Program—Faculty Advisor and Volunteer

Selected Awards
Indiana Governor's Distinguished Service Medal: 2010
Indiana Hospital Association Merit Award: 2009
Association of Family Medicine Residency Directors Program Director Gold Award: 2005

SAMUEL L. ODLE, FACHE

Education
Master of Science—Hospital Administration
Indiana University
Indianapolis, Indiana

Selected Work Experience
Executive Vice President and Chief Operating Officer
Indiana University Health
Indianapolis, Indiana

President and CEO
IU Health Methodist and University Hospitals
Indianapolis, Indiana

Vice President, Professional Services and Medical Staff Affairs
Director, School of Radiology Technology
Winona Memorial Hospital
Indianapolis, Indiana

Selected Community Service & Associations: Present & Past
American College of Healthcare Executives, Chairman & Fellow
Boy Scouts of America, Crossroads of America Council—Chairperson
National Association of Health Services Executive—Member
Robert Wood Johnson National Advisory Committee—Member
United Way of Central Indiana—Chairperson
Rehabilitation Hospital of Indiana—Board Member
American Registry of Radiologic Technologists—Member
Black and Minority Health Advisory Committee—Member
Governor's Family and Social Services Advisory Committee—Member
Governor's Technology Roundtable—Member
Governor's Indiana Adult Literacy Coalition—Member
Health Administrators' Forum—President
Mayor's Task Force on Housing—Co-Chairperson
National Advisory Council for Emerging Leaders/Healthcare Forum—Member

Select Awards
IHA Distinguished Service Award: 2009
Most Powerful People in Healthcare: 2006
National Emerging Leader in Healthcare Award: 1990

JOHN C. RENDER, J.D.

Education

J.D.
Indiana School of Law
Indianapolis, Indiana

Selected Work Experience

Partner
Hall, Render, Killian, Heath & Lyman, P.C.
Indianapolis, Indiana

Adjunct Instructor, MHA Program
Indiana University
Indianapolis, Indiana

Selected Community Service & Associations: Past & Present

Indiana State Bar Association—Member
Michigan Bar Association—Member
District of Columbia Bar Association—Member
American Bar Association—Member
American Health Lawyers Association—Member
Advisory Board of Indiana University Robert H. McKinney School of Law—Member
Indiana Hospital Association—General Council
State of Indiana Health Policy Advisory Committee—Member
State of Indiana Health Finance Advisory Committee—Member
Board of Visitors of Indiana University Robert H. McKinney School of Law—Member

Selected Awards

Indianapolis Bar Foundation Distinguished Fellow Award
IU School of Law Distinguish Alumni Award
Indiana Hospital Association Award of Merit
Sagamore of the Wabash
IU MHA Program Outstanding Professor Award

KENNETH G. STELLA, FACHE

Education

Master of Health Administration
Indiana University
Indianapolis, Indiana

Selected Work Experience

Chairman
Board of Directors
St. Vincent Hospital
Indianapolis, Indiana

President
Indiana Hospital Association
Indianapolis, Indiana

Administrator
Morgan County Hospital
Martinsville, Indiana

Selected Community Service & Associations: Past & Present

American College of Healthcare Executives (ACHE)—Fellow
ACHE Health Associations Committee—Member
ACHE Public Policy Committee—Member
Indiana University Alumni Association—Member
AHAPAC Steering Committee—Member
American Hospital Association's State Issues Forum—Member
Lincoln National Life Insurance Company Variable Annuity Fund—Member
Harris Bank—Advisory Board Member
BSA LifeStructures—Advisory Board Member
Regenstrief Center for Healthcare Engineering—Board Member
Indiana University School of Public and Environmental Affairs
Board of Visitors—Member

Selected Awards

American Hospital Association Board of Trustees Award: 2006
Indiana Hospital Association Award of Merit: 2006
Sagamore of the Wabash: 1990

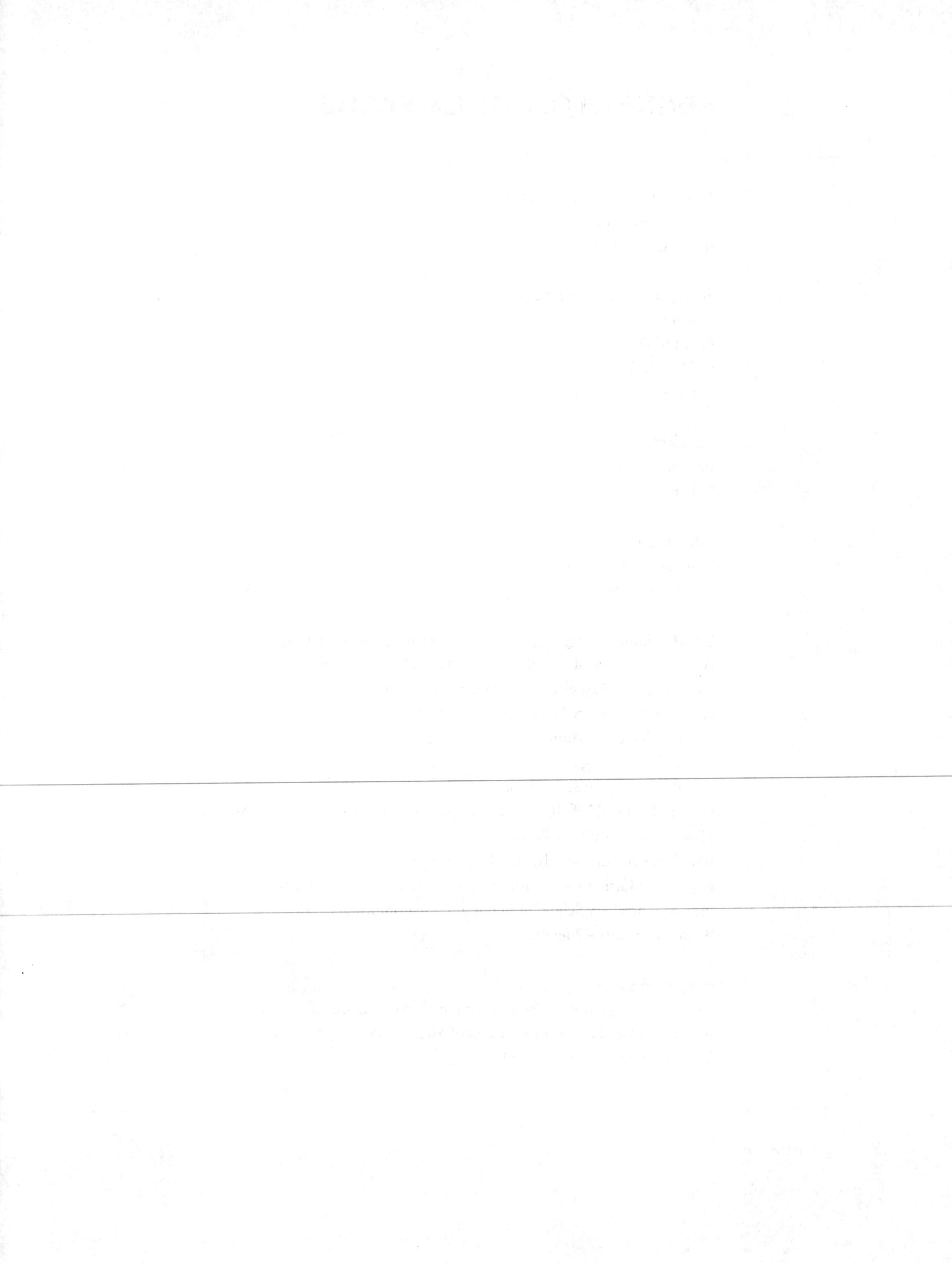

What Would You Do?

- The highest performing Department Manager, who reports directly to you as the hospital Assistant Administrator, has been seen recently by several employees out on the town and intoxicated several times. This manager hasn't caused any problems or gotten into any trouble. Approximately 6 months ago, this manager was divorced by his wife of 20 years. What do you do?
- You've taken a new job at a large hospital to help analyze and manage its readmissions and develop an initiative to reduce readmissions. The hospital's overall readmission rates are higher than approximately 70% of hospitals in the state. Identify key steps you'd take in the first 30 days.
- You are the new CEO of a community health center. Your administrative assistant has been in her role for approximately 18 years. After the first month, you realize she doesn't have the proficiency or skills to help you perform at the high level you'll need to. She is slow, unreliable, and doesn't take initiative. You constantly have to give her detailed instructions on everything. What do you do?
- You are the CEO of a small hospital. You are having a problem with office computers being stolen. Your maintenance supervisor thinks one of the housekeeping employees is taking these

computers at night (when he works). You have installed a video camera and have someone on tape taking a computer out of an office during the night; however, you don't have a good, clear picture of the person's face. The maintenance supervisor states the video positively identifies the housekeeping employee as the thief. You aren't sure it does. What do you do?

- You are the COO of a medium-size hospital. Six months ago, the hospital went with a smoke-free campus policy. However, the sidewalk around the hospital is city property. Some of the employees stand on the sidewalk on breaks and smoke and encourage patients and families who smoke to do the same. It looks bad. What do you do?
- You are the COO of a medium-size hospital. The hospital's customer service is "average." You have been driving an initiative to get employees engaged and improve customer service. You are convinced that employee roleplaying and coaching at the department level is critical to enhancing employee engagement and accountability for customer service. Moreover, there hasn't been a culture of accountability for department managers or vice presidents regarding customer service. What do you do to make this happen?
- You are the CEO of a small, proprietary hospital. The hospital needs to improve its financial performance and cash flow in order to meet its budget. The problem is there hasn't been a culture of accountability at the department level for financial performance. Identify key steps to take to address this situation.
- You are COO of a medium-size hospital and responsible for all operations, including human resources. The hospital's employee recognition program involves an annual dinner whereby employees are recognized for their length of service. Vice presidents, department heads, and supervisors are expected to attend. Everyone complains about the program, and managers don't want to attend, because it is boring and just routine. The same format has been used for 15 years. Moreover, you believe that employee performance and service should also be recognized, not just length of service. What do you do?
- You are hired as the new COO of a medium-size hospital to direct a project to replace the old, outdated facility. You believe the hospital should develop a 10-year master site and facility plan. Identify the major steps you should take to get this initiative organized and underway.
- You are the CEO of a small proprietary hospital in an urban area. Your boss at corporate is putting pressure on you to get your accounts receivable (A/R) days down from 65 to 50 days within the next 90-day period. Your business office manager seems to make a logical argument for why A/R days are at 65; however, corporate wants a plan on how you'll get A/R days to 50 within 90 days. What do you do?
- You are the COO of a medium-size hospital and responsible for operations. 6 months into your new fiscal year, the hospital is way off budget (income from operations is $2 million below budget on an annual income budget of $10 million). What steps do you take to get your hands around the main problems and turn things around?

- You are the hospital CEO of a medium-size hospital. Your top admitting surgeon may start his own ambulatory surgery center with 10 other surgeons on staff. Surgical services provide the largest contribution to your hospital's bottom line than any service. What do you do?
- You are the CEO of a small suburban hospital. The hospital has touted its "Sanctuary of Healing," which features patient-centered care. Patient satisfaction is high; however, you want to drive action to strengthen the culture of caring in the hospital. What do you do?
- You are the COO of a 350-bed hospital. You recently moved the CNO out who had been working at the hospital for 18 years and was close to retirement. You are in the hiring process for the new CNO with one candidate internal and the other external. Both candidates appear to be equally qualified. What process and factors should you consider in this hiring decision?
- You are the CEO of a medium-size hospital. The hospital's Medical Director is an excellent physician and good friend; however, he continues to make subtle passes at female nurses and tells them dirty jokes after you have spoken with him about this and he agreed to stop. What do you do?
- You are the CEO of a small hospital. Your board chairman has started allowing himself to get "sucked in" to employee complaints and then periodically asking you about them. Some of the complaints are just incidents of employee manipulation. What do you do?
- You are the assistant administrator at a medium-size hospital and responsible for quality/performance improvement. The hospital's top admitting general surgeon's clinical outcomes aren't very good, and the hospital gets periodic complaints from patients. The medical staff supports the general surgeon (with a few exceptions). You really can't tell exactly what is happening with the care by reviewing the medical record, as you feel the surgeon isn't accurately documenting his care and interactions with the patients (for example, the documentation may misrepresent the level of pain the patient is experiencing). The documentation in the medical record is thorough and complete, but it may not be accurate. What do you do?
- You are the hospital CEO of a 50-bed hospital and desperate to recruit an additional orthopedic surgeon. You currently have one orthopedic surgeon who is ultra-selective and very conservative when it comes to operating on patients (i.e., he doesn't do much surgery). Also, although this physician's outcomes are good, he is slow, and the hospital is losing market share in orthopedics because of him. However, you have approached him about recruitment, and he is threatened and won't assist the hospital in recruiting. Moreover, he tells orthopedic candidates there isn't enough business for another orthopedic surgeon and recruits are scared away. What do you do?
- You are the new Vice President of Planning and Marketing at a 200-bed, community hospital. The hospital is in a market with a number of competitors. You discover the current strategic plan is five years old, isn't being followed, and isn't very good. There doesn't seem to be much emphasis on planning, change, or innovation within the hospital. Market share is eroding. What steps do you take to address this situation?
- You are the Director of Environmental Services at a mid-size hospital. One of your employees is chronically late to work and excessively absent. This situation negatively impacts the department and all the employees. You've talked to the employee repeatedly and have given this employee

several verbal and written warnings. Nothing has changed. You feel it is past time to terminate this employee per hospital policy; however, this employee is good friends with your boss, the Vice President of Support Services. When you've talked with your boss about the situation, he has clearly stated ***"Do whatever you think you should; however, don't fire that employee."*** What do you do?

- As the Vice President of Professional Services at a mid-size hospital, you are administratively responsible for surgical services. The morale in surgery has recently dropped off and several good, long-term surgical nurses have resigned due to the behavior of a new neurosurgeon. The new physician has outstanding credentials and provides excellent care. He has a good bedside manner and is personable with patients. However, he is egotistical, overbearing, demanding, and inappropriate with the staff. What should you do?
- You are the new Administrator of a 100-bed skilled nursing facility. When you interviewed for the position, you were made aware of the poor morale and high turnover of staff, so coming in, you knew this would be a top priority in the first few months on the job. You are now in your second week. Identify some of the initial steps you should take to address this problem.
- You are the Practice Administrator for a group of six family physicians. One of the physicians has now turned 80 years old and is still practicing four days per week. There are growing rumblings that his quality is really starting to slip, and he is becoming forgetful. The other physicians are reluctant to address the situation, because this physician has been with the group for 30 years and is well liked and respected. What do you do?
- You are Director of Human Resources of a large, multi-specialty group practice. The practice has 75 physicians and 350 employees. You provide health insurance under a fully-insured group health plan with a large carrier who has quoted rates for the new plan year that are 17% above the current year. The carrier says the rate increase is attributed to plan experience: high utilization of services and higher costs incurred by the plan. This rate increase is way beyond your budget or what will work financially. What do you do?
- You are the Director of Materials Management at a mid-size hospital. One of your buyers, who has been in the department for about a year, is performing at an acceptable level; however, you believe this employee has much more potential to work harder and perform at a much higher level. Identify what steps you should take to address this situation.
- You've just started a new position as the CEO of a community mental health center is a mid-size community. You are excited as this is your first CEO position. Within the first 30 days, you realize there has been no vision for the organization and its future. Employees, managers, and physicians in all areas have expressed they don't know where the organization is heading or what the priorities are. People seem to be de-motivated by this. The organization does not have a strategic plan or goals it strives to achieve. What do you do?

References

Healthcare Strategic Planning, Second Edition, by Alan M. Zuckerman.

Strategic Management of Health Care Organizations, Sixth Edition, by Linda A. Swayne, W. Jack Duncan, and Peter M. Ginter.

Effective Management, Fourth Edition, by Chuck Williams.

A Framework For Marketing Management, Third Edition, by Philip Kotler and Kevin Lane Keller.

www.wikipedia.org

Yorker, Beatrice, Kenneth W. Kizer, Paula Lampe, A.R.W. Forrest, Jacquetta Lannan, and Donna Russell. "Serial Murder by Healthcare Professionals." *Forensic Science 51.6* (2006): 1362–1371

https://en.wikipedia.org/wiki/Employee Retirement Income Security Act of 1974

Ray Martin, *MoneyWatch*, October 24, 2017

Stephen Miller, "2018 FSA Contribution Cap Rises to $2,650," *Society for Human Resource Management*, October 23, 2017.

https://www.zanebenefits.com/blog/how-to-tell-if-your-high-deductible-health-plan-is-hsa-qualified

Indiana Hospital Association. "Eleven Ways Indiana Businesses Are Attempting to Cut Health Care Costs." *Harmony*.

Glossary

ACCOUNTABILITY: Being responsible for one's own actions to another person or governing body.

ACTION PLAN: A concrete, detailed list of steps to take in order to accomplish a goal or objective.

ACTIVE LISTENING: The process of paying close attention to a speaker or the sender of a message in order to fully understand and engage with the communication.

ADJOURNING: The final stage of teamwork, during which team members review outcomes, analyze methodologies, provide feedback, and disband.

APPROPRIATENESS OF CARE: An approach to evaluating whether specific medical care is warranted. It is a potential-costs / -benefits analysis weighing receiving the treatment vs. not receiving the treatment.

AUTHORITY: The power or right to give and enforce commands, to make decisions on behalf of a larger group.

AUTONOMY: The ability to self-govern, free of the controlling influence of others.

AVAILABLE MARKET: Potential clientele, identified to have the income and interest that would align with a company's products or services.

BALANCED SCORECARD: Organizational performance measured typically within four equally important areas: customers, finances, internal operations, and innovation/learning.

BECOMING: An adjective to describe something as appropriate, fitting, worthy, or compatible, but can also mean attractive, enhancing, or flattering.

BENCHMARKING: A tactic for improving business processes by comparing internal operations to competitors' operations.

BEST PRACTICES: Processes and procedures that are relied on because they are believed to produce the best outcomes.

BIAS: Adjusting behavior or thought toward a person or within a situation because of one's own prejudices, which may or may not necessarily be obvious internally or externally.

BRAINSTORMING: A method in which members of a group try to generate as many ideas as possible using open, quick communication to build off of each other and inspire and provoke new thoughts.

BRAND EQUITY: The perceived value and quality of a particular product or service offered by a particular company, as opposed to the product or service in of itself. For example, a popular, brand-name drug may be perceived as higher in quality than a generic drug, even if both drugs can clinically be shown to be equally effective.

BRAND IMAGE: An identity or impression crafted by a company to influence the behavior of consumers. Active and potential consumers can also shape brand image based on their perceptions or beliefs toward the company or even a company's signature product or service.

BRANDING: The creation of a unique way for a consumer to recognize and remember goods and services offered by a business or organization.

BRAND KNOWLEDGE: The cumulative emotional and physical experiences, including thoughts, feelings, memories, and beliefs, associated with a particular brand.

BRAND LOYALTY: The habit or propensity for a consumer to return to a particular product or company to fulfill a need.

BRAND PROMISE: The perceived or explicit commitment to a consumer of what a company offers to the market, consistency and integrity in how a company operates.

BUDGET: The financial parameters in which a person, group, or company can operate for a set period of time.

CAPITAL BUDGET: The plan for how an organization will invest in its development. Examples of major capital expenditure items that would be budgeted include research and development, opening new offices, or upgrading manufacturing machinery.

CENTERS FOR DISEASE CONTROL AND PREVENTION (CDC): An agency of the U.S. Department of Health and Human Services that works to promote good health and high quality of life by preventing and controlling disease through vaccines, research, and education. This agency also tracks disease and illness outside of the U.S. and provides information to travelers.

CENTERS FOR MEDICARE AND MEDICAID SERVICES (CMS): A federal agency within the Department of Health and Human Services that oversees Medicare, Medicaid, and health insurance exchanges.

CENTRALIZED DECISION MAKING CULTURE: An environment in which most or all decisions are made by one person or a small group of people at the top of a company's hierarchy.

CHAIN OF COMMAND: The order in which authority is structured within a company or organization.

CHANGE AGENT: A person formally or informally appointed to make sure planned change occurs.

CHANNEL: The means used to deliver or convey a marketing message. A direct channel refers to the message going straight to the consumer or client.

CHARGEMASTER: The complete, thorough, itemized listing of all services and prices charged, especially for medical treatment.

CIRCULATION: The number of people reached through a particular medium, especially a magazine or newspaper.

CODE OF ETHICS: A written statement describing the set of moral principles and values a company strives to follow in its business practices.

COERCION: The use of force or the threat of force to compel action.

COGNITIVE DISSONANCE: A mental state of anxiety and uncertainty resulting in inconsistent, unpredictable behavior.

COLLABORATION: Promoting cohesiveness or the extent to which team members are attracted to a team and motivated to remain with it and work together with others

COMMUNICATION: The interaction between entities in which information is shared, verbally or otherwise.

COMPETENCY: Having the skills and abilities to function in an efficient, successful manner.

COMPETITIVE ADVANTAGE: A unique strength or distinction of an organization that provides an added value or benefit to consumers.

CONCEPTUAL SKILLS: The ability to think abstractly or creatively to understand and explain complex ideas.

CONCEPTUAL SKILLS: The ability to think in more abstract, creative ways in order to better analyze and address issues, challenges, and opportunities. Such skills are particularly important in management and leadership roles where a holistic or bird's-eye-view perspective is critical to the success of the business or organization as a whole.

CONFLICT OF INTEREST: When someone has a responsibility to another person or organization but decision-making with respect to that duty would affect one's own welfare as well, thus calling into question the ability to truly act neutrally and dutifully with the other person's or organization's best interest at heart.

CONSTRUCTIVE FEEDBACK: Feedback meant to be helpful and encouraging.

CONSULTATIVE SELLING: An approach to selling goods or services by focusing on consumer needs, which often results in a customized solution for a more personal seller-buyer relationship.

CONSUMER DECISION-MAKING PROCESS: Typically characterized by recognizing a need, gathering information, weighing options, choosing an option, and then evaluating the decision.

CONSUMER GOODS: Products purchased for the intended purpose of being used by the consumer directly, such as food or clothing, rather than goods that are purchased for the creation or manufacturing of other goods.

CONTINGENCY PLAN: An alternative plan that can be put into use should existing factors, needs, or goals suddenly change.

CONTINUOUS QUALITY IMPROVEMENT (CQI): Based on the idea that there is always room for improvement, this process focuses on routinely striving to make better a service or product. It is also sometimes known as Performance and Quality Improvement (PQI).

CONTINUUM OF CARE: The concept of tracking a patient's history of medical care in order to better understand and predict patient needs. Refers also to a program (CoC) started in 1995 through the Department of Housing and Urban Development that provides services to the homeless.

CONTRACTUAL ALLOWANCE: The discrepancy between what hospitals bill and what they are paid by third parties such as Medicare.

CONTROL: A process in which performance or goods are compared to established standards as a means to check for quality.

CONTROLLING: A core function of management in which performance is monitored, compared to expected performance, and corrected as necessary.

CONTROLLING: A management function that involves monitoring progress as it compares to set standards and goals and taking corrective action as needed to keep an organization's plans on track.

CORE COMPETENCY: A concept in management theory that encourages businesses to seek out a key, unique aspect of itself that would be difficult for competitors to imitate.

CORPORATE COMMUNICATION: Communication representing the business or organization as a whole.

CORPORATE COMPETENCIES: A company's expertise, techniques, and abilities that shape and produce critical organizational strengths.

CORPORATE CULTURE: The values, beliefs, and behaviors that become common within an organization. New people brought into the corporate culture tend to take on and express the surrounding values, beliefs, and behaviors.

CRITICAL INTANGIBLES OF LEADERSHIP: Aspects or characteristics of a leader that are crucial for success, yet are difficult to clearly define and measure, such as wisdom, integrity, and good judgment.

CUSTOMER LOYALTY: The level of customer commitment toward a business and the expectation that the customer will patronize the business again.

CUSTOMER RELATIONSHIP MANAGEMENT: The process of managing customer information and business-customer interactions to maximize customer loyalty.

DASHBOARD REPORT: A report that brings the most important information together to one main source for easy readability and understanding, often color-coded and with additional features like charts and graphs.

DATA MINING: The distillation or extraction of useful information from a wider source of knowledge.

DECENTRALIZED DECISION MAKING CULTURE: An environment in which people within different levels of authority are able to influence what's going on.

DECISION CRITERIA: Variables or qualities considered when trying to compare several options against each other to pick the best option.

DECISION FREEDOM: The idea that people tend to feel happier when they have—or perceive to have—more choices.

DECODING: Interpreting or analyzing the words and sometimes hidden symbols or meanings of a message.

DEDUCTIBLE: A specified amount of spending that goes toward health services for which an individual or a family is responsible before health insurance coverage takes over.

DEFENSIVE MEDICINE: Treatment or service recommended by a doctor having more to do with the intention of minimizing the risk for litigation rather than providing a patient with medical care that is truly necessary.

DEFINED CONTRIBUTION: A type of financial plan, usually for retirement, in which the employer and employee both provide consistent monetary input for the employee's benefit.

DELEGATION: The act of exercising authority to assign tasks and responsibilities. This word can also refer to a group of people who act as representatives for a larger entity such as a school, company, or even country.

DESTRUCTIVE FEEDBACK: Feedback given without any clear intention of being helpful, criticism that may even be used to provoke a negative or defensive reaction from the recipient of the feedback.

DIFFERENTIATION: The positioning strategy of a product or service that stands out among the competition, often at a higher price that consumers are willing to pay for due to perceived increased value.

DIRECT COSTS: Costs that are related to a specific activity of an organization. Contrast with *indirect costs.*

DIRECTION OF EFFORT: Refers to the choices people make in how they use their time and energy and for what outcomes.

DISCOUNTED FEE-FOR-SERVICE: A plan member pays for a medical provider's service but receives a discount on the fee. The provider typically offers a discount to plan members in an effort to increase the volume of patients.

DISCRETIONARY EFFORT: The level of involvement and focus an employee is generally willing to give or happens to be giving at any given time beyond the minimum requirements for a task.

DISPARATE TREATMENT: Intentional discrimination that occurs when someone is purposely not given the same hiring, promotion, membership, or other opportunities due to their race, age, gender, religious beliefs, etc.

DISTINCTION: The way in which someone or something stands out.

DIVERSIFICATION: A risk-reducing investment strategy where money is spread across multiple sectors or businesses within a sector so that a failure does not wipe out the entirety of the investment.

DIVERSITY: Variety, often in relation to characteristics such race, ethnicity, religion, gender, age, physical ability, educational level, and socioeconomic status.

DURABLE GOOD: A product that is able to last over a longer period of time.

DURABLE POWER OF ATTORNEY: Power of attorney assigns the power for one person to legally act on behalf of the other. The power is durable if the power granted persists when the grantor has become mentally incapacitated. An agent with durable power of attorney could make financial and medical decisions for the incapacitated, if they were so empowered.

ECONOMIC RESPONSIBILITY: An aspect of social responsibility wherein a company strives to establish stable longevity and continue to make a profit, contributing to the overall wellness of the economy.

EFFECTIVENESS: The level of success in a product, service, or action.

EFFICIENCY: Maximum results with minimum effort, cost, or waste.

EMERGENCY MEDICAL TREATMENT AND ACTIVE LABOR ACT (EMTALA): A statute requiring hospitals to treat people who come into their emergency rooms with a medical issue regardless of ability to pay. Created as a legislative response to "patient-dumping" in which hospitals would refuse to treat patients based on their ability to pay and would transfer them to a different medical institution.

EMOTIONAL INTELLIGENCE (EI) / Emotional Quotient (EQ): An individual's ability to differentiate and accurately recognize emotions in themselves and others and to appropriately identify the connection between inferred emotion and observed behavior. Empathy is a key aspect of emotional intelligence.

EMOTIONAL INTELLIGENCE (EQ): A person's level of self-awareness and the emotional states of others, as well as the ability to see the link between feelings and behaviors and the ability to control one's own emotions.

EMPATHETIC LEADERSHIP: A style of leadership where the leader is in touch with and responsive to the emotional needs and dynamics of their followers.

EMPATHETIC LISTENING: The process in which the listener aims to understand the speaker by considering the speaker's perspective and background and possibly suspending the listener's own perspective and bias.

EMPLOYEE ENGAGEMENT: A measurement of an employee's level of motivation and involvement within the work environment for personal, interpersonal, and company-wide success.

EMPOWERMENT: Granting others the ability to exercise some level of autonomy or be more involved in decision-making, creative thinking, and problem solving.

ENCODING: Converting meaning into words or symbols.

ENVIRONMENTAL SCANNING: Searching and analyzing surrounding external factors and how they might affect a business or organization.

EQUITY THEORY: The idea that people are motivated when they operate within a system they believe to be fair. If an employee perceives to be treated unfairly, the employee will seek out ways to return to a level of fairness.

ETHICAL BEHAVIOR: Behavior that follows accepted social principles and standards of what is moral and decent.

ETHICAL CULTURE: Within an organization, the shared beliefs about what it means to behave ethically.

ETHICAL DILEMMA: A challenging situation that requires a decision or action that is not obvious or clear-cut. These situations often have negative and positive aspects to any of the possible choices, or where the actor in the situation could be tempted to reap benefit while harming others.

ETHICAL RESPONSIBILITY: The premise that organizations should be considering the morality of their actions and not simply acting in a purely self-interested way.

ETHICS: The set of moral principles or values that shapes the behavior of a person or group.

ETHICS TRAINING: Educational sessions to teach employees to consider the ethical consequences of their decisions and actions. Typically includes ethical dilemmas and explores the consequences of potential responses to a situation. The goal is to increase how ethically the organization behaves.

EXCHANGE: A core marketing concept describing a transaction between two parties who each have something desirable to the other.

EXPECTANCY THEORY: A theory popularized by Victor Vroom from the Yale School of Management that states a person's behavior is, at its most simplistic level, motivated to maximize pleasure and minimize pain, and therefore employees will be motivated to perform well if they believe good effort will lead to good performance, that good performance will be rewarded, and that the rewards will be worthwhile.

EXPENSE: A cost incurred in daily operations.

EXTRINSIC REWARD: A reward that is tangible and visible to others, such as a bonus, prize, or certificate of excellence, and serves as a source of motivation.

FEEDBACK: Assessment provided for review of an action to determine strengths and weaknesses of the situation.

FIRST DOLLAR COVERAGE: Health insurance that covers every cost associated with an insured event. The coverage typically has a maximum, but below this maximum, the insured will incur no costs (such as the deductible).

FIXED COSTS: Expenses that do not change with growth or amount of production. See *variable costs*.

FLOW: A state of mind popularized by positive psychologist Mihály Csíkszentmihályi in which focus and productivity come effortlessly.

FOCUS GROUPS: A number of people with particular backgrounds or experiences who are interviewed by a trained facilitator in order to gather feedback that then helps shape a business's offerings or behavior.

FOLLOWERSHIP: The capacity of a subordinate to effectively follow a leader and to skillfully work toward the goals set by the leader.

FOOD AND DRUG ADMINISTRATION (FDA): A federal agency of the United States government tasked with protecting the public health. The FDA exercises regulatory authority over foods, drugs, medical devices, biologics (e.g. vaccines and blood products), devices that produce radiation, cosmetics, veterinary products, and tobacco.

FORECASTING: Projections or estimates for the short term as well as the long term, the anticipation of buyer or consumer behavior based on collected information.

FORMAL POWER: The authority granted by possessing a role or title within an organization. Contrast with *informal power*.

FORMING: The first stage of teamwork where members of a team identify their collective purpose and goals.

FOSTERING: Encouragement or promotion to develop, nurture, initiate, or revitalize something.

FRAUD AND ABUSE: Intentional billing on the part of health providers at a cost that is higher than normal or for services not rendered at all in order to unfairly profit from the patient. According to the CMS, abuse refers here to when health providers incorrectly charge a patient *by mistake*, with no deliberate ill-will.

FREQUENCY: The amount of times information or communication is conveyed to the recipient within a particular time frame.

GATEKEEPING: The role of a patient's main health service provider, such as a primary care physician (PCP), in establishing the patient's plan for care and for access to medical specialists.

GENERAL ENVIRONMENT: Any external factors, including political, technological, economic, and cultural factors, that may influence a company's operations.

GOAL-SETTING THEORY: The idea that people can become and remain motivated to reach a goal if they receive feedback and see indication of progress toward that goal.

GOAL: A desired outcome or intended result for a course of action.

GROSS RATING POINTS: A standard measure used in advertising to gauge reach and an advertisement's effectiveness.

GROSS REVENUE: Revenue reflecting full charge for services and products without regard to discounts or refunds that occurred.

GROUPTHINK: When a group reaches a level of decision-making and communication that begins to shut out the input of an individual within the group, thus creating a work environment that diminishes creativity and individual responsibility.

GROWTH STRATEGY: A strategy focusing on increased revenues, market share, profit, and reach.

HEALTH CARE OUTCOMES: The resultant change in a patient's health due to the care they received.

HEALTH PROMOTION: Individual, social, and environmental programs and services that help people improve their physical and mental well-being. Such efforts aim to reduce health risks and increase self-care skills.

HOSTILE WORK ENVIRONMENT: When recurring behavior in the workplace creates an uncomfortable, intimidating, or even unsafe professional setting.

INCOME STATEMENT: A report showing the financial activities of an organization or individual.

INCREMENTAL CHANGE: Small, generally non-disruptive or threatening adjustments to an existing process or policy that, over time, guide a company to a larger shift in behavior.

INDIRECT COSTS: A cost of doing business that is not tied to any narrow or specific activity. Liability insurance is an example of an indirect cost. Contrast with *direct costs.*

INFORMAL POWER: The ability to lead and influence by virtue of skill or personality. Contrast with *formal power.*

INITIATION OF EFFORT: The analysis of how employees decide which tasks to prioritize and when.

INSTITUTIONAL ADVERTISING: Promotes the company or organization itself, rather than any specific product or service the company or organization offers.

INTERDISCIPLINARY TEAM: A group of diverse individuals representing different disciplines working together to accomplish a mutual goal.

INTERNAL MARKETING: The process of strengthening loyalty and satisfaction with customers more directly from within the company by, for example, building long-term customer relationships and facilitating trust.

INTERNAL RECRUITING: Filling new or newly vacant positions with existing employees rather than hiring people from outside the company.

INTERPERSONAL SKILLS: Skills that demonstrate a person's ability to communicate and otherwise interact with others. Also known as social skills or people skills, strong interpersonal skills often play a critical role not just in employment but in job retention.

INVISIBLE VALUE: Value not explicitly seen or perceived by the customer but can nonetheless influence a positive experience for the customer and encourage brand loyalty.

JOB ANALYSIS: The identification of details related to a job, details that include the skills needed to do the job well, any tools or equipment needed for the job, and environmental and other working conditions of the job. Such analysis helps shape employment need and performance evaluation.

JOB DESCRIPTION: The tasks, responsibilities, expectations, etc. associated with a particular employment position and typically defined clearly in a document.

JOB EVALUATION: A process in which the job and the skills and knowledge required to perform it successfully are identified and analyzed, used to measure expectations, growth, and need. Companies typically use job evaluations to, for example, set pay scales and offer promotions.

LEADERSHIP STYLE: The approach taken to inspire, motivate, and organize others in order to achieve a mutual goal.

LEADING: Guiding, motivating, and inspiring others to achieve defined goals.

LEGACY: Important and persisting consequences that continue beyond the entity that created them.

LEVEL OF AUTHORITY: Concerns one's hierarchical level in an organization.

LINE AUTHORITY: A person empowered by his or her organization to direct the work activity of others. The essential authority that establishes a superior-subordinate relationship

LINE FUNCTION: Any activity within an organization that contributes to generating income.

MALPRACTICE: Negligence by a health care provider.

MANAGED CARE: A type of health care plan in which the central organization providing the plan restricts the healthcare choices the covered can make. The stated goal of managed care is to reduce costs and increase quality of care.

MANAGEMENT: The process of coordinating, organizing, and supervising the tasks of a company or group in order to achieve the company or group's collective goals.

MANAGEMENT BY OBJECTIVES: A managerial approach popularized in 1954 by Peter Drucker in which employees at all levels within a company create group objectives and then remain involved in monitoring and reviewing work done to achieve those objectives.

MARKETING AUDIT: A thorough, independent examination of a company's objectives, strategies, processes, behaviors, target market, and marketing environment, among other things.

MARKETING CHANNELS: A series of interdependent organizations involved in the process of making a product or providing a service to consumers.

MARKETING FUNCTION: The approach a company takes to analyze its role for consumers and what else or how else it might offer goods or services for continued growth.

MARKETING MANAGEMENT: The process of acquiring and keeping new customers through specialized initiatives and strategies targeted at particular segments in the marketplace.

MARKETING METRICS: A way of measuring a company's performance in its marketing efforts.

MARKETING MIX: The variety of ways a company tries to acquire new clients, from product design and packaging to pricing, discounting, promotions, and availability.

MARKETING ORIENTATION: A philosophy in which meeting consumer needs and wants are the primary sources of motivation for a company.

MARKETING PLAN: A concise plan summarizing the existing marketplace, a company's marketing objectives, and the strategies and initiatives a company intends to follow for successful marketing efforts.

MARKETING RESEARCH: The gathering and analysis of consumer buying habits.

MARKETING TOUCH POINTS: Interactions or situations in which a customer experiences communication with a company or organization that then influence the customer's attitude toward the company or organization.

MARKETPLACE: A physical as well as figurative territory within which buyers and sellers interact for the exchange of goods, where products and services compete.

MARKET SEGMENT: A particular group of consumers who have similar wants or needs based on such characteristics like income, age, gender, geographic location, etc.

MARKET SEGMENTATION: The process in which consumers are grouped by similar wants or needs.

MARKET SHARE: A part of the market or clientele base belonging to a specific company or organization.

MASLOW'S HIERARCHY OF NEEDS: A psychological theory first proposed in 1943 by Abraham Maslow that organizes basic human needs into five categories within the shape of a pyramid, ascending in priority.

The needs are, starting from the bottom of the pyramid: psychological, safety, love/belonging, esteem, and self-actualization.

MASS MARKETING: Appealing to the largest group of consumers possible without segmentation or differentiation.

MEANINGFUL USE: Also known as the Electronic Health Records (EHR) Incentive Program, this term refers to a process in which medical history information is streamlined in order to create more easily accessible, thorough, and transparent medical records to facilitate clear communication among providers, insurers, and patients.

MEDIUM: A mechanism or tool, such as TV, magazines, radio, email, text messaging, art, and music, used to convey information and facilitate communication.

MESSAGE: A concise amount of information communicated from one entity to another.

MILESTONES: Formalized role or project review points used to assess performance and growth.

MISSION STATEMENT: A succinct, official summary describing the organization's purpose or reason for being, generally outward-facing and accessible to the public.

MOTIVATION: The reason that compels a particular behavior or action.

NEEDS: The physical or psychological requirements for survival and well-being.

NEEDS SATISFACTION SELLING: A sales approach that focuses on identifying and meeting a customer's needs.

NEGATIVE REINFORCEMENT: An approach described by psychologist B. F. Skinner in which behavior is strengthened when something is removed or stopped, such as when a source of distraction is taken away or altered to increase productivity. Also known as avoidance learning.

NET REVENUE: The money an organization has taken in. Can differ from gross revenue because it accounts for everything that affects revenue, such as discounts and refunds.

NON-DURABLE GOOD: An item with a short shelf-life, one that needs to be consumed or used within a defined period of time.

NONVERBAL COMMUNICATION: Conveying information without expressing words.

NONVERBAL CUES: Facial expressions, body language, gestures, tone and volume of voice, clothing, and other outlets for conveying information without words.

NORMING: The third stage of teamwork in which the team overcomes internal conflict and agree upon working styles and approaches to communication. During this stage, the team's goals and processes may be redefined or further shaped.

NORMS: Agreed-upon standards, usually casual, that regulate team behavior.

NOSOCOMIAL INFECTION: An infection or illness acquired while at a hospital, also referred to as HAIs. Common HAIs include urinary tract, skin, and respiratory infections.

OBJECTIVE PERFORMANCE MEASURES: Job performance measurements that are easily and clearly quantified.

OPERATIONAL PLANS: The day-to-day processes and strategies developed and implemented within an organization to ensure a regular production schedule, such as within a 30-day period.

OPERATION BUDGET: An appraisal of expected revenue and costs for a given time period.

OPERATIONS MANAGEMENT: Developing and executing the processes that create an organization's product or service output.

OPERATIONS MANAGEMENT: Management of routine practices and the regular production of goods and/or services.

ORGANIZATIONAL CHART: Shows the formal structure, hierarchy, and chain of command within an organization.

ORGANIZATIONAL CULTURE: The patterns of behavior reflecting the shared values, beliefs, and attitude of members within an organization.

ORGANIZATIONAL DEVELOPMENT: Planned effort and the study of an organization's current and expected growth and performance.

ORGANIZATIONAL ETHICS: Guiding standards of behavior that an organization adopts. The intent is to produce ethical or moral behavior, which may be at odds with maximizing financial outcomes.

ORGANIZATIONAL FIT: An employee's compatibility with the values, mission statement, and work environment of a company or organization.

ORGANIZING: Identifying needs and goals and creating a clearly defined structure or process to ensure those needs and goals are met as efficiently as possible.

OUT-OF-POCKET PAYMENT: The amount one is expected to pay personally, without insurance or other financial assistance, for health services.

OUTSIDE INSIGHT: Feedback used to help us see and understand what we don't know about ourselves. This kind of data often identifies areas of growth for an existing business or can help shape the direction of a start-up.

PARTICIPATORY LEADERSHIP: A style of management in which the leader encourages and values employee input toward decision-making.

PATH-GOAL LEADERSHIP THEORY: The way in which leaders motivate followers to successfully achieve their goals, thus creating a mutually beneficial and inspiring environment.

PATIENT SATISFACTION: Measurements attained often through direct-to-patient surveys that help indicate the quality of medical care.

PAY-FOR-PERFORMANCE (P4P): Payment models, also known as value-based purchasing, that offer financial incentives to healthcare providers for achieving certain pre-determined performance goals.

PERCEPTION: The ability to use sensory information to achieve understanding or awareness.

PERFORMANCE APPRAISAL/EVALUATION: A formal process of employee evaluation carried out by a superior. Sometimes an employee's colleagues provide input for the evaluation. The employee is given feedback on performance. Compensation and promotions can be tied to performance evaluations.

PERFORMANCE APPRAISAL/EVALUATION: Work behavior and efforts reviewed and analyzed to document an employee's professional growth.

PERFORMING: The fourth stage of teamwork marked by progress and reaching goals without conflict, when team members are producing results and showing dedication and commitment.

PERSISTENCE OF EFFORT: An analysis of how long and with what intensity employees stay on task.

PLANNING: The process of developing a strategy to achieve a goal.

PLANNING HORIZON: The length of time into the future an organization considers in its strategic planning.

POINT-OF-SERVICE (POS) PLAN: With a POS health care plan, the insured has reduced costs for less control over from whom they receive care. The insured has a primary care physician (PCP) who is always the first point of contact for any health issue. If the PCP refers the patient to out-of-network providers, then the insurance company pays far less of the resulting medical bill. It is a type of managed-care plan (see *managed care*).

POINTS-OF-DIFFERENCES (PODS): Aspects of a product or service that differentiate it from others on the market. Such aspects can create for the consumer positive, strong associations with a brand that encourage brand loyalty.

POINTS-OF-PARITY (POPS): Aspects of a product or service that connect it or make it similar to existing options on the market. These similarities are used as an advantage to gain customers, such as a cleaning product that is as effective as a leading brand but costs less, therefore creating a more favorable incentive for the customer to switch brands or try something new.

POLICY: A formal strategy or plan of action that guides decision-making in particular events or situations.

POSITIONING: The act of shaping a company's identity and what it offers to consumers so that the company occupies a distinctive place on the market.

POSITIVE REINFORCEMENT: An approach to strengthen desired behavior or outcomes by adding or increasing something favorable, such as installing more lights for better working conditions or providing praise for a job well done.

POST-PURCHASE EVALUATION: A consumer's review or assessment of a product or service after purchase that influences his or her likelihood to purchase the product or service again. This assessment can also greatly influence the shopping decisions of other consumers.

PRACTICE VARIATION: Ideally, clinical care would be standard and of high quality across practitioners and geography. However, clinical care does vary, and this is a measure of that variance.

PRIMARY DATA: Information acquired or collected first-hand to address the main purpose of the research.

PROCEDURE: A specific series of steps to be taken in response to a particular event or situation, focused on completing a task.

PROCESS: A methodology put into place with the intention of achieving a specific outcome. A process can be made up of procedures, though individual procedures don't necessarily need to be completed successfully in order for the process to be successful.

PRODUCT ADVERTISING: Promotion centered on a particular good or service that typically is factual (providing basic information on the use and availability), persuasive (comparing to other options), and/or functions as a reminder or follow-up to catch the customer's attention.

PRODUCTIVITY: A measure of performance based on the ratio of input to output. Greater output with lesser input indicates higher productivity.

PRODUCT LIFE CYCLE: The full lifespan of a product. Spans from its initial introduction to the market to its eventual withdrawal.

PRODUCT MIX: The sum of all product lines that a company offers its customers.

PRODUCT POSITIONING: Where a particular product fits in to the marketplace. Marketers may analyze competition, needs of likely buyers and other factors to determine where they can best position their product to sell.

PROJECT TEAM: A team of people who don't usually work together who come together to complete specific, one-time projects or tasks within a limited time.

PROMOTIONAL MIX: The particular variety of advertising approaches an organization is using (e.g. classified ads, paid social media testimonials, and infomercials)

PROTECTED HEALTH INFORMATION (PHI): Data pertaining to a patient's health providers, payment for care, and health status that can easily identify the patient. This kind of information is considered private and must be handled appropriately as defined by the Health Insurance Portability and Accountability Act (HIPAA) of 1996.

PSYCHOLOGICAL READINESS: An employee's own level of self-confidence and ambition for performing his or her job.

PUBLICITY (PUBLIC RELATIONS): Dissemination of information about a company, usually through the media. Of concern to an organization because it affects how the organization is viewed.

PULL STRATEGY: Trying to induce customers to seek you out. For example, advertising on the radio. Contrast with *push strategy*.

PUSH STRATEGY: Trying to put your product in front of your customer. For example, soliciting door-to-door. Contrast with *pull strategy*.

QUALITY IMPROVEMENT (QI): A formal process of data gathering and analysis to measure the improvement in health care services and patient health status.

RATIONAL DECISION-MAKING: A process of defining issues or problems, considering alternative options, and choosing what is neutrally assessed to be the best course of action.

REACH: The unique count of individuals accessible through an advertising vehicle.

RECEIVER: The recipient of a communication.

REINFORCEMENT: The process in which behavior is changed or affected based on the consequences following the behavior.

REINFORCEMENT THEORY: The idea that behavior is a function of its consequences, also sometimes known as behaviorism or operant conditioning.

RELATIONSHIP MARKETING: Advertising activity whose goal is customer engagement and brand loyalty, rather than inducing purchasing behavior.

RESISTANCE TO CHANGE: The hesitation or outright refusal to comply with an operational shift in the workplace, often expressed out of misunderstanding, distrust, or fear of the shift and its potential outcomes.

RESOURCES: The skills, money, tools, capabilities, processes, and other material and non-material assets an organization has in order to improve efficiency and growth and to create and sustain competitive advantage.

RESULTS-DRIVEN CHANGE: Innovation or revision driven by the implementation of many small, measurable goals within a larger objective.

RETENTION RATE: In the insurance world, the amount an insurance provider can hold onto as profit once all eligible claims have been paid.

RETURN ON INVESTMENT (ROI): A description of the financial return with the original investment as the basis. Usually expressed as a ratio or percentage. If a stock is purchased for $20 and sold for $30, it would have a 50% ROI.

RISK ADJUSTMENT: Compensation or incentives generally given to insurance companies from the government to incentivize taking on a larger proportion of high-risk individuals in order to increase coverage across a population.

RISK ASSESSMENT: Evaluating behaviors, medical status, and lifestyle to determine how much risk a person is in. The approach can also be used to assess the risk that medical providers are in when serving a given population.

RISK MANAGEMENT: The process in which known risks are planned for and prioritized in terms of their likelihood and their potential damage. Resources can then be allocated on that basis to minimize the impact of adverse events.

RISK POOLING: An agreement by a group to collectively assume risk and share the burden of paying for a negative consequence. When an adverse event is variable or unpredictable, pooling risk makes the financial consequences smaller and more regular across time on a group level. For example, insurance companies group together and pool risk to prevent unpredictable events like natural disasters from being financially ruinous.

ROOT CAUSE ANALYSIS: An attempt to identify the causal factor or factors that lead to a particular situation. Often carried out as a response to a negative event in an effort to prevent its recurrence.

S.M.A.R.T. GOALS: An approach to managing personal or professional development, stands for Specific, Measurable, Attainable, Realistic, and Timely.

SALES PROMOTION: A discount or offer meant to entice a consumer to make a purchase.

SCENARIO ANALYSIS: The consideration of multiple possible outcomes of an action, which can lead to problem-solving breakthroughs and a better state of preparedness.

SECONDARY DATA: Info that was collected by someone other than the user (e.g. a purchased mailing list).

SELF-ACTUALIZATION: The fulfillment or striving toward fulfillment of one's own potential.

SENDER: The person or entity from whom communication is initiated.

SERVANT LEADERSHIP: A style of leadership in which leaders focus on serving those around them, sharing power, and facilitating others' work, rather than accumulating power for themselves and wielding that power by directing others.

SERVICE DEMAND: The demand for service-based offerings. In the context of medical service, a measure of the number of patients a provider sees during a particular period of time.

SERVICE RECOVERY SYSTEM: A process that anticipates customer dissatisfaction and strives to make amends so that the relationship remains positive.

SHAREHOLDER MODEL: A business philosophy which holds that the primary and overriding corporate responsibility is to maximize shareholder profit.

SITUATIONAL ANALYSIS: An assessment of an organization's standing in order to better understand how it can improve or change, especially in regards to policy-making. An example of a specific type of situational analysis is the SWOT analysis, which identifies and considers an organization's strengths, weaknesses, opportunities, and threats.

SITUATIONAL LEADERSHIP: An approach to leadership in which the leader adjusts his or her style to the particular needs or aspects of the followers, placing importance on job readiness as well as psychological readiness.

SOCIAL LOAFING: Behavior within a team when an individual withholds his or her efforts and does not contribute evenly or performs a fair share of the work.

SOCIAL RESPONSIBILITY: The obligation an individual, business, or organization has to follow or create policies and otherwise behave in such a way that benefits society as a whole.

SPECIFIC ENVIRONMENT: Regulations, suppliers, advocacy groups, and other influential factors within a particular industry.

SPOT: A single placement of an ad on TV or radio.

STAGES OF TEAMWORK:

STAKEHOLDER: A person or entity with an interest in the success and failure of an organization. See *stakeholder model.*

STAKEHOLDER MODEL: A business philosophy stating that a corporation should consider the welfare of a multitude of stakeholders, such as employees and vendors, related to the company. This model contrasts with the more traditional and narrow view of considering only owners' and shareholders' financial welfare (the *shareholder model*).

STORMING: The second stage of teamwork, during which team members become more familiar with each other. Conflict, disagreement, and tension characterize this stage, and the team's ability to work through its issues is critical to the team's growth and success.

STRATEGIC MANAGEMENT: The process of conscientiously prioritizing company goals and plans by assessing resources. Typically done by upper levels of management.

STRATEGIC MOMENTUM: An organization's consistency in planning and execution of a strategy.

STRATEGIC PLANNING: The process of defining a company's approach in order to accomplish its goals, developing decision-making guidelines and steps so that a concrete plan can be set into motion.

STRATEGIC THINKING: An intellectual process or analysis that encourages looking at "the bigger picture" and into the future to craft a path of action in order to arrive at desirable results for both personal and professional gain.

STRATEGY: A determined policy, plan, or methodology used by a business to achieve success.

SUBOPTIMIZATION: A situation in which a process or company is not as successful or efficient as it could be because there is too much focus or emphasis on one aspect and it does not perform as a cohesive whole.

TACTICAL PLANS: Unlike strategic plans, which look further out to the future, tactical plans tend to focus on short-term goal achievement through specific steps and clearly defined processes.

TARGET AUDIENCE; The segment of the population a company is targeting media toward.

TARGET MARKET: The segment of the population to which an organization is marketing a product or service.

TEAM DIVERSITY: The differences in experience, ability, personality, or any other factor among individuals who are part of a team.

TEAM LEADERS: Managers of a team, responsible for facilitating and maintaining team efforts in order to accomplish a goal.

TECHNICAL SKILLS: The abilities to perform specific, often practical, tasks successfully. Such tasks often require knowledge of physical or technological tools such as mechanical equipment or a computer program.

TRANSACTIONAL LEADERSHIP: A leadership style centered on the exchange of behavior or goods, promoting compliance through rewards and punishments.

TRANSFORMATIONAL LEADERSHIP: A leadership style focusing on working with others to identify needs, using four main elements (motivation, stimulation, consideration, and influence) to achieve desired outcomes.

TRANSFORMATIONAL LEADERSHIP: A leadership style that creates organizational cohesion, enhances cooperation, encourages development of followers, promotes greater morality, and striving for ideals.

TREND: A general tendency, inclination, direction, or movement that reflects the preferences and attitudes of a particular period of time.

VALUE: The perceived benefit, usefulness, or worth of a good or service.

VALUE CHAIN: An analysis of production that considers each step from receiving raw materials to producing a product as adding value. The goal of the analysis is to increase efficiency, maximize value for the customer, and reduce costs.

VALUES STATEMENT: A list of core principles and beliefs that guide a company's actions and goals.

VARIABLE COSTS: Expenses that change with growth or amount of production. See *fixed costs*.

VEHICLE: The specific channel that advertising will go through within a media class. For example, an ad may be on the radio. The specific local country music station would be the vehicle for the ad.

VISIBLE VALUE: The benefits that are perceptible and tangible to the customer.

VISIONARY LEADERSHIP: A style of leadership that is focused on seeing possible outcomes that are not obvious. Visionary leaders share their vision of a possible future and help followers see how they can contribute to making it a reality.

VISION STATEMENT: A company or organization's manifesto that speaks to its longterm goals and typically is meant more for employees rather than clients or partners. Whereas a mission statement might focus more on the "who" and "what" of a company, a vision statement usually addresses the "why" and "how."

WORKER READINESS: The ability and willingness for directing one's own behavior at work.

WORKERS' COMPENSATION INSURANCE: A type of insurance that some states can require employers to carry in order to protect employees in the event of a work-related injury. When such an injury occurs, employers are not held responsible for what happened.

WRONGFUL DISCHARGE: When an employee is fired without appropriate cause as stipulated by contract or law.

Index

D

E

Q

R

S

T

U

V

W

CPSIA information can be obtained
at www.ICGtesting.com
Printed in the USA
LVHW020231080722
722987LV00003B/29

9 781516 529001